Clinical Aspects of Electroporation

Stephen T. Kee · Julie Gehl · Edward W. Lee
Editors

Clinical Aspects of Electroporation

Springer

Editors
Stephen T. Kee, MD
Ronald Reagan Medical Center at UCLA
Division of Interventional Radiology
Department of Radiology
Los Angeles, California
USA
skee@mednet.ucla.edu

Edward W. Lee, MD, PhD
Division of Interventional Radiology
Department of Radiology
David Geffen School of Medicine at UCLA
Los Angeles, California
USA
EdwardLee@mednet.ucla.edu

Julie Gehl, MD, DMSc
Center for Experimental Drug and
Gene Electrotransfer (C*EDGE)
Department of Oncology
Copenhagen University Hospital Herlev
Herlev
Denmark
juge@heh.regionh.dk

ISBN 978-1-4939-3960-2 ISBN 978-1-4419-8363-3 (eBook)
DOI 10.1007/978-1-4419-8363-3
Springer New York Dordrecht Heidelberg London

Softcover re-print of the Hardcover 1st edition 2011

Printed on acid-free paper

Springer is part of Springer Science+Business Media (www.springer.com)

Preface

In just a few decades, electroporation has moved from being an interesting idea to being offered to patients as part of treatment strategies. This development has involved physicists, biochemists, biologists, eventually medical doctors, as well as engineers and technicians. And what's more, this development is likely to continue at rapid speed. Electroporation is a platform technology; pulse characteristics may be changed to perform various functions. Tumor ablation by strong electric fields (so-called irreversible electroporation, IRE) may be used in the treatment of cancer. Reversible electroporation (RE) works at lower field strengths and enables transient opening of cell membranes which allows for diffusion of otherwise nonpermeating drugs. The obvious use of this technology is to greatly enhance the efficacy of chemotherapy (Electro Chemotherapy). Indeed, the technologies may overlap as tumor treatment may be a result of both processes.

A major avenue ahead will be the use of gene electrotransfer, where therapeutic genes may be transferred to all kinds of different tissues by local injection and application of electric pulses. This methodology is far safer than other delivery methods, and the transfection may be directed at a small area and have either local or systemic effects. We are only beginning to see the contours of what this technology may bring to patients suffering from a variety of diseases.

IRE and electrochemotherapy are now being offered to patients suffering from a variety of cancer histologies, treating tumors in different organs, and gene therapy is offered in clinical trials.

This book is the first book published on electroporation-based technologies seen *from the medical doctors' perspective*. What's the scientific background for this technology? The terminology? How do you proceed? What equipment do you use? What is the experience gained?

In editing this book, we have sought to create the clinicians' guide to electroporation-based technologies.

In addition to the authors contributing to this book, we would like to acknowledge the particular efforts of Daphne Wong and Susanne Husted Nielsen for invaluable assistance in the editing process.

Los Angeles, CA, USA — Stephen T. Kee
Herlev, Denmark — Julie Gehl
Los Angeles, CA, USA — Edward W. Lee

Contents

Contributors

Birgit Agerholm-Larsen
Glostrup Research Institute, Copenhagen University Hospital Glostrup, Glostrup, Denmark

Marco Alberghini
SSD Anatomia ed Istologia Patologica, Rizzoli Orthopaedic Institute, Bologna, Italy

Giuseppe Bianchi
Clinica Ortopedica e Traumatologica IV a Prevalente Indirizzo Oncologico,
Rizzoli Orthopaedic Institute, Bologna, Italy

Michael G. Bourke
Cork Cancer Research Centre, Leslie C. Quick Jnr. Laboratory, BioSciences Institute,
University College Cork, Cork, Ireland

Ruggero Cadossi
Laboratory of Clinical Biophysics, IGEA, Carpi, Italy

Laura Campanacci
Clinica Ortopedica e Traumatologica IV a Prevalente Indirizzo Oncologico,
Rizzoli Orthopaedic Institute, Bologna, Italy

Francesco Cavani
Department of Anatomy and Histology, University of Modena and Reggio Emilia, Modena, Italy

Maja Cemazar
Department of Experimental Oncology, Institute of Oncology Ljubljana, Ljubljana, Slovenia

Francesca de Terlizzi
Laboratory of Clinical Biophysics, IGEA, Carpi, Italy

David A. Dean
Department of Pediatrics, University of Rochester, Rochester, NY, USA

Jean-Michel Escoffre
Centre Nationale de la Recherche Scientifique (CNRS), IPBS (Institut de Pharmacologie
et de Biologie Structurale), Université de Toulouse, UPS, Toulouse, France

Paolo Fagone
Department of Pathology and Laboratory Medicine, University of Pennsylvania
School of Medicine, Philadelphia, PA, USA

Milena Fini
Laboratory of Preclinical and Surgical Studies, Rizzoli Orthopaedic Institute, Bologna, Italy

Patrick F. Forde
Cork Cancer Research Centre, Leslie C. Quick Jnr. Laboratory, BioSciences Institute, University College Cork, Cork, Ireland

Jean-Remy Garbay
Department of Surgery, Institut Gustave-Roussy, Villejuif, France

Julie Gehl
Center for Experimental Drug and Gene Electrotransfer (C*EDGE), Department of Oncology, Copenhagen University Hospital Herlev, Herlev, Denmark;
University of Copenhagen, Copenhagen, Denmark

Richard Gilbert
Department of Chemical and Biomedical Engineering, University of South Florida, Tampa, FL, USA

Hanne Gissel
Institute of Physiology and Biophysics, Aarhus University, Aarhus C, Denmark

Anita Gothelf
Center for Experimental Drug and Gene Electrotransfer (C*EDGE), Department of Oncology, Copenhagen University Hospital Herlev, Herlev, Denmark

Loree C. Heller
Frank Reidy Research Center for Bioelectrics, Old Dominion University, Norfolk, VA, USA

Richard Heller
Frank Reidy Research Center for Bioelectrics, Old Dominion University, Norfolk, VA, USA

Pernille Hojman
Centre of Inflammation and Metabolism at Department of Infectious Diseases, Rigshospitalet, University of Copenhagen, Copenhagen, Denmark

Helle K. Iversen
Glostrup Research Institute, Copenhagen University Hospital Glostrup, Glostrup, Denmark;
Department of Neurology, Copenhagen University Hospital Glostrup, Glostrup, Denmark

Stephen T. Kee
Ronald Reagan Medical Center at UCLA, Division of Interventional Radiology, Department of Radiology, David Geffen School of Medicine at UCLA, Los Angeles, CA, USA

Stephen Kemmerer
Inovio Biomedical Corporation, San Diego, CA, USA

Tadej Kotnik
Department of Biomedical Engineering, University of Ljubljana, Ljubljana, Slovenia

Edward W. Lee
Division of Interventional Radiology, Department of Radiology, David Geffen School of Medicine at UCLA, Los Angeles, CA, USA

Raphael C. Lee
Center for Molecular Regeneration, Department of Surgery, The University of Chicago, Chicago, IL, USA

Mette Linnert
University of Copenhagen, Copenhagen, Denmark;
Center for Experimental Drug and Gene Electrotransfer (C*EDGE), Department of Oncology, Copenhagen University Hospital Herlev, Herlev, Denmark

Faisal Mahmood
Center for Experimental Drug and Gene Electrotransfer (C*EDGE), Department of Oncology, Copenhagen University Hospital Herlev, Herlev, Denmark

Louise W. Matthiessen
Center for Experimental Drug and Gene Electrotransfer (C*EDGE), Department of Oncology, Copenhagen University Hospital Herlev, Herlev, Denmark

Mario Mercuri
Clinica Ortopedica e Traumatologica IV a Prevalente Indirizzo Oncologico, Rizzoli Orthopaedic Institute, Bologna, Italy

Damijan Miklavčič
Department of Biomedical Engineering, University of Ljubljana, Ljubljana, Slovenia

Lluis M. Mir
Unité Mixte de Recherche (UMR), Centre Nationale de la Recherche Scientifique (CNRS), Institut Gustave-Roussy, Univ Paris-Sud, Villejuif, France

Tobian Muir
Department of Plastic Surgery, The James Cook University Hospital, Middlesbrough, UK

Gerald C. O'Sullivan
Cork Cancer Research Centre, Leslie C. Quick Jnr. Laboratory, BioSciences Institute, University College Cork, Cork, Ireland

Gorazd Pucihar
Department of Biomedical Engineering, University of Ljubljana, Ljubljana, Slovenia

Dietmar Rabussay
Inovio Biomedical Corporation, San Diego, CA, USA

Marie-Pierre Rols
Centre Nationale de la Recherche Scientifique (CNRS), IPBS (Institut de Pharmacologie et de Biologie Structurale), Université de Toulouse, UPS, Toulouse, France

Mattia Ronchetti
Laboratory of Clinical Biophysics, IGEA, Carpi, Italy

Slawomir Salwa
Cork Cancer Research Centre, Leslie C. Quick Jnr. Laboratory, BioSciences Institute, University College Cork, Cork, Ireland

Gregor Sersa
Department of Experimental Oncology, Institute of Oncology Ljubljana, Ljubljana, Slovenia

Devon J. Shedlock
Department of Pathology and Laboratory Medicine, University of Pennsylvania School of Medicine, Philadelphia, PA, USA

Aude Silve
Unité Mixte de Recherche (UMR), Centre Nationale de la Recherche Scientifique (CNRS), Institut Gustave-Roussy, Univ Paris-Sud, Villejuif, France

Marko Snoj
Department of Experimental Oncology, Institute of Oncology Ljubljana, Ljubljana, Slovenia

Declan M. Soden
Cork Cancer Research Centre, Leslie C. Quick Jnr. Laboratory, BioSciences Institute, University College Cork, Cork, Ireland

Lasse G. Staal
Sonion Medical, Roskilde, Denmark

Ken Thomson
Department of Radiology, The Alfred Hospital, Monash University, Prahran, Melbourne, VIC, Australia

Matilde Tschon
Laboratory of Preclinical and Surgical Studies, Rizzoli Orthopaedic Institute, Bologna, Italy

David B. Weiner
Department of Pathology and Laboratory Medicine, University of Pennsylvania School of Medicine, Philadelphia, PA, USA

Daphne Wong
Division of Interventional Radiology, Department of Radiology, David Geffen School of Medicine at UCLA, Los Angeles, CA, USA

Part I
Introductory

Chapter 1
Introduction to Electroporation

Edward W. Lee, Julie Gehl, and Stephen T. Kee

Abstract Electroporation refers to the ability of electric fields to cause the formation of reversible or irreversible pores in the membranes of cells. Reversible electroporation (RE) is now in widespread use as a method of delivering chemicals and large molecules to cells, both as a research tool and a clinical technique. Recently, irreversible electroporation (IRE) has garnered interest as a stand-alone ablation device that may have a role in the treatment of various cancers. This book attempts to illustrate the current state of the art of electroporation and authors a number of areas of growing interest currently being studied.

Keywords Electroporation • Reversible electroporation • Irreversible electroporation • Electrochemotherapy • Gene delivery • Ablation

Electroporation

Electroporation is an innovative minimally invasive technique that uses microsecond length electric pulses to alter the permeability of cell membranes forming nanoscale defects or pores [1, 2]. The use of electrical fields at certain parameters temporarily permeabilize the membrane, allowing the cells to return to its natural state afterwards, a process known as reversible electroporation (RE) [2]. The RE technology platform allows us to *rethink* drug and gene delivery, thereby altering the sensitivity of certain cancers to chemotherapy and gene therapy.

Stronger electric fields can cause the cell membrane to permanently permeabilize, leading to cell death, in a process called irreversible electroporation (IRE) [2]. The delivery of this energy can be used to kill cancer cells and spare adjacent tissues from damage.

History of Electroporation

Electroporation has lately garnered enthusiasm in the fields of biotechnology and medicine. This technique has been observed as early as the 1750s; however, the recent 30 years has seen increased research leading to implementation for medical purposes [2]. The first theoretical experiments using

E.W. Lee (✉)
Division of Interventional Radiology, Department of Radiology, David Geffen School of Medicine at UCLA, 10833 Le Conte Avenue, B2-168, Los Angeles, CA 90095-1721, USA
e-mail: EdwardLee@mednet.ucla.edu

S.T. Kee et al. (eds.), *Clinical Aspects of Electroporation*,
DOI 10.1007/978-1-4419-8363-3_1, © Springer Science+Business Media, LLC 2011

electroporation on the lipid bilayer were conducted in 1970's [3–5]. As a result of these studies, Neumann et al. authored the first publication on electroporation in 1982 on gene transfer into murine cells [6]. Shortly afterwards, pulse electroporators were developed, and the phenomenon of electroporation for the delivery of molecules into cells became widespread [7–9]. In 1993, investigations by Belehradek et al. reported the first use of electroporation to increase the uptake of chemotherapeutic agents in tumors [10]. Since then, numerous studies and publications have been made on the various clinical practices of electroporation, which includes the induction of drugs and genes into cells and electrochemotherapy for the treatment of cancer [11–15]. These various applications of "reversible" electroporation require cells to survive postprocedure, and therefore the occurrences of IRE, in which the cell dies, had been considered undesirable.

In more recent years, IRE has emerged as an important medical technique in a field that has previously been dominated by RE [2]. Since 1961, IRE has been used in the food industry for sterilization purposes [16] and in 1987, the electrical injury of a cell by a nonthermal mechanism was investigated [17, 18]. The most recent research conducted by Lee et al. has have demonstrated the potential of using IRE for tumor ablation [19].

Reversible Electroporation Vs. Irreversible Electroporation

Electroporation energy is delivered using square wave direct current (DC) pulse generators. It is possible to independently change the pulse amplitude, length, number of pulses delivered, and the frequency of delivery. It has been shown that with increasing amplitude, the *area* of the cell membrane that is permeabilised is increased. For electrotransfer of drugs or genes, a degree of permeabilisation sufficient to allow diffusion of molecules is the goal. Following the treatment the cells recover. For permanent destruction of tumor cells using electroporation alone, a massive permeation of the cell membrane is desired, in order to allow long-term loss of membrane integrity and thus ion homeostasis. This can be achieved by altering the DC pulses delivered.

In both RE and IRE, the delivery of an electric field across a cell alters its transmembrane potential. Therefore, the lipid bilayer structure is disrupted, and small, transient nanopores are created to allow the transportation of micro and macromolecules into and out of the cell [19]. The mechanism by which the electric field permeabilizes the cell membrane is similar for the two methods; however, in RE, the pores are formed on the membrane during electroporation, and are resealed after the procedure [12]. This temporary pore opening allows the cell to survive after the application of the electric field; however, this requires that the electrical parameters are much lower than in IRE [12]. The goal of RE is to expose the cell to the external electric field, which allows genes, drugs, dyes, and proteins that normally do not penetrate the membrane, to enter the cell [12]. As a result, RE has been used for a variety of clinical and medicinal applications, such as the introduction of drugs into cells, electrochemotherapy, gene delivery to tissue, and transdermal delivery of drugs and genes [2, 20]. RE is also being used to treat cancer cells by permeabilizing the cell and allowing chemotherapeutic agents to enter the cell at greater, more effective concentrations to kill the target cell – in a process called electrochemotherapy [1].

On the other hand, the phenomenon termed as "irreversible" electroporation uses the electric field to directly destroy the cell – without the intervention of drugs [2]. While electrical pulses are delivered at only hundreds of voltages in RE, IRE requires a sufficiently high voltage of at least 1,000 V and up to 3,000 V to exceed the threshold required for creating permanent pores in the cell [1]. High voltages are generated and applied through electrodes inserted under ultrasound guidance [1]. IRE uses the applied electric field to induce cell death by creating pores that are unable to reseal after the procedure, therefore destroying the cell's ability to maintain homeostasis [19]. While RE requires the supplemental use of drugs to kill tumor cells, IRE uses the electrical field to create cell death through the mechanism of apoptosis.

Reversible Electroporation

Silve et al. demonstrated that reversible cell electropermeabilization increases the cellular uptake of bleomycin, a nonpermeant anticancer drug possessing high cytotoxicity. Sersa et al. validated these claims by asserting that bleomycin and cisplatin, along with electric pulses delivered to treat tumors, plays a crucial role in the local control of cancers. The author claims that the treatment is easy to perform, and is effective for the treatment of skin melanoma, breast cancer, and other tumor skin metastases. The capability of RE being used for electrochemotherapy has also been confirmed by the research of Matthiessen et al., whose study concluded that electrochemotherapy for larger malignant tumors has promise as a palliative treatment and may be a good alternative or supplement to surgery. However, for this study, the author claims that further investigation is needed in order to make more evident guidelines for such treatment. Besides having a direct cytotoxic effect on tumor cells, electrochemotherapy also has a vascular disrupting effect.

As shown by the many reported cases in the research of Sersa et al., electrochemotherapy can be beneficially used in the treatment of bleeding metastases.

Another development has also been made in the application of drugs and genes to brain tissue in humans using RE, as demonstrated by Agerholm-Larsen et al. Because of the blood brain barrier, the access of agents from the blood into brain tissue is restricted. This could theoretically be overcomed by the use of RE. This technique is a new and developing field of research and drug and gene electrotransfer in the brain has promising outlooks for clinical applications. The concept of gene electrotransfer to the lung is also new to RE; however, Dean et al.'s research has developed an effective treatment for several pulmonary diseases in their study. Research by several different parties and institutions has also shown strides in gene electrotransfer to muscle tissue and skin, as well as tumors, as described by Heller et al.

Irreversible Electroporation

Preclinical IRE studies have shown promising results. Lee et al. [19] recently published a study on radiologic–pathologic correlation of IRE-induced cell death. US-guided IRE of normal liver was performed on Yorkshire pigs, imaged with US, MR, and CT, and evaluated with immunohistochemical analysis. Neal et al. [21] orthotopically implanted human breast cancer tumors in the mammary fat pad of Nu/Nu mice and treated with IRE. Tumor regression was observed in five out of seven of the MDA-MB231 human mammary tumors four weeks after treatment, with continued growth in controls measured by calipers, bioluminescent imaging of tagged cancer cells from the tumor, and histological examination [21]. Onik et al. [22] also recently studied IRE ablation in the normal prostate of dogs using transrectal ultrasound guidance. Rubinsky et al. [23] studied IRE of prostate adenocarcinoma cells in vitro to determine the number, length, and field strength of the IRE pulses required to produce complete human cancer cell ablation. Ellis et al. [24] studied the safety of IRE in normal canine brain tissue. Ultrasonography, MR imaging, and histological analyzes were used. Charpentier et al. [25] demonstrated IRE of normal pancreas in swine showing evidence of irreversible ablation by gross appearance and triphenyltetrazolium chloride (TTC) staining [25]. These studies all demonstrated IRE to be a fast, safe, and potent ablative method, causing complete tissue death with full preservation of periablative zone structures, including blood vessels, bile ducts, and neighboring nonablated tissues [19]. Lastly, IRE can now be delivered in real time, unlike RFA and cryoablation. Lee et al. [26] demonstrated this with observation and measurements of the treated area acquired during real-time monitoring. Ablation with IRE allows the visualization of IRE effects with real-time ultrasound, making it possible to adjust protocol parameters in real time to achieve desired results. Thermal ablation modalities create hyperechoic microbubbles from the thermally injured tissue in US images, hindering the possibility of real-time monitoring [27, 28]. Lee et al. [19, 26] showed that

IRE creates a spherical hypoechoic area of ablation during and immediately after IRE, with no lesion-obscuring gas, lasting up to 24 h after which the area becomes hyperechogenic. They postulate that the initial hypoechogenicity is likely caused by increased intra/extracellular water as a result of the disruption of cellular homeostasis [19, 26]. Granot et al. [29] recently described using 3D electrical impedance tomography (EIT) for real time monitoring of IRE [29].

Conclusion and Perspectives

Electroporation is a platform technology that has unlimited potential for innovation. RE using electrotransfer can be used to allow for the transfer of *any* molecule or *any* gene to *any* tissue, and is already in widespread clinical use for delivery of chemotherapy, with a wide therapeutic window, currently mostly for skin cancers; however, developments will shortly see this treatment being used for other cancers including brain cancer.

IRE with the application of very intense electric pulses is being used clinically in the USA, Australia, and Europe for ablation purposes at this time. Early developments have focused on liver and kidney cancers with research into treatments in the pancreas and lung underway. The equipment used and the techniques being applied are still in development and there is considerable excitement in the Oncology community that this technique will become the dominant tumor ablation method in the near future.

References

1. Bertacchini C, Margotti PM, Bergamini E, Lodi A, Ronchetti M, Cadossi R. Design of an irreversible electroporation system for clinical use. Technol Cancer Res Treat. 2007;6:313–20.
2. Rubinsky B. Irreversible electroporation in medicine. Technol Cancer Res Treat. 2007;6:255–60.
3. Crowley JM. Electrical breakdown of bimolecular lipid membranes as an electromechanical instability. Biophys J. 1973;13:711–24.
4. Zimmermann U, Pilwat G, Riemann F. Dielectric breakdown of cell membranes. Biophys J. 1974;14:881–99.
5. Kinosita Jr K, Tsong TT. Hemolysis of human erythrocytes by transient electric field. Proc Natl Acad Sci USA. 1977;74:1923–7.
6. Neumann E, Schaefer-Ridder M, Wang Y, Hofschneider PH. Gene transfer into mouse lyoma cells by electroporation in high electric fields. EMBO J. 1982;1:841–5.
7. Wong TK, Neumann E. Electric field mediated gene transfer. Biochem Biophys Res Commun. 1982;107: 584–7.
8. Orlowski S, Mir LM. Cell electropermeabilization: a new tool for biochemical and pharmacological studies. Biochim Biophys Acta. 1993;1154:51–63.
9. Weaver JC. Electroporation: a general phenomenon for manipulating cells and tissues. J Cell Biochem. 1993;51:426–35.
10. Belehradek M, Domenge C, Luboinski B, Orlowski S, Belehradek Jr J, Mir LM. Electrochemotherapy, a new antitumor treatment. First clinical phase I-II trial. Cancer. 1993;72:3694–700.
11. Nanda GS, Sun FX, Hofmann GA, Hoffman RM, Dev SB. Electroporation therapy of human larynx tumors HEp-2 implanted in nude mice. Anticancer Res. 1998;18:999–1004.
12. Gehl J. Electroporation: theory and methods, perspectives for drug delivery, gene therapy and research. Acta Physiol Scand. 2003;177:437–47.
13. Gothelf A, Mir LM, Gehl J. Electrochemotherapy: results of cancer treatment using enhanced delivery of bleomycin by electroporation. Cancer Treat Rev. 2003;29:371–87.
14. Bloquel C, Fabre E, Bureau MF, Scherman D. Plasmid DNA electrotransfer for intracellular and secreted proteins expression: new methodological developments and applications. J Gene Med. 2004;6 Suppl 1:S11–23.
15. Maxim PG, Carson JJ, Ning S, et al. Enhanced effectiveness of radiochemotherapy with tirapazamine by local application of electric pulses to tumors. Radiat Res. 2004;162:185–93.
16. Doevenspeck H. Influencing cells and cell walls by electrostatic impulses. Fleishwirtshaft. 1961;13:986–7.

17. Lee RC, Kolodney MS. Electrical injury mechanisms: electrical breakdown of cell membranes. Plast Reconstr Surg. 1987;80:672–9.
18. Lee RC, Kolodney MS. Electrical injury mechanisms: dynamics of the thermal response. Plast Reconstr Surg. 1987;80:663–71.
19. Lee EW, Chen C, Prieto VE, Dry SM, Loh CT, Kee ST. Advanced hepatic ablation technique for creating complete cell death: irreversible electroporation. Radiology. 2010;255:426–33.
20. Mir LM, Morsli N, Garbay JR, Billard V, Robert C, Marty M. Electrochemotherapy: a new treatment of solid tumors. J Exp Clin Cancer Res. 2003;22:145–8.
21. Neal 2nd RE, Singh R, Hatcher HC, Kock ND, Torti SV, Davalos RV. Treatment of breast cancer through the application of irreversible electroporation using a novel minimally invasive single needle electrode. Breast Cancer Res Treat. 2009;123:295–301.
22. Onik G, Mikus P, Rubinsky B. Irreversible electroporation: implications for prostate ablation. Technol Cancer Res Treat. 2007;6:295–300.
23. Rubinsky J, Onik G, Mikus P, Rubinsky B. Optimal parameters for the destruction of prostate cancer using irreversible electroporation. J Urol. 2008;180:2668–74.
24. Ellis TL, Garcia PA, Rossmeisl JH, Henao-Guerrero N, Robertson J, Davalos RV. Nonthermal irreversible electroporation for intracranial surgical applications. J Neurosurg. 2010.
25. Charpentier KP, Wolf F, Noble L, Winn B, Resnick M, Dupuy DE. Irreversible electroporation of the pancreas in swine: a pilot study. HPB (Oxford). 2010;12:348–51.
26. Lee EW, Loh CT, Kee ST. Imaging guided percutaneous irreversible electroporation: ultrasound and immunohistological correlation. Technol Cancer Res Treat. 2007;6:287–94.
27. Carey RI, Leveillee RJ. First prize: direct real-time temperature monitoring for laparoscopic and CT-guided radiofrequency ablation of renal tumors between 3 and 5 cm. J Endourol. 2007;21:807–13.
28. Mast TD, Pucke DP, Subramanian SE, Bowlus WJ, Rudich SM, Buell JF. Ultrasound monitoring of in vitro radio frequency ablation by echo decorrelation imaging. J Ultrasound Med. 2008;27:1685–97.
29. Granot Y, Ivorra A, Maor E, Rubinsky B. In vivo imaging of irreversible electroporation by means of electrical impedance tomography. Phys Med Biol. 2009;54:4927–43.

Chapter 2
Electroporation and Cellular Physiology

Hanne Gissel, Raphael C. Lee, and Julie Gehl

Abstract Structural integrity of the cellular membrane is of critical importance for cellular viability. The membrane acts as a regulatory barrier for transport into and out of the cell and thereby enables the cell to build up chemical and electrical gradients important for cellular function. A large part of the metabolic energy required for cell function, used in the form of ATP catalysis, is invested in maintaining the transmembrane concentration gradients. If the membrane becomes hyperpermeable due to structural breakdown, the amount of ATP required to maintain normal osmotic balance and prevent fluid and electrolyte shifts would exceed the capability of cellular ATP generation. Thus, the cell faces metabolic energy exhaustion which may lead to cellular calcium (Ca^{2+}) overload, Ca^{2+}-mediated enzymatic breakdown, and increased superoxide generation. This may lead to further breakdown of the cellular membrane and a further influx of Ca^{2+}, thus activating a vicious cycle. Most cells are very apt at repairing membranes, which makes it possible for the cell to regain control. Therefore, in many cases cell survival becomes dependent on the balance between degradative mechanisms (activated by Ca^{2+} and reactive oxidative species (ROS)) and the membrane repair mechanisms and thus on the metabolic demand on the cell. Depending on the electrical pulses used, cell membranes may reseal spontaneously or become permeabilized indefinitely. It is therefore important to exercise care when pulses are chosen for a given application. When cell survival and tissue recovery is important, it is possible to assist resealing and recovery from electroporation through the use of, for example, surfactants, antioxidants, and stimulation of the Na^+, K^+ pump.

Keywords Cell membrane • ATP • Calcium • Permeabilization • Resealing

Introduction

In order to appreciate the many opportunities offered by electroporation (EP) in the treatment of patients and to efficiently use this platform technology in the clinic, it is necessary to understand how electroporation affects cellular physiology. Over the past few years, a large amount of time and effort has been put to understand how permeabilization of the membrane affects cellular function and viability. To set the stage for the following chapters, basic cellular physiology in regards to membrane permeabilization and the consequences thereof will be covered.

H. Gissel (✉)
Institute of Physiology and Biophysics, Aarhus University, Ole Worms Allé 4, 8000 Aarhus C, Denmark
e-mail: hgh@fi.au.dk

S.T. Kee et al. (eds.), *Clinical Aspects of Electroporation*,
DOI 10.1007/978-1-4419-8363-3_2,

The Cellular Membrane and Membrane Integrity: A Prerequisite for Cell Survival

The cellular membrane constitutes the barrier that separates the cell interior from the exterior, both chemically and electrically. In essence, the cellular membrane plays the crucial role as the gatekeeper, acting as a regulatory barrier for transport into and out of the cell. The membrane consists of a lipid bilayer permeable to water, O_2, and CO_2. It is also relatively permeable to hydrophobic molecules but only permeable to polar compounds (e.g., amino acids, DNA, RNA, carbohydrates, proteins, and ions) to a very small degree. These substances are moved across the membrane by endocytosis (macromolecules) or by the aid of proteins embedded in the membrane. Transport occurs as facilitated diffusion through pores and channels or by active transport. The presence of ion channels in the membrane allows for controlled permeability to specific ions, for example, Na^+, K^+, Ca^{2+}, and Cl^-. This, in combination with ion pumps and exchangers, enables the cells to build up chemical and electrical gradients important for cellular function. A large part of the energy required to sustain cellular function is expended in maintaining the large differences in electrolyte ion concentration across the cell membrane due to the action of ATP-dependent membrane transport enzymes, the Ca^{2+}- and Na^+, K^+-ATPases. In skeletal muscle, the cost of maintaining the Na^+ and K^+ gradients accounts for 4–10% of the total energy turnover both at rest and during activity, whereas the pumping of Ca^{2+} accounts for 5% at rest and up to 50% during contractile activity [1]. Electroporation (also known as electropermeabilization) permeabilizes the cellular membrane, thus allowing an uncontrolled diffusion of ions and molecules to occur. This, in turn, vastly increases the work of maintaining the transmembrane concentration gradients by an amount that scales with the increase in membrane permeability. A summary of how cells may respond to electroporation is presented in Fig. 2.1.

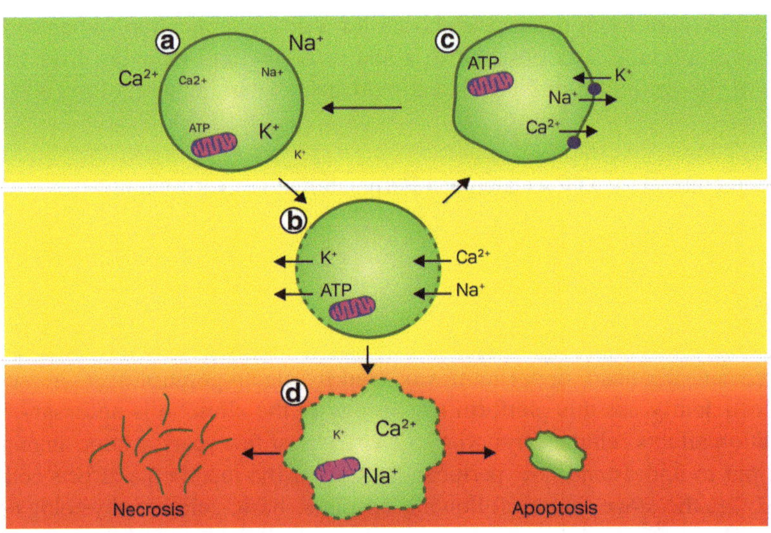

Fig. 2.1 Effects of permeabilization on the cell. (**a**) The cell under normal conditions. Note the gradients for Na^+, K^+, and Ca^{2+} across the membrane as well as the high content of ATP. (**b**) The permeabilized cell. Increases in membrane permeability lead to the influx of Ca^{2+} and Na^+ and the loss of K^+ and ATP. (**c**) The resealed cell. Resealing of the membrane allows the cell to recover ion gradients by utilizing ion pumps (the Ca^{2+}- and Na^+, K^+-ATPases). (**d**) The damaged cell. If the permeabilized membranes do not reseal or reseal too slowly, cellular Ca^{2+} overload will occur, leading to further membrane damage and mitochondrial Ca^{2+} overload. Depending on the circumstances, the cell dies by either necrosis or apoptosis

The Cell Under Normal Conditions

The healthy cell is characterized by chemical gradients for Na^+ and K^+ across the cell membrane, giving rise to the membrane potential important for many cell functions. The Ca^{2+} signaling system controls the majority of cellular reactions. It is therefore necessary that the concentration of free Ca^{2+} in the cytoplasm is under strict control. Thus, Ca^{2+} signaling occurs within tightly regulated temporal and spatial domains. Due to a very low permeability for Ca^{2+} and constant clearance of Ca^{2+} from the cytoplasm by ATPases, the concentration of free intracellular Ca^{2+} can be kept very low (around 0.1 μM), in striking contrast to the concentration of free Ca^{2+} outside the cell (around 1.3 mM). Finally, a steep gradient for ATP is maintained across the membrane, with high levels of ATP being kept inside the cell, readily available to sustain energy-dependent cellular processes.

The Permeabilized Cell

Electroporation greatly increases the permeability of the cellular membrane, leading to the loss of ionic homeostasis and the disturbance of normal cell function. In particular, it will lead to a rundown of the Na^+ and K^+ gradients and, accordingly, depolarization of the membrane potential [2]. Electroporation will also lead to a large influx of Ca^{2+} due to the very large gradient for Ca^{2+} across the membrane [3]. The loss of cell membrane integrity quickly drains the cell's energy resources due to high energy expenditure as the cell attempts to maintain the normal transmembrane ion gradients, using the Ca^{2+}- and Na^+, K^+-ATPases [1], and due to direct loss of ATP out of the cell. Finally, following cell membrane damage, the production of reactive oxygen species (ROS) increases by many orders of magnitude [4], leading to membrane injury as well as protein denaturation.

The influx of Ca^{2+} combined with a loss of ATP poses a potential threat to cell viability. Ca^{2+} functions as an important signaling molecule; thus, if control of Ca^{2+} is lost, pathological signals can be activated, leading to necrotic or apoptotic cell death. Control of Ca^{2+} is dependent on availability of ATP, since the very low concentration of Ca^{2+} in the cytoplasm is maintained by the pumping of Ca^{2+} into Ca^{2+} storage in the sarcoplasmic or endoplasmic reticulum (SR or ER) or out across the membrane by ATPases. Even though a large amount of Ca^{2+} can be stored in internal storage compartments (ER/SR and mitochondria), the storage capacity of these organelles can be exceeded, resulting in an increase of intracellular free Ca^{2+}.

Thus, the fate of the permeabilized cell depends on the degree and duration of the permeabilization, all of which depends partly or in full on the pulses used for EP. If resealing occurs before control of Ca^{2+} is lost, the cell recovers (C in Fig. 2.1); on the other hand, if control of Ca^{2+} is lost, the cell dies (D in Fig. 2.1).

The Resealed Cell

Whereas pore formation occurs in the microsecond time frame, membrane resealing has a much longer timeframe. Resealing of transient pores happens over a range of minutes, depending on the electrical parameters used and the temperature [5–7]. Once the membrane is resealed, it is the status of Ca^{2+} and ATP that determines whether cellular homeostasis can be recovered.

Assuming sufficient availability of ATP, the Na^+ and K^+ gradients and the membrane potential are recovered by the action of the Na^+, K^+-ATPase, and intracellular free Ca^{2+} is recovered by the action of the Ca^{2+}-ATPases in the SR/ER and cellular membranes [1, 8].

Although the membrane is resealed, it might still be slightly perturbed. Eventually, however, the membrane is believed to recover completely.

The Damaged Cell

In some cases, cells are permeabilized indefinitely, and the ensuing Ca^{2+} overload and ROS production leads to a secondary breakdown of the membrane. This activates a vicious cycle of continued influx of Ca^{2+}, production of ROS, and the depletion of ATP eventually leading to the destruction of the cell. Cell death may either occur by apoptosis (a controlled process requiring ATP) or by necrosis [9].

Cell Damage

Having a permeabilized membrane is perilous to the cell, as it may lead to the loss of osmotic balance and the influx of fluids and ions, as well as the loss of proteins, enzymes, coenzymes, and ribonucleic acids. The cells may also leak metabolites which are vital for the reconstitution of ATP, thus further depleting net content of intracellular high-energy phosphates. Most cells are very apt at membrane repair, with resealing being an effective emergency response among different species and cell types [10]. Thus, in many cases, cell survival becomes dependent on the balance between degradative mechanisms (activated by Ca^{2+} and ROS) and the membrane repair mechanisms. If the repair mechanisms overcome the damage before metabolic depletion occurs, the cell may regain control and survive the insult; however, if the degradative mechanisms take over, the cell dies.

Ca^{2+} is the main agent involved in cell damage. Since the permeability of the membrane can increase 1,000-fold with electroporation, the ATP demand may increase to the same degree and exceed ATP synthesis rates. This leads to an accumulation of Ca^{2+}, which will become available in cellular environments normally protected from excess Ca^{2+} [8]. The increase in ATP synthesis also leads to an increase in the production of superoxide, which may also cause damage to the cell.

Apart from producing ATP, the mitochondria play a central role in the cellular Ca^{2+} signaling by shaping and buffering cellular Ca^{2+} signals [11]. Mitochondria have a finite capacity for Ca^{2+}. However, in the presence of inorganic phosphate, calcium phosphate precipitation occurs within the mitochondria. This facilitates a total accumulation of Ca^{2+} approaching 1 M, while maintaining a low concentration of free Ca^{2+} within the mitochondria [12]. This allows the mitochondria to form a significant cellular Ca^{2+} buffer, more so than the ER or SR [13].

A small uptake of Ca^{2+} by the mitochondria has a positive effect on oxidative phosphorylation. However, larger uptakes of Ca^{2+} may result in mitochondrial Ca^{2+} overload, which serves as the primary stimulus for the opening of the permeability transition pore (PTP) [13]. Although multiple destructive processes are activated by Ca^{2+}, lethal outcomes are determined largely by Ca^{2+}-induced mitochondrial permeability transition leading to cell death by apoptosis or necrosis [8].

The threshold for when cells survive electroporation will vary with the kind and state of tissue used, as well as the type of application (in vitro, ex vivo, and in vivo).

Death by Apoptosis and Necrosis

Irreversibly injured cells invariably undergo morphological changes that are recognized as cell death. Previously, two major types of cell death were recognized: necrosis and apoptosis. However, it is now clear that this is a simplified view, and probably a number of different pathways exist that lead to cell death – pathways that differ in their morphology, mechanisms, and roles in disease and physiology.

Apoptosis is a controlled reaction which requires ATP and turns the cell into encapsulated apoptotic bodies that are easily removed by macrophages without leaving a trace. Necrosis, on the other hand, may be the result of several pathways leading to cell lysis and release of cellular components, triggering inflammatory reactions. Apoptosis and pathways leading to necrosis are interrelated; without ATP, cells committed to apoptosis die by necrosis [8]. Death following electroporation most likely follows a necrotic pathway due to the large expenditure of ATP in the attempt to recover cellular ion homeostasis.

To Seal or Not to Seal: A Question of Survival

Whether the cell survives permeabilization depends on the degree of permeabilization and resealing of the membrane.

It has been shown in rat skeletal muscle that transmembrane potentials above 340 mV result in the formation of transient electropores in the cell membrane. These pores reseal spontaneously in a matter of minutes, and resealing time does not depend on the field strength used. Above a certain threshold (540 mV) stable pores start to form [7]. The thresholds for transient and stable pore formation are very likely to be dependent on membrane composition. Resealing of stable pores possibly depends on membrane repair mechanisms where vesicles are transported to the membrane, thus lowering the membrane tension and allowing resealing of the defect. The existence of the cytoskeleton increases membrane tension. Activation of calpain (a Ca^{2+}-dependent protease) is necessary for membrane repair [14, 15]. Calpain degrades cytoskeletal components, thereby lowering membrane tension and clearing the way for the vesicles. CaMK (a Ca^{2+}-dependent protein kinase) likewise seems to be involved in wound-induced exocytosis [16]. And finally, PKC (protein kinase C) has been shown to have a potentiating effect on wound healing in the short term by stimulating gene expression via CREB (cAMP response element-binding protein) [17] and by increasing the vesicle pool [18].

As shown in Fig. 2.2, permeabilization and resealing can be investigated using nonpermeating tracers. Under normal conditions, the tracer drug does not enter the cell, but as the membrane becomes permeabilized, the tracer drug gains access to the interior of the cell. When the membrane reseals, the tracer drug is caught inside and does not disappear as the remaining tracer drug is cleared from the extracellular space. If resealing does not occur, the tracer drug will not be retained.

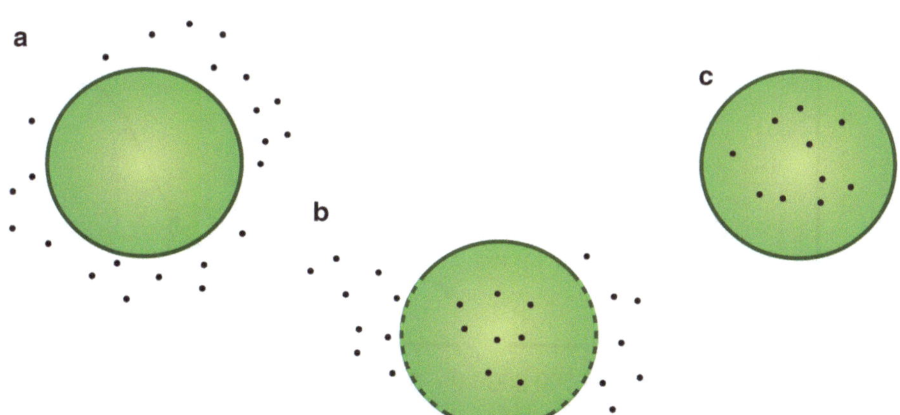

Fig. 2.2 Uptake of tracer drug in permeabilized cells. An impermeable tracer drug is added, and at first, there is no uptake into the intact cell (**a**). Permeabilization allows uptake of the tracer drug into the cell (**b**). When the membrane is resealed, the tracer drug is caught inside the cell and does not wash out as the extracellular tracer drug is removed (**c**)

Using this technique, resealing following electroporation was shown in isolated rat skeletal muscle (Fig. 2.3). The radioactive tracer ^{45}Ca was added with increasing delay from electroporation. ^{45}Ca is taken up both in the resting control and in the permeabilized muscle. The uptake is larger in the permeabilized muscle; thus, the electroporation-induced uptake can be calculated by subtracting the uptake in the resting control from the uptake in the permeabilized muscle. The immediate uptake of ^{45}Ca is very large, but the uptake decreases exponentially, and after 10 min, the uptake is reduced to less than 20%. After 60 min, the membrane is completely resealed.

Permeabilization and resealing can also be studied in vivo. Figure 2.4 shows the uptake of the tracer ^{51}Cr-EDTA into mouse *tibialis cranialis* (TC) muscle in vivo [19]. ^{51}Cr-EDTA-administered

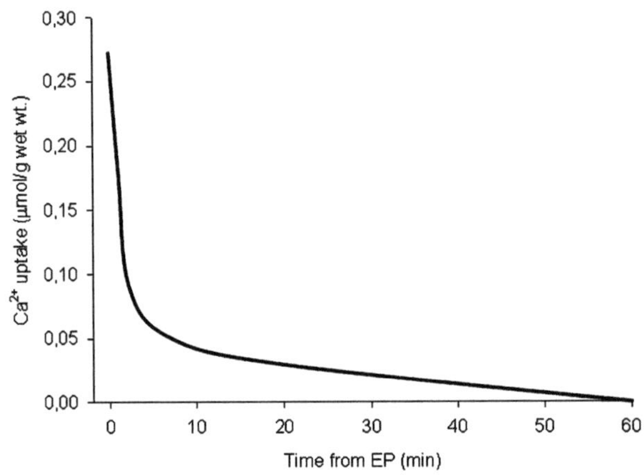

Fig. 2.3 Uptake of radioactive ^{45}Ca in isolated rat muscle following electroporation using 8–100 μs pulses of 250 V/cm

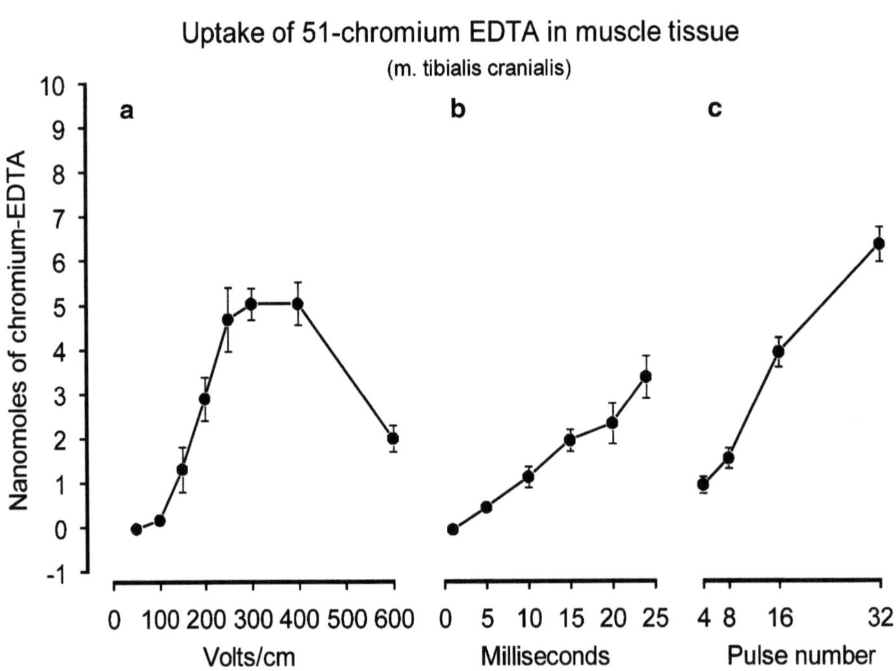

Fig. 2.4 Uptake of radioactive ^{51}Cr-EDTA into mouse TC muscle. (**a**) Effect of increasing field strength, using 8 pulses of 20 ms duration. (**b**) Effect of pulse duration, using 8 pulses at 200 V/cm. (**c**) Effect of number of pulses, using 20-ms pulses at 200 V/cm. Reproduced with permission from the authors from [19]

I.V. is normally not taken up by the muscle and is quickly cleared from plasma. However, as shown in Fig. 2.4, if the muscle cells are permeabilized, ^{51}Cr-EDTA gains access to the cell interior, and subsequent resealing traps the ^{51}Cr-EDTA in the cells. If the membrane does not reseal, ^{51}Cr-EDTA is lost.

^{51}Cr-EDTA uptake increases with increasing field strength up to 300 V/cm, possibly due to permeabilization of an increasing fraction of cells in the muscle. Above 300 V/cm, ^{51}Cr-EDTA shows a plateau which can be explained by a further increase in the fraction of permeabilized cells combined with a fraction of cells not resealing. At 600 V/cm, a large fraction of the cells do not reseal, resulting in a smaller uptake of ^{51}Cr-EDTA. Panels b and c in Fig. 2.4 show that increasing pulse duration or number of pulses increases permeabilization but has no apparent detrimental effect on resealing.

In situations where cell recovery is desired, resealing of the membrane is of primary concern. Several strategies can be employed as given below:

1. One strategy is to directly assist the resealing. A group of triblock copolymers have proven to be effective for this purpose. Poloxamer 188 (P188) has been used widely in medical applications since 1957, mainly as an emulsifier and antisludge agent in blood [20]. Due to its already-established safety record, P188 has been the focus of most investigations. P188 is a biocompatible polymer consisting of two hydrophilic side chains attached to a hydrophobic center core. It has been shown to be capable of sealing stable defects in cell membranes after various types of trauma [21, 22], significantly inhibiting apoptosis and preventing necrosis [23].
2. A second strategy could be the use of antioxidants. Electroporation is associated with ROS production [4], and since ROS contributes to the damage process, antioxidant treatment could reduce tissue damage. This was indeed shown in CHO (Chinese hamster ovary) cells, where cell survival after electroporation was markedly increased by the presence of antioxidants [4].
3. Finally, stimulation of the Na^+,K^+ pump (e.g., by β_2 agonists) has been shown to improve membrane potential and force recovery following electroporation of skeletal muscle [2]. Since many β_2 agonists have been used for years in asthma treatment, safety of this type of drug has been proven. Thus, treatment with β_2 agonists may prove to be a safe strategy for faster recovery of tissue function.

In reality, a combination of these three strategies may prove beneficial in increasing cell survival and tissue function after electroporation.

How Different Pulses Affect the Tissue

Recently, a comprehensive study was undertaken to investigate the manner in which different pulses affect membrane permeability and cell physiology [3]. Figure 2.5 shows Na^+ and K^+ content in mouse TC muscle exposed to EP. Three different pulsing regimes were used. The first consisted of eight short high voltage pulses (100 μs, 1,000 V/cm) (8 HV), the second consisted of one short high voltage pulse and one long low voltage pulse (100 μs, 1,000 V/cm + 400 ms, 100 V/cm) (HV + LV), and the third consisted of eight low voltage pulses (20 ms, 200 V/cm) (8 LV) [3]. As can be seen in Fig. 2.5, the 8 HV pulses resulted in a high degree of permeabilization, allowing a rather large flux of Na^+ and K^+. In contrast, HV + LV pulses only caused a mild perturbance in muscle Na^+ and K^+ content, allowing the cell to return to normal values after 1 week. Eight LV pulses resulted in slightly larger disturbances in Na^+ and K^+ contents than HV + LV, in the presence of DNA. Note that the presence of DNA results in larger changes in ion content.

From these studies, it is clear that careful consideration should be given when choosing the electroporation pulses, as amplitude, duration, and the number of pulses have large effects on permeabilization and resealing, and thus on the recovery from electroporation.

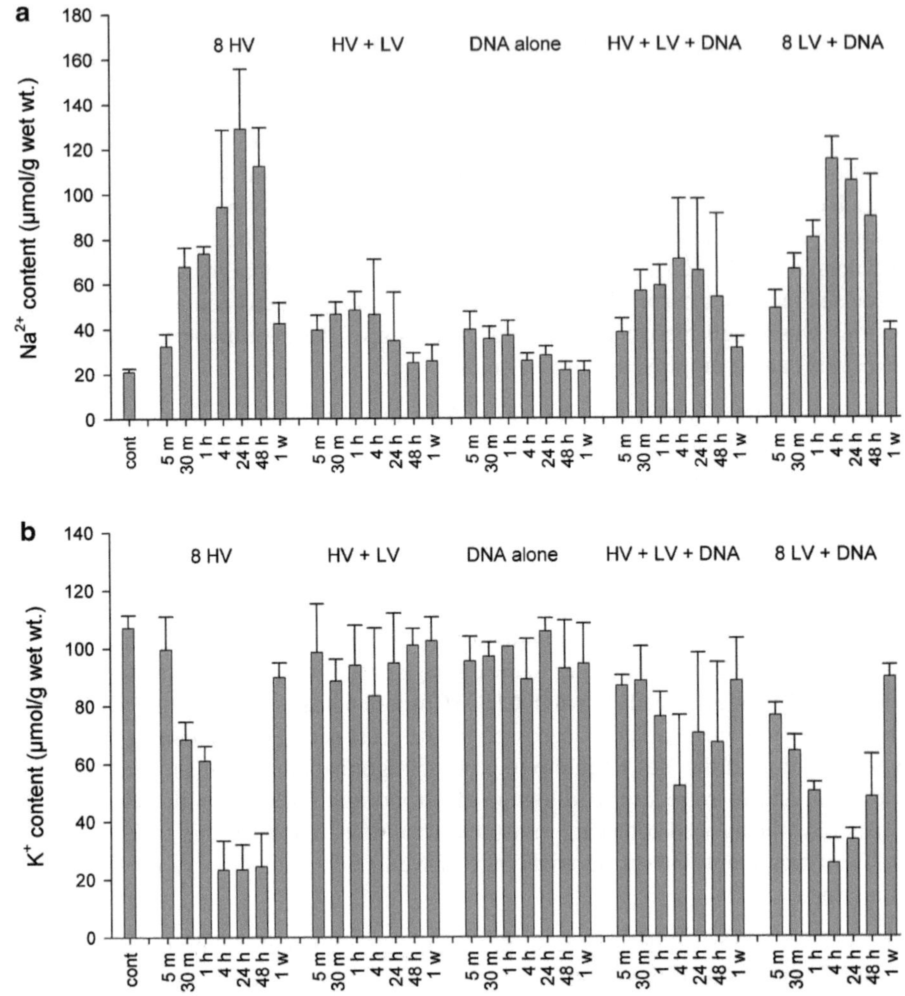

Fig. 2.5 Na^+ (**a**) and K^+ (**b**) content in mouse TC muscle exposed to electroporation (8 HV or HV + LV), DNA injection (DNA alone), or a combination of electroporation and DNA injection (HV + LV + DNA and 8 LV + DNA). For each treatment, muscles were isolated with increasing delay from electroporation (5 min to 1 week) and total muscle Na^+ and K^+ content was determined. Reproduced with permission from the authors from [3]

Conclusion

Increasing the permeability of the membrane is perilous for a cell. This may prove to be an advantage when electroporation is used for ablation. In most other cases, however, cell survival is essential. In these situations, it is important to choose the right pulse combination, giving rise to as little tissue damage as possible, while still efficiently introducing the drug of choice into the cell. Finally, certain actions can be taken to minimize the detrimental effects of permeabilization, such as ensuring an adequate ATP level in the cells of the target tissue (to maintain cellular functions and sustain repair processes) and actively assisting recovery from electroporation.

References

1. Clausen T, Van Hardeveld C, Everts ME. Significance of cation transport in control of energy metabolism and thermogenesis. Physiol Rev. 1991;71(3):733–74.
2. Clausen T, Gissel H. Role of Na+, K+ pumps in restoring contractility following loss of cell membrane integrity in rat skeletal muscle. Acta Physiol Scand. 2005;183:263–71.
3. Hojman P, Gissel H, Andre F, et al. Physiological effects of high- and low-voltage pulse combinations for gene electrotransfer in muscle. Hum Gene Ther. 2008;19:1249–60.
4. Gabriel B, Teissie J. Generation of reactive-oxygen species induced by electropermeabilization of Chinese hamster ovary cells and their consequence on cell viability. Eur J Biochem. 1994;223(1):25–33.
5. Rols MP, Teissie J. Electropermeabilization of mammalian cells. Quantitative analysis of the phenomenon. Biophys J. 1990;58(5):1089–98.
6. Saulis G. Pore disappearance in a cell after electroporation: theoretical simulation and comparison with experiments. Biophys J. 1997;73(3):1299–309.
7. Bier M, Hammer SM, Canaday DJ, Lee RC. Kinetics of sealing for transient electropores in isolated mammalian skeletal muscle cells. Bioelectromagnetics. 1999;20(3):194–201.
8. Dong Z, Saikumar P, Weinberg JM, Venkatachalam MA. Calcium in cell injury and death. Annu Rev Pathol. 2006;1:405–34.
9. Orrenius S, Zhivotovsky B, Nicotera P. Regulation of cell death: the calcium-apoptosis link. Nat Rev Mol Cell Biol. 2003;4(7):552–65.
10. Han R, Campbell KP. Dysferlin and muscle membrane repair. Curr Opin Cell Biol. 2007;19(4):409–16.
11. Duchen MR. Mitochondria in health and disease: perspectives on a new mitochondrial biology. Mol Asp Med. 2004;25(4):365–451.
12. Nicholls DG. Mitochondria and calcium signaling. Cell Calcium. 2009;38(3–4):311–7.
13. Feissner RF, Skalska J, Gaum WE, Sheu SS. Crosstalk signaling between mitochondrial Ca2+ and ROS. Front Biosci. 2009;14:1197–218.
14. Godell CM, Smyers ME, Eddleman CS, Ballinger ML, Fishman HM, Bittner GD. Calpain activity promotes the sealing of severed giant axons. Proc Natl Acad Sci USA. 1997;94(9):4751–6.
15. Mellgren RL, Zhang W, Miyake K, McNeil PL. Calpain is required for the rapid, calcium-dependent repair of wounded plasma membrane. J Biol Chem. 2007;282(4):2567–75.
16. Steinhardt RA, Bi G, Alderton JM. Cell membrane resealing by a vesicular mechanism similar to neurotransmitter release. Science. 1994;263(5145):390–3.
17. Togo T. Long-term potentiation of wound-induced exocytosis and plasma membrane repair is dependent on cAMP-response element-mediated transcription via a protein kinase C- and p38 MAPK-dependent pathway. J Biol Chem. 2004;279(43):44996–5003.
18. Togo T, Alderton JM, Bi GQ, Steinhardt RA. The mechanism of facilitated cell membrane resealing. J Cell Sci. 1999;112(Pt 5):719–31.
19. Gehl J, Mir LM. Determination of optimal parameters for in vivo gene transfer by electroporation, using a rapid in vivo test for cell permeabilization. Biochem Biophys Res Commun. 1999;261(2):377–80.
20. Schmolka IR. Physical basis for poloxamer interactions. Ann N Y Acad Sci. 1994;720:92–7.
21. Lee RC, River LP, Pan FS, Ji L, Wollmann RL. Surfactant-induced sealing of electropermeabilized skeletal muscle membranes in vivo. Proc Natl Acad Sci USA. 1992;89(10):4524–8.
22. Collins JM, Despa F, Lee RC. Structural and functional recovery of electropermeabilized skeletal muscle in-vivo after treatment with surfactant poloxamer 188. Biochim Biophys Acta. 2007;1768(5):1238–46.
23. Serbest G, Horwitz J, Jost M, Barbee K. Mechanisms of cell death and neuroprotection by poloxamer 188 after mechanical trauma. FASEB J. 2006;20(2):308–10.

Chapter 3
The Cell in the Electric Field

Tadej Kotnik, Gorazd Pucihar, and Damijan Miklavčič

Abstract An exposure of a cell to an external electric field results in the induced transmembrane voltage ($\Delta\Psi_m$) that superimposes to the resting voltage. This can have a range of effects, from modification of the activity of voltage-gated channels to membrane electroporation, and accurate knowledge of spatial distribution and time course of $\Delta\Psi_m$ is important for the understanding of these effects. In this chapter, we present the analytical, numerical, and experimental methods of determination of $\Delta\Psi_m$, and combine them with the monitoring of electroporation-induced transmembrane molecular transport (TMT) in Chinese Hamster Ovary (CHO) cells. Potentiometric measurements are performed using di-8-ANEPPS, and TMT is monitored using propidium iodide. In isolated cells, we combine analytical derivation (for spherical cells) and numerical computation of $\Delta\Psi_m$ (for irregularly shaped cells) with potentiometric measurements to show that the latter are accurate and reliable. Monitoring of TMT in these same cells shows that it is confined to the regions with the highest $|\Delta\Psi_m|$. We then review other parameters influencing electroporation of isolated cells, and proceed, through the intermediate case of dense suspensions, to cells in direct contact with each other. We use the scrape-loading test to show that the CHO cells in a monolayer are interconnected, and then study $\Delta\Psi_m$ and TMT in a cluster of four such cells. With low pulse amplitudes, the cluster behaves as one big cell, with $\Delta\Psi_m$ continuous along its outer boundary, reflecting the interconnections. With interconnections inhibited, the cells start to behave as individual entities, with $\Delta\Psi_m$ continuous along the plasma membrane of each cell. With the cluster exposed to porating (higher amplitude) pulses, TMT occurs in the membrane regions for which computations predict the highest $|\Delta\Psi_m|$ if the cells are modeled as insulated, suggesting that the interconnections are blocked by supraphysiological $\Delta\Psi_m$, either directly by voltage gating or indirectly through changes in ionic concentrations caused by electroporation.

Keywords Induced transmembrane voltage • Potentiometric dyes • Electroporation • Molecular transport

Introduction

The spatial distribution of the voltage on the plasma membrane of biological cells has a number of theoretical and experimental implications, such as the activation of voltage-gated membrane channels, cardiac cell stimulation, and plasma membrane electroporation [1–7]. In studies of these phenomena, cells are usually exposed to an external electric field, which induces a voltage across the cell membrane,

---

T. Kotnik (✉)
Department of Biomedical Engineering, University of Ljubljana, Trzaska 25, 1000 Ljubljana, Slovenia
e-mail: tadej.kotnik@fe.uni-lj.si

S.T. Kee et al. (eds.), *Clinical Aspects of Electroporation*,
DOI 10.1007/978-1-4419-8363-3_3, © Springer Science+Business Media, LLC 2011

termed the induced transmembrane voltage and denoted by $\Delta\Psi_m$ [8, 9]. Unlike the resting transmembrane voltage, which is always present and constant everywhere on the plasma membrane, $\Delta\Psi_m$ only lasts for the duration of the exposure and varies with the position on the membrane. Consequently, it is often important to accurately determine not only its amplitude, but also its spatial distribution.

Many studies imply that plasma membrane electroporation and the resulting molecular flow across the membrane occur in the regions of the membrane exposed to a sufficiently high $\Delta\Psi_m$ [10–14]. Although formation and stabilization of each pore in the membrane is a stochastic process, on the scale of cells and tissues, the effects of membrane electroporation only become detectable at $\Delta\Psi_m$ exceeding a certain "critical" value, $\Delta\Psi_{mC}$ (typically several hundred mV), which treats electroporation as a deterministic process. Thus, for efficient applications of electroporation and understanding of the phenomenon, accurate determination of the distribution of $\Delta\Psi_m$ on the cell membrane is important.

Isolated Cells

Spherical Cells in a Homogeneous Field

In exposures of cells to a direct current (DC) homogeneous electric field, $\Delta\Psi_m$ is determined by solving Laplace's equation. Although biological cells are not perfect spheres, in theoretical treatments they are usually considered as such – a spherical interior (the cytoplasm) surrounded by a concentric spherical shell of uniform thickness (the membrane). For certain types of cells, and particularly for cells in suspensions, this is a reasonable assumption. In the first approximation, the plasma membrane can also be treated as nonconductive. Under these assumptions, the solution of Laplace's equation leads to the formula for $\Delta\Psi_m$ often referred to as the (steady-state) Schwan's equation [15],

$$\Delta\Psi_m = 1.5\, ER\cos\theta, \tag{3.1}$$

where E is the electric field in the region where the cell is situated, R is the cell radius, and θ is the angle measured from the center of the cell with respect to the direction of the field. Thus, $\Delta\Psi_m$ is proportional to the applied electric field and the cell radius. Furthermore, it has extremal values at the points where the field is perpendicular to the membrane, that is, at θ=0° and θ=180° (the "poles" of the cell), and in between these poles it varies proportionally to the cosine of θ, as shown in Fig. 3.1b.

$\Delta\Psi_m$, as given by (3.1) is typically established several microseconds after the onset of the electric field. With exposures to a DC field lasting hundreds of microseconds or more, this formula can safely be applied to yield the maximal, steady-state value of the induced transmembrane voltage. To describe the transient behavior during the initial microseconds, one uses the first-order Schwan's equation [8]:

$$\Delta\psi_m = 1.5\, ER\cos\theta\left(1 - e^{-t/\tau_m}\right), \tag{3.2}$$

where τ_m is the time constant of the membrane charging and is expressed as:

$$\tau_m = \frac{R\varepsilon_m}{2d\dfrac{\sigma_i\sigma_e}{\sigma_i + 2\sigma_e} + R\sigma_m}, \tag{3.3}$$

with σ_i, σ_m and σ_e as the conductivities of the cytoplasm, cell membrane, and extracellular medium, ε_m the dielectric permittivity of the membrane, d the membrane thickness, and R again the cell radius.

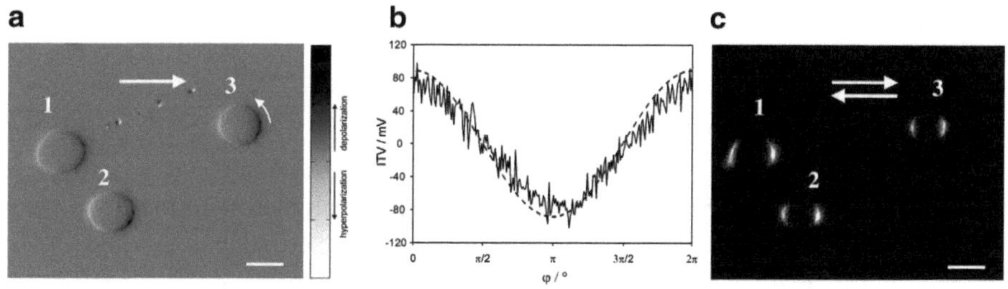

Fig. 3.1 $\Delta\Psi_m$ and electroporation of three spherical CHO cells. (**a**) Changes in fluorescence of di-8-ANEPPS proportional to $\Delta\Psi_m$ caused by a nonporating, 100 V/cm, 50 ms electric pulse. (**b**) Spatial distribution of $\Delta\Psi_m$ as measured on the cell #3 in (**a**) along the path shown by the *arrow* (*solid*), and as predicted by the steady-state Schwan's equation (*dashed*). (**c**) Electroporation obtained on the same cells with an exposure to a 650-V/cm, 750+750 μs bipolar pulse, as visualized by inflow of propidium iodide through the porated membrane regions 100 ms after the exposure. The detected areas of poration imply $\Delta\Psi_{mC} \approx 540$ mV. The bar in (**a**) and (**c**) corresponds to 10 μm

Equations (3.2) and (3.3) are applicable to exposures to sine (alternating current, AC) electric fields with frequencies below 1 MHz and to rectangular electric pulses longer than 1 μs. To determine the time course of $\Delta\Psi_m$ induced by even higher field frequencies or even shorter pulses, the second-order extension of Schwan's equation must be used, in which dielectric permittivities of the cytoplasm and the cell exterior also have to be taken into account [16–18].

An alternative to the analytical derivation of $\Delta\Psi_m$ are the experimental techniques. These include the measurements of $\Delta\Psi_m$ with microelectrodes and with potentiometric fluorescent dyes. The invasive nature of microelectrodes, their low spatial resolution and physical presence, which distorts the electric field, are considerable shortcomings of this approach. In contrast, measurements by means of potentiometric dyes are noninvasive, offer higher spatial resolution, and moreover do not distort the field and thus $\Delta\Psi_m$. As a consequence, during the last decade the potentiometric dyes, such as di-8-ANEPPS [19–22] have become the preferred tool in experimental studies and measurements of $\Delta\Psi_m$.

In Fig. 3.1, the measurements of $\Delta\Psi_m$ on spherical CHO cells are compared to the analytical solution given by (3.1), and a correlation between $\Delta\Psi_m$ and the location of the electroporated membrane regions through which molecular flow occurs is demonstrated. Figure 3.1a, b shows that the measured $\Delta\Psi_m$ correlates well with the theoretical predictions, with the highest values of $\Delta\Psi_m$ found in the membrane regions facing the electrodes (the "poles"). Figure 3.1c shows that the molecular flow through the membrane, and thus membrane electroporation, is confined to these same regions, that is, the areas for which $\Delta\Psi_m > \Delta\Psi_{mC}$.

Nonspherical Geometrically Regular Cells

When suspended, many cells have a shape close to spherical, but for some cell types this is clearly not the case. Among the few generalizations of the cell shape that still allow for analytical derivation of $\Delta\Psi_m$, the most useful are cylinders (e.g., for muscle cells and axons of nerve cells), oblate spheroids (e.g., erythrocytes), and prolate spheroids (e.g., bacilli). To obtain the analogs of Schwan's equation for such cells, one solves Laplace's equation in a suitable coordinate system [23–25]. For a circular cylinder with the axis perpendicular to the field, this yields

$$\Delta\Psi_m = 2ER\cos\theta. \tag{3.4}$$

For an oblate spheroid with the axis of rotational symmetry aligned with the field, we get

$$\Delta\Psi_{\mathrm{m}} = E\frac{R_2^2 - R_1^2}{\left(\frac{R_2^2}{\sqrt{R_2^2-R_1^2}}\right)\operatorname{arcctg}\left(\frac{R_1}{\sqrt{R_2^2-R_1^2}}\right) - R_1} \times \frac{R_2\cos\theta}{\sqrt{R_1^2\sin^2\theta + R_2^2\cos^2\theta}} \quad (3.5)$$

and for a prolate spheroid with the axis of rotational symmetry aligned with the field, we get

$$\Delta\Psi_{\mathrm{m}} = E\frac{R_1^2 - R_2^2}{R_1 - \left(\frac{R_2^2}{\sqrt{R_1^2-R_2^2}}\right)\ln\left(\frac{R_1+\sqrt{R_1^2-R_2^2}}{R_2}\right)} \times \frac{R_2\cos\theta}{\sqrt{R_1^2\sin^2\theta + R_2^2\cos^2\theta}} \quad (3.6)$$

where R_1 and R_2 are the radii of the spheroid in the directions parallel and perpendicular to the field, respectively.

A description of a cell is geometrically realistic if the thickness of its membrane is uniform. This is the case if the membrane represents the space between two concentric spheres, but not with two confocal spheroids or ellipsoids. As a result, the thickness of the membrane modeled in spheroidal or ellipsoidal coordinates is necessarily nonuniform. By solving Laplace's equation in these coordinates, we thus obtain the spatial distribution of the electric potential in a nonrealistic setting. However, under the assumption that the membrane conductivity is zero, the induced transmembrane voltage obtained in this manner is still realistic. Namely, the shielding of the cytoplasm is then complete, and hence the electric potential everywhere inside the cytoplasm is constant. Therefore, the geometry of the inner surface of the membrane does not affect the potential distribution outside the cell, which is the same as if the cell were a homogeneous nonconductive body of the same shape. A more rigorous discussion of the validity of this approach can be found in Kotnik and Miklavčič [24].

For nonspherical cells, it is generally more revealing to express $\Delta\Psi_{\mathrm{m}}$ as a function of the arc length along the membrane than as a function of the angle θ (for a sphere, the two quantities are directly proportional). For uniformity, the normalized version of the arc length is used, increasing from 0 to 1 equidistantly along the arc of the membrane.

Irregularly Shaped Cells

Cells in tissues have markedly irregular shapes, deviating considerably from the regular shapes described above. For many such cases, an analytical solution for $\Delta\Psi_{\mathrm{m}}$ cannot be derived. In practice, there are two approaches for obtaining accurate estimates of $\Delta\Psi_{\mathrm{m}}$ on irregularly shaped cells: experimental determination and numerical computation. Experimentally, $\Delta\Psi_{\mathrm{m}}$ can be measured by means of a potentiometric fluorescent dye, as already presented above (see Fig. 3.1). The numerical approach, on the other hand, requires the construction of a model of the cell and subsequent computation of the electric potential inside and outside the cell.

The simplest approach in numerical modeling of an irregularly shaped cell is to compose it from several simple geometrical objects, such as hemispheres and cylinders [26–28]. However, this can only yield a rough approximation of the actual situation, and can thus lead to considerable error. A more realistic three-dimensional model of an irregularly shaped cell can be constructed from a sequence of cross sections of the cell under consideration, as shown in Fig. 3.2 and explained in more detail in Pucihar et al. [29, 30].

In a suitable numerical software package, such as COMSOL Multiphysics, the distribution of the electric potential Ψ in such a model of the cell and its vicinity is then easily computed and the induced transmembrane voltage is determined as the difference between electric potentials on both

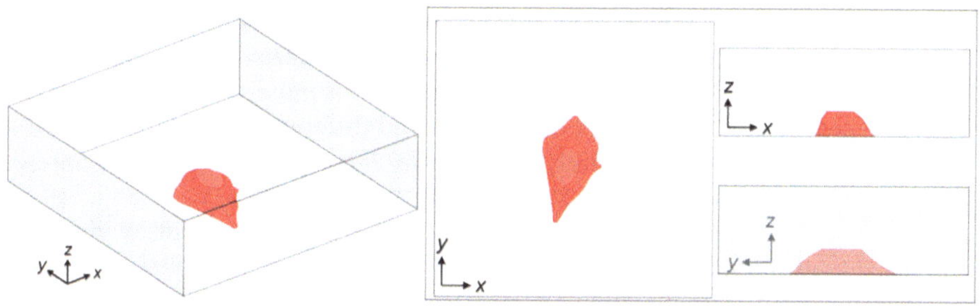

Fig. 3.2 Finite-elements model of a CHO cell attached to a cover glass. The interior of the rectangular block represents the extracellular medium, and the *gray*-shaded faces are the electrodes generating the electric field

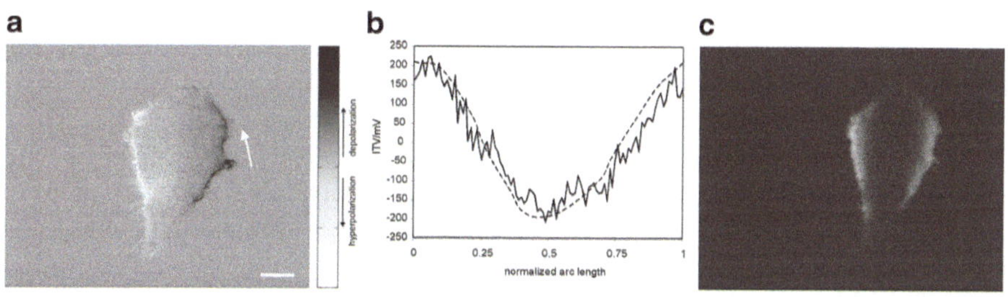

Fig. 3.3 $\Delta\Psi_m$ and electroporation of the CHO cell shown in Fig. 3.2. (**a**) Changes in fluorescence of di-8-ANEPPS proportional to $\Delta\Psi_m$ caused by a nonporating, 100 V/cm, 50 ms electric pulse. (**b**) Spatial distribution of $\Delta\Psi_m$ as measured on a cell in (**a**) along the path shown by the *arrow* (*solid*), and as computed on a model shown in (**a**) (*dashed*). (**c**) Electroporation obtained on the same cell with an exposure to a 1,000 V/cm, 200 μs unipolar pulse, as visualized by inflow of propidium iodide through the porated membrane regions 100 ms after the exposure. The detected areas of poration imply $\Delta\Psi_{mC} \approx 650$ mV. The bar in (**a**) and (**c**) corresponds to 10 μm

sides of the membrane. In analogy to Fig. 3.1, Fig. 3.3a, b demonstrate close correlation between the measured and the numerically computed $\Delta\Psi_m$, while Fig. 3.3c shows that also in irregular cells electroporation occurs in the membrane regions with the highest absolute value of $\Delta\Psi_m$. These regions are generally located in the areas of the membrane closest to (i.e., facing) the electrodes. This is most obvious in cells with pronounced protrusions, where electroporation occurs at their very tips [31].

The results shown in Figs. 3.1 and 3.3 confirm the finding that electroporation is limited to the membrane regions in which the absolute value of $\Delta\Psi_m$ exceeds a certain critical level, $\Delta\Psi_m > \Delta\Psi_{mC}$. With nonspherical shapes, the maximal $\Delta\Psi_m$ attained also depends on the orientation of the cell with respect to the field. Therefore, by exposing the cells to several different orientations of the field, the efficiency of electroporation can be increased significantly, which is also confirmed by experiments [28].

Parameters Influencing Electroporation of Isolated Cells

Pulse Parameters

Electroporation of isolated cells and dilute suspensions in vitro is influenced by both the parameters of the electric pulse(s) and the experimental conditions. Investigations of the role of the amplitude, number, and duration of unipolar rectangular pulses have been the subject of several comprehensive studies [32–36]. These studies show that electroporation only becomes detectable above a certain pulse amplitude, $\Delta\Psi_{mC}$. With further increases in pulse amplitude, the percentage of porated cells increases, while the percentage of cells surviving the treatment decreases. The average amount of molecules introduced into a cell reaches a peak at some intermediate pulse amplitude. It has also been shown that both poration and cell survival as functions of pulse amplitude vary significantly between various types of cells [37]. Some of the observed differences can be attributed to differences in cell size, but several studies imply that the differences in membrane composition and structure can also play an important role [38, 39].

Experiments show that increasing the number and/or duration of the pulses yields detectable electroporation at a lower minimal pulse amplitude, and that the average amount of molecules introduced into a cell generally increases with an increase of the number of pulses applied [32, 34]. Several studies have demonstrated that for macromolecules such as DNA, electrophoresis plays an important role in the transmembrane transport, and sufficiently long pulse duration is crucial for adequate uptake [33, 34, 40]. Typically, pulse durations for the uptake of smaller molecules are in the range of hundreds of microseconds, while for macromolecules, pulses lasting from several milliseconds to several tens of milliseconds are usually required. Combinations of shorter (electroporating) and longer (electrophoretic) pulses have also been shown to improve the efficiency of gene electrotransfer [41, 42].

At least two studies have focused on a comparison of the efficiency of unipolar and bipolar rectangular pulses in vitro, demonstrating that with bipolar pulses, detectable electroporation is obtained with lower pulse amplitudes, while substantial cell death occurs at similar amplitudes as when unipolar pulses of the same duration are applied [43, 44]. Moreover, contamination of the medium through electrolytical release of metal ions from the electrodes is also lower with bipolar than with unipolar pulses [45].

Unlike the role of the amplitude, number, duration, and polarity of pulses, a hypothetical role of pulse dynamics, or the "pulse shape," has been a subject of relatively few studies. Two reports by the same authors have claimed an improved efficiency of electroporation and gene electrotransfer when a sine wave was superimposed to a rectangular pulse [46, 47]. In another study, rectangular, sine, and triangular waves of the same amplitude were compared, obtaining the most efficient transfection for rectangular, less for sine, and the least for triangular waves [48]. This is in agreement with a later systematic study showing that among the parameters describing the pulse shape, by far the most important for the efficiency of electroporation is the time during which the pulse amplitude exceeds a certain critical value [49]. In another study, it was shown that the efficiency of electroporation is roughly the same for pulse repetition frequencies ranging from 1 Hz (i.e., one pulse per second) up to several kHz, provided that the same total number of pulses is delivered [50].

Experimental Conditions

Electroporation and cell death caused by exposure to high voltage electric pulses also depend on the composition of the extracellular medium. Since electroporation results in substantial exchange of ions between the medium and the cytosol, care must be taken to avoid possible detrimental effects. In particular, in electroporation media, potassium ions are often used instead of the sodium ions of the typical culture media [14, 34, 51]. Also, the calcium ions typically present in culture media should be avoided, as electroporation provides them with a pathway for entering cytosol, leading to supraphysiological intracellular concentrations of Ca^{2+} that can result in cytotoxic effects [52] (as described in Chap. 2).

The electrical conductivity of the extracellular medium also plays a role in electroporation. In media with a conductivity several orders of magnitude below the physiological levels, Schwan's equation as given by (3.1) or (3.2) must be modified by lowering the multiplication factor 1.5 accordingly, as explained in detail in Kotnik et al. [9] and confirmed experimentally in Pucihar et al. [51]. Due to this, in a low-conductivity medium, $\Delta\Psi_m$ induced by a pulse of a given amplitude is lower than in a physiological medium, and somewhat higher pulse amplitudes must, in general, be applied to obtain the same extent of poration. The decrease in medium conductivity also leads to a lower heating of the cell suspension during the exposure to electroporating pulses [51].

Among the other experimental conditions that influence electroporation are the osmotic pressure and the temperature of the suspension. It was reported that osmotic pressure is not an important factor in transmembrane transport of small molecules, but use of a hypoosmolar buffer during pulsation allows for more efficient uptake of large proteins [53]. With respect to the temperature, postporational incubation at 37°C results in a faster membrane recovery and thus in a higher fraction of cells surviving the treatment. It was also observed that in vitro, the highest uptake of DNA is obtained by incubating the cells before poration at 4°C and after poration at 37°C [54].

Dense Suspensions and Monolayers

In natural situations the cells are rarely isolated, and when sufficiently close to each other, the mutual distortion of the field caused by their proximity cannot be overlooked. Often, the cells are also in direct contact, forming two-dimensional (monolayers attached to the bottom of a dish) or three-dimensional (tissues) structures, and they can even be interconnected.

In dilute cell suspensions, the distance between the cells is much larger than the cell sizes themselves, and the local field outside each cell is practically unaffected by the presence of other cells. Thus, for cells representing less than 1% of the suspension volume (for a spherical cell with a radius of 10 μm, this means up to two million cells/mL), the deviation of the induced transmembrane voltage, $\Delta\Psi_m$, from the prediction given by (3.1) is negligible. However, for larger volume fractions occupied by the cells, the distortion of the local field around each cell by the adjacent cells becomes more pronounced. As the volume fraction occupied by the cells increases beyond 10% and approaches 50%, the spatial distribution of $\Delta\Psi_m$ starts to deviate significantly from that given by (3.1), as the factor 1.5 gradually decreases towards 1, and the distribution also starts to diverge from the ideal cosine shape, as shown in detail in Susil et al. [55], Pavlin et al. [56], and Pucihar et al. [57]. Due to the lower $\Delta\Psi_m$, the efficiency of electroporation with the same pulse parameters is typically lower in dense suspensions than in dilute ones [57].

For even larger volume fractions, the cells come into direct contact, and the electrical properties of the suspension start to resemble that of a tissue, but only to a certain extent. Namely, cells can form specific structures, such as layers, and moreover in tissues they can also be directly electrically coupled, for example, through gap junctions. The amplitude and the spatial distribution of $\Delta\Psi_m$ on these cells can differ considerably from $\Delta\Psi_m$ observed on single isolated cells. This is because dense cell packing shields the cells electrically to some extent, and intercellular pathways can connect adjacent cells electrically. Due to the nature of the tissue structure, it is difficult to observe these effects experimentally in individual tissue cells. As a more feasible alternative, we can study clusters of cells growing in monolayers, which present a simple model for examining the behavior of cells in tissues. As in tissues, cells in clusters also have complex geometrical shapes, are densely packed, and are often connected with intercellular pathways. Thus, the only significant deviation is their two-dimensional arrangement, as opposed to typically three-dimensional cellular structures of tissues.

Intracellular pathways, also termed gap junctions, are small protein channels that allow for the exchange of ions between neighboring cells. The opened or closed state of the gap junctions renders the cells electrically connected or electrically insulated, respectively, and in this manner it can affect $\Delta\Psi_m$ and electroporation considerably.

Figure 3.4 shows that CHO cells form gap junctions allowing for exchange of ions and smaller molecules between the cells, and that these gap junctions are inhibited (blocked) effectively using oleamide. Figures 3.5 and 3.6 show a numerical model and an experiment performed on a cluster of four such cells attached to a cover glass.

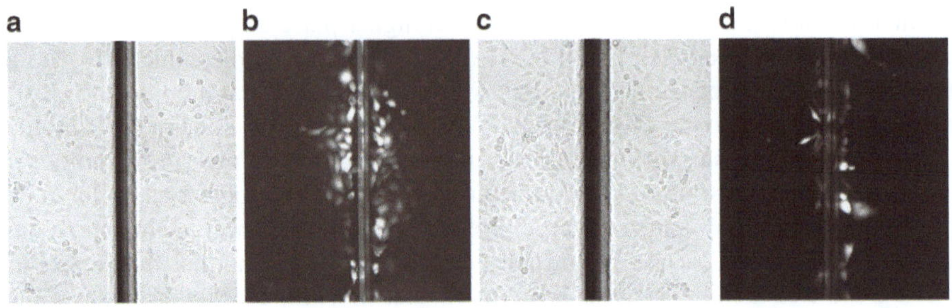

Fig. 3.4 Scrape loading test with 1 mM Lucifer Yellow performed on CHO cells. (**a**) Phase contrast image of the cells scraped with a needle (*black vertical* in the *middle*). (**b**) Fluorescence of the cells 5 min later. The dye entered the damaged cells and quickly diffused into the neigboring, undamaged cells. (**c**) Same as (**a**), but with the cells preincubated for 45 min with 200 μM oleamide, a gap junction inhibitor. (**d**) Fluorescence 5 min later. The dye only entered the cells directly damaged by scraping

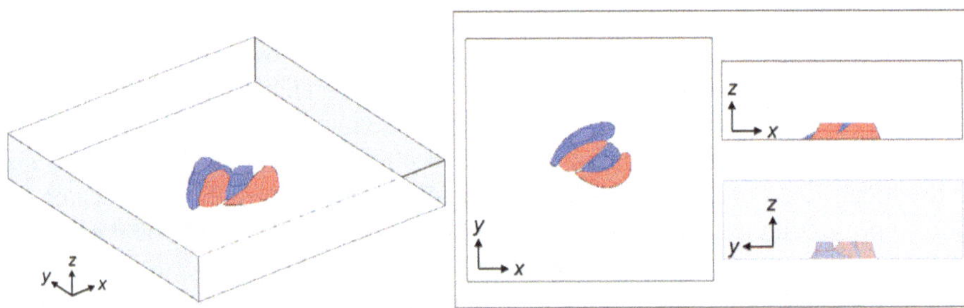

Fig. 3.5 Finite-elements model of a cluster of CHO cells forming a monolayer cluster attached to a cover glass. By changing the electrical conductivity of the membrane regions forming contacts between the cells, cells in clusters can be modeled as either electrically interconnected or electrically insulated

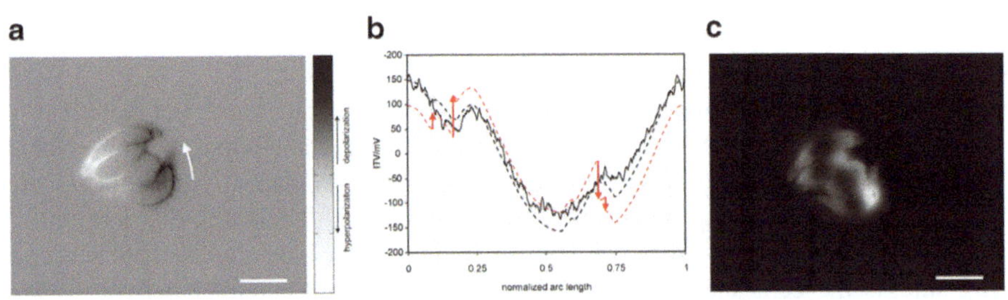

Fig. 3.6 $\Delta\Psi_m$ and electroporation of a cluster of the four attached CHO cells shown in Fig. 3.5. (**a**) Changes in fluorescence of di-8-ANEPPS proportional to $\Delta\Psi_m$ caused by a nonporating, 75 V/cm, 50 ms electric pulse. (**b**) Spatial distribution of $\Delta\Psi_m$ as measured on the cluster in (**a**) along its outer boundary as shown by the *arrow* (*solid*), and numerically computed $\Delta\Psi_m$ for electrically interconnected (*dashed black*) and electrically insulated cells (*dashed gray*). The *arrows* show the discontinuities of $\Delta\Psi_m$ along the outer cluster boundary with insulated cells. (**c**) Electroporation obtained on the same cluster with an exposure to a 1,000 V/cm, 750+750 μs bipolar pulse, as visualized by inflow of propidium iodide through the porated membrane regions 500 ms after the exposure. The bar in (**a**) and (**c**) corresponds to 20 μm

With nonelectroporating pulses (lower amplitude, longer duration) and without inhibition of the gap junctions, $\Delta\Psi_m$ induced on the membranes of the cells was continuous when traced along the outer boundary of the cluster (Fig. 3.6b, solid curve). This correlates well with the numerically computed $\Delta\Psi_m$ for the case of electrically interconnected cells (Fig. 3.6b, dashed black). In other words, the cluster behaved as if it was one big cell, reflecting the interconnections of the cells by gap junctions.

Applying the same pulse parameters, but with the gap junctions inhibited, the cells started behaving as individual entities (i.e., as electrically insulated), so that $\Delta\Psi_m$ was continuous along the plasma membrane of each individual cell, yet discontinuous when traced along the outer boundary of the cluster (Fig. 3.6b, dashed gray, with discontinuities marked by arrows).

When the cluster was exposed to electroporating pulses (higher amplitude, shorter duration), however, the molecular transport occurred in the membrane regions for which numerical computations predicted the highest $\Delta\Psi_m$ if the cells were modeled as insulated. The results were unaffected by the presence or absence of oleamide, suggesting that with $\Delta\Psi_m$ substantially above the physiological levels, the gap junctions can also be blocked by another mechanism, perhaps directly by voltage gating, or indirectly as a consequence of changes in ionic concentrations caused by electroporation. The ongoing investigations should cast additional light on these observations.

Within clusters of cells, in a similar fashion to isolated nonspherical cells, the efficiency of electroporation depends on the orientation of the field with respect to the cells. If a single pulse is used for electroporation, the appropriate field orientation with respect to the cell should be chosen for optimal effects. For applications in which the aim is to achieve electroporation, but the size of the porated area is unimportant, it is advisable to orient the field along the larger dimension of the cell, for example, so that the longest protrusions face the electrodes. For such an orientation, a moderate external field will induce $\Delta\Psi_m > \Delta\Psi_{mC}$ only at the very ends of these protrusions. In contrast, if the aim is to maximize the size of the porated area, the field should generally be oriented perpendicularly to the larger dimension of the cell (see e.g., Fig. 3.3). With several pulses applied, an improved efficiency can be obtained by changing the field orientation between consecutive pulses. As this approach renders a higher electroporated area of the membranes, it allows the use of a somewhat lower pulse amplitude, resulting in reduced loss of cell viability [58, 59].

In addition to the variability of cell shapes, a recent study suggests that also $\Delta\Psi_{mC}$ can vary considerably even between cells of the same type [60]. As a consequence, numerical modeling can be useful for analyzing the spatial distribution of $\Delta\Psi_m$ on the membranes of the cells under consideration when planning an efficient electroporation protocol, but the location and size of the porated membrane regions can only be estimated [30].

References

1. Bedlack RS, Wei M, Fox SH, et al. Distinct electric potentials in soma and neurite membranes. Neuron. 1994;13:1187–93.
2. Cheng DKL, Tung L, Sobie EA. Nonuniform responses of transmembrane potential during electric field stimulation of single cardiac cells. Am J Physiol. 1999;277:H351–62.
3. Neumann E, Kakorin S, Toensing K. Fundamentals of electroporative delivery of drugs and genes. Bioelectrochem Bioenerg. 1999;48:3–16.
4. Teissié J, Eynard N, Gabriel B, et al. Electropermeabilization of cell membranes. Adv Drug Deliv Rev. 1999;35:3–19.
5. Burnett P, Robertson JK, Palmer JM, et al. Fluorescence imaging of electrically stimulated cells. J Biomol Screen. 2003;8:660–7.
6. Sharma V, Tung L. Ionic currents involved in shock-induced nonlinear changes in transmembrane potential responses of single cardiac cells. Pflugers Arch. 2004;449:248–56.
7. Huang CJ, Harootunian A, Maher MP, et al. Characterization of voltage-gated sodium-channel blockers by electrical stimulation and fluorescence detection of membrane potential. Nat Biotechnol. 2006;24:439–46.
8. Pauly H, Schwan HP. Über die Impedanz einer Suspension von kugelformigen Teilchen mit einer Schale. Z Naturforsch B. 1959;14:125–31.
9. Kotnik T, Bobanović F, Miklavčič D. Sensitivity of transmembrane voltage induced by applied electric fields – a theoretical analysis. Bioelectrochem Bioenerg. 1997;43:285–91.

10. Hibino M, Shigemori M, Itoh H, et al. Membrane conductance of an electroporated cell analyzed by submicrosecond imaging of transmembrane potential. Biophys J. 1991;59:209–20.
11. Hibino M, Itoh H, Kinosita Jr K. Time courses of cell electroporation as revealed by submicrosecond imaging of transmembrane potential. Biophys J. 1993;64:1789–800.
12. Tekle E, Astumian RD, Chock PB. Selective and asymmetric molecular-transport across electroporated cell-membranes. Proc Natl Acad Sci USA. 1994;91:11512–6.
13. Gabriel B, Teissié J. Direct observation in the millisecond time range of fluorescent molecule asymmetrical interaction with the electropermeabilized cell membrane. Biophys J. 1997;73:2630–7.
14. Gabriel B, Teissié J. Time courses of mammalian cell electropermeabilization observed by millisecond imaging of membrane property changes during the pulse. Biophys J. 1999;76:2158–65.
15. Schwan HP. Electrical properties of tissue and cell suspensions. Adv Biol Med Phys. 1957;5:147–209.
16. Grosse C, Schwan HP. Cellular membrane potentials induced by alternating fields. Biophys J. 1992;63: 1632–42.
17. Kotnik T, Miklavčič D, Slivnik T. Time course of transmembrane voltage induced by time-varying electric fields – a method for theoretical analysis and its application. Bioelectrochem Bioenerg. 1998;45:3–16.
18. Kotnik T, Miklavčič D. Second-order model of membrane electric field induced by alternating external electric fields. IEEE Trans Biomed Eng. 2000;47:1074–81.
19. Fluhler E, Burnham VG, Loew LM. Spectra, membrane binding, and potentiometric responses of new charge shift probes. Biochemistry. 1985;24:5749–55.
20. Gross D, Loew LM, Webb W. Optical imaging of cell membrane potential changes induced by applied electric fields. Biophys J. 1986;50:339–48.
21. Loew LM. Voltage sensitive dyes: measurement of membrane potentials induced by DC and AC electric fields. Bioelectromagnetics. 1992;Suppl 1:179–89.
22. Pucihar G, Kotnik T, Miklavčič D. Measuring the induced membrane voltage with di-8-ANEPPS. J Visual Exp 2009;33:1659.
23. Bernhard J, Pauly H. Generation of potential differences across membranes of ellipsoidal cells in an alternating electrical field. Biophysik. 1973;10:89–98.
24. Kotnik T, Miklavčič D. Analytical description of transmembrane voltage induced by electric fields on spheroidal cells. Biophys J. 2000;79:670–9.
25. Gimsa J, Wachner D. Analytical description of the transmembrane voltage induced on arbitrarily oriented ellipsoidal and cylindrical cells. Biophys J. 2001;81:1888–96.
26. Fear EC, Stuchly MA. Modeling assemblies of biological cells exposed to electric fields. IEEE Trans Biomed Eng. 1998;45:1259–71.
27. Buitenweg JR, Rutten WL, Marani E. Geometry-based finite-element modeling of the electrical contact between a cultured neuron and a microelectrode. IEEE Trans Biomed Eng. 2003;50:501–9.
28. Valič B, Golzio M, Pavlin M, et al. Effect of electric field induced transmembrane potential on spheroidal cells: theory and experiment. Eur Biophys J. 2003;32:519–28.
29. Pucihar G, Kotnik T, Valič B, et al. Numerical determination of transmembrane voltage induced on irregularly shaped cells. Ann Biomed Eng. 2006;34:642–52.
30. Pucihar G, Miklavčič D, Kotnik T. A time-dependent numerical model of transmembrane voltage inducement and electroporation of irregularly shaped cells. IEEE Trans Biomed Eng. 2009;56:1491–501.
31. Teruel MN, Meyer T. Electroporation-induced formation of individual calcium entry sites in the cell body and processes of adherent cells. Biophys J. 1997;73:1785–96.
32. Rols MP, Teissié J. Electropermeabilization of mammalian cells. Quantitative analysis of the phenomenon. Biophys J. 1990;58:1089–98.
33. Wolf H, Rols MP, Boldt E, et al. Control by pulse duration of electric-field mediated gene transfer in mammalian cells. Biophys J. 1994;66:524–31.
34. Rols MP, Teissié J. Electropermeabilization of mammalian cells to macromolecules: control by pulse duration. Biophys J. 1998;75:1415–23.
35. Canatella PJ, Karr JF, Petros JA, et al. Quantitative study of electroporation-mediated molecular uptake and cell viability. Biophys J. 2001;80:755–64.
36. Maček-Lebar A, Miklavčič D. Cell electropermeabilization to small molecules *in vitro*: control by pulse parameters. Radiol Oncol. 2001;35:193–202.
37. emažar M, Jarm T, Miklavčič D, et al. Effect of electric-field intensity on electropermeabilization and electrosensitivity of various tumor-cell lines *in vitro*. Electro Magnetobiol. 1998;17:261–70.
38. Troiano GC, Tung L, Sharma V, et al. The reduction in electroporation voltages by the addition of a surfactant to planar lipid bilayers. Biophys J. 1998;75:880–8.
39. Kandušer M, Fošnarič M, Šentjurc M, et al. Effect of surfactant polyoxyethylene glycol ($C_{12}E_8$) on electroporation of cell line DC3F. Colloid Surface A. 2003;214:205–17.

40. Sukharev SI, Klenchin VA, Serov SM, et al. Electroporation and electrophoretic DNA transfer into cells. Biophys J. 1992;63:1320–7.
41. Satkauskas S, André F, Bureau MF, et al. Electrophoretic component of electric pulses determines the efficacy of *in vivo* DNA electrotransfer. Human Gene Ther. 2005;16:1194–201.
42. Kandušer M, Miklavčič D, Pavlin M. Mechanisms involved in gene electrotransfer using high- and low-voltage pulses – an *in vitro* study. Bioelectrochemistry. 2009;74:265–71.
43. Tekle E, Astumian RD, Chock PB. Electroporation by using bipolar oscillating electric field: an improved method for DNA transfection of NIH 3T3 cells. Proc Natl Acad Sci USA. 1994;88:4230–4.
44. Kotnik T, Mir LM, Flisar K, et al. Cell membrane electropermeabilization by symmetrical bipolar rectangular pulses. Part I. Increased efficiency of permabilization. Bioelectro-chemistry. 2001;54:83–90.
45. Kotnik T, Miklavčič D, Mir LM. Cell membrane electropermeabilization by symmetrical bipolar rectangular pulses: Part II. Reduced electrolytic contamination. Bioelectrochemistry. 2001;54:91–5.
46. Chang DC. Cell poration and cell fusion using an oscillating electric field. Biophys J. 1989;56:641–52.
47. Chang DC, Gao PQ, Maxwell BL. High efficiency gene transfection by electroporation using a radio-frequency electric field. Biochim Biophys Acta. 1991;1092:153–60.
48. Xie TD, Tsong TY. Study of mechanisms of electric field-induced DNA transfection. II. Transfection by low-amplitude, low-frequency alternating electric fields. Biophys J. 1990;58:897–903.
49. Kotnik T, Pucihar G, Reberšek M, et al. Role of pulse shape in cell membrane electropermeabilization. Biochim Biophys Acta. 2003;1614:193–200.
50. Pucihar G, Mir LM, Miklavčič D. The effect of pulse repetition frequency on the uptake into electropermeabilized cells *in vitro* with possible applications in electrochemotherapy. Bioelectrochemistry. 2002;57:167–72.
51. Pucihar G, Kotnik T, Kandušer M, et al. The influence of medium conductivity on electropermeabilization and survival of cells *in vitro*. Bioelectrochemistry. 2001;54:107–15.
52. Nicotera C, Bellomo G, Orrenius S. Calcium-mediated mechanisms in chemically induced cell death. Annu Rev Pharmacol Toxicol. 1992;32:449–70.
53. Golzio M, Mora MP, Raynaud C, et al. Control by osmotic pressure of voltage-induced permeabilization and gene transfer in mammalian cells. Biophys J. 1998;74:3015–22.
54. Rols MP, Delteil C, Serin G, et al. Temperature effects on electrotransfection of mammalian cells. Nucleic Acids Res. 1994;22:540.
55. Susil R, Šemrov D, Miklavčič D. Electric field induced transmembrane potential depends on cell density and organization. Electro Magnetobiol. 1998;17:391–9.
56. Pavlin M, Pavšelj N, Miklavčič D. Dependence of induced transmembrane potential on cell density, arrangement, and cell position inside a cell system. IEEE Trans Biomed Eng. 2002;49:605–12.
57. Pucihar G, Kotnik T, Teissié J, et al. Electroporation of dense cell suspensions. Eur Biophys J. 2007;36: 173–85.
58. Reberšek M, Faurie C, Kandušer M, et al. Electroporator with automatic change of electric field direction improves gene electrotransfer *in vitro*. Biomed Eng Online. 2007;6(25):1–11.
59. Trontelj K, Reberšek M, Kandušer M, et al. Optimization of bulk cell electrofusion *in vitro* for production of human–mouse heterohybridoma cells. Bioelectrochemistry. 2008;74:124–9.
60. Towhidi L, Kotnik T, Pucihar G, et al. Variability of the minimal transmembrane voltage resulting in detectable membrane electroporation. Electromagn Biol Med. 2008;27:372–85.

Chapter 4
Understanding Electric Fields for Clinical Use

Faisal Mahmood

Abstract For physicians or researchers from the biological sciences, it is usually not necessary to deal with the in-depth scientific theory of the electric field in order to handle procedures involving electrotransfer. On the other hand, it is very often of utmost importance to know the basic concept, from a pragmatic point of view, to understand simple electric field distributions. In this chapter, we initially address the basic physics and definitions of electrostatics in order to prepare the reader for the practical topics that follow. The electric field strength and the electric vector field are explained in connection with tissue characteristics, especially heterogeneity and anisotropy. The role of the pulse generator and the electrode geometry is addressed in relation to electric field distributions and electric field strength. The reader is provided with electric field visualization methods, which are important for both comprehension and interpretation of otherwise complicated data. Finally, critical steps for ensuring the intended delivery of the appropriate electric field for treatment procedures are proposed. It is stressed that numerical derivation of the electric field is the only reasonable way of handling individual nonstandardized electrotransfer procedures.

Keywords Electrostatics • Electric field • Electric potential • Electrode geometry • Tissue heterogeneity • Treatment planning • Electric field plot

Introduction

Understanding the nature of the electric field is important for any physician or researcher who wants to make use of electroporation on a preclinical or clinical basis. In fact, the clinician's level of comprehension of this technology should match that of the established treatment technologies, such as external beam radiation therapy in cancer irradiation.

The aim of this chapter is to:

1. Provide the reader with the tools to understand the basic physics of the electric field.
2. Discuss and clarify some issues concerning nomenclature and physical concepts.
3. Give an overview of factors that affect the electric field.

F. Mahmood (✉)
Center for Experimental Drug and Gene Electrotransfer (C*EDGE), Department of Oncology, Copenhagen University Hospital Herlev, Herlev Ringvej 75, 2730 Herlev, Denmark
e-mail: fama@heh.regionh.dk

S.T. Kee et al. (eds.), *Clinical Aspects of Electroporation*,
DOI 10.1007/978-1-4419-8363-3_4, © Springer Science+Business Media, LLC 2011

4. Give examples of the visualization of electric field distribution of common electrode configurations.
5. Describe the necessary steps in treatment planning of clinical electroporation to ensure optimized delivery of the electric field to the target volume.

Basic Concept and Definitions

Coulomb's Law

Electrical force emerges from the presence of charge, and acts between charges only. It is one of the four fundamental interactions known to physics, and the most precisely determined. Here, we shall only consider charges that do not move; we then speak of an electrostatic force, described by Coulomb's law. It states that between two charges at rest, there is a force **F** directly proportional to the product of the charges and inversely proportional to the square of the distance between them. The mathematical equivalence is:

$$\mathrm{F} = K \cdot \frac{q_1 q_2}{r^2} \hat{r}$$

where K is a proportionality factor which is usually written as $1/4\pi\varepsilon_0$ and has a value of 9.0×10^9 and the unit Vm/C. q_1 and q_2 are two point charges, r is the distance between the charges, and "r-hat" is a unit vector parallel to the line connecting the charges. (The concept of vectors is described in Section "**E**: A Vector").

The Principle of Superposition

When there are more than two charges present, which is always the case in macroscopic systems, we supplement Coulomb's law with one other fact of nature: "The principle of superposition". It states that the force on any charge is the sum of the Coulomb forces from each of the other charges.

The combination of Coulomb's law and the principle of superposition is all there is to electrostatics, which is electromagnetics in its most simple form. We can, in theory, solve any problem of static charge distributions (electrode configurations) by applying these two principles.

The Electric Field

The concept of the electric field is merely a matter of definition: If we divide the electric force by charge, we get **F/q**, which we call the electric field **E**. We understand this new quantity, the electric field, which is introduced for practical reasons, as a force per charge "exerted" at a point with no charge. The unit of the electric field is thus N/C (Newton per charge), or more conveniently, V/m (volt per meter). When we speak of for example, 100 V/m, it is a measure of the strength, or intensity, of the electric field at a particular point. As a result, we call it the electric field strength or the electric field intensity.

$$\mathbf{E} = \mathbf{F} / q \quad \text{(Unit is Newton / charge } [\mathrm{N/C}] \text{ or volt / meter } [\mathrm{V/m}]).$$

The Electrostatic Approximation

The electric field is generally a function of space and time, i.e., $\mathbf{E} = \mathbf{E}(x,y,z,t)$. However, if the response of the system, where the electric field is to be determined, is governed by a time constant that is much smaller than the duration of the exposure to the electric field, we can assume steady state, that is, $\mathbf{E} = \mathbf{E}(x,y,z)$. This condition is satisfied in polarization of the cell membrane, where the time constant is about 1 μs [1], which is much smaller than the typical voltage pulse duration in clinical applications of electroporation (0.1–10 ms). Moreover, as the electromotive force of the pulse generator ensures a constant potential difference across the electrodes, electrostatic conditions can be assumed (net amount of charge on the electrodes is kept constant).

The Maxwell Equations

In many research papers in this field, the authors derive expressions for various quantities from the basic equations of electrostatics; that is, the Maxwell equations in electrostatic condition. These equations are the mathematical formulations of the physics just described, and we bring them here only for the sake of completeness. For a thorough discussion of these equations, please refer to a text book on the electromagnetic theory (e.g., [2]):

$$\nabla \cdot \mathrm{E} = \frac{\rho}{\epsilon_0}$$

$$\nabla \times \mathrm{E} = 0$$

The Electric Potential

The electric potential, also denoted as voltage, is yet another quantity that is invented for convenience. It emerges from the second Maxwell equation of electrostatics, and relates to the electric field as:

$$-\nabla\varphi = \mathrm{E}$$

The electric potential φ has the unit energy per charge (volt); that is, it represents the work (energy) required to bring charges together. For example, an electrode with the potential 100 V carries charges each having the energy of 100 J. From the definition of the potential, it follows that the electric field scales linearly with the potential.

Calculation of the Electric Field

To state the laws of electrostatics (the Maxwell equations of electrostatics) is one thing, to use them easily and with a certain amount of ingenuity is another. The calculation of the electric field is simple, but only in theory. Therefore, we shall not try to provide the reader with examples of the calculation of various electrode geometries, as it will require introduction to many more concepts from electromagnetics, which is not the aim of this chapter. Medical doctors should not concern themselves with how the electric field is calculated; rather, they should be able to interpret the numbers of a calculation and to a certain extent be able to point out parameters that could alter the electric field from one clinical situation to another. In the remainder of this chapter, we shall therefore give attention to concrete issues of the electric field from a practical point of view.

E, a Vector

In the previous section, we denoted the electric field by a boldface letter, **E**. Here, we will explain what is the difference between E and **E**, and why this has clinical relevance.

The "electric field" is often referred to by stating a number (e.g., 100 V/m), that is, as a scalar quantity. Mostly, this "short cut" does not lead to confusion or error, but in some situations one must be more precise to avoid misunderstandings.

The electric field can be specified at every point in space; therefore we call it a field. A field is any physical quantity that takes on different values at different points in space. Temperature is an example of a field which can be fully described by measuring the internal thermal energy of each point; that is, a single number can be assigned to every point in space. This is known as a scalar field. In contrast, the electric field is made up of vectors; one at each point in space. So in addition to a number, the electric field also has a direction at every point in space. This is known as a vector field **E**. The size of each vector is denoted as $|\mathbf{E}|$ or E and defines the electric field strength. The electric field strength (size of the vector) is, in most cases, the adequate information for the researcher or physician. The difference is illustrated in Fig. 4.1 showing one point in space depicted with its temperature and its electric vector, respectively.

In clinical situations, however, the orientation of the electric vectors is not always insignificant. The reason is that most biological tissue is anisotropic (e.g., muscle and skin), making it sensitive to the direction of the electric vectors. In Fig. 4.2, two different hypothetical tissue samples are illustrated along with the applied electric field, which for illustrative purposes is perfectly uniform.

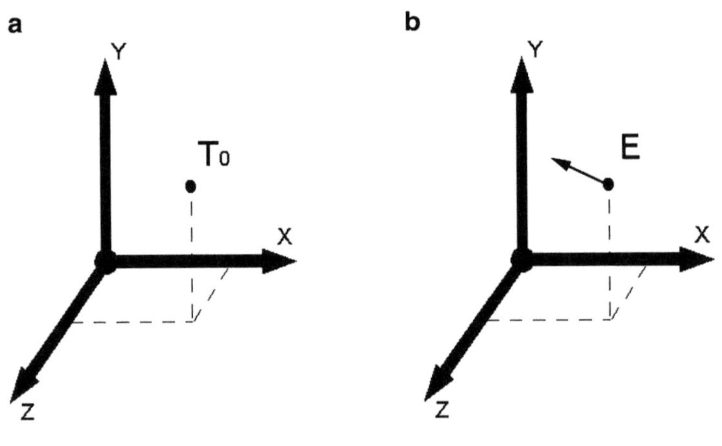

Fig. 4.1 An arbitrary point in space described by its temperature and electric field vector. (**a**) The temperature is described by only a number, T_0; hence temperature is a scalar field. (**b**) The electrostatic force is described by the electric field vector **E**; hence electric field is a vector field

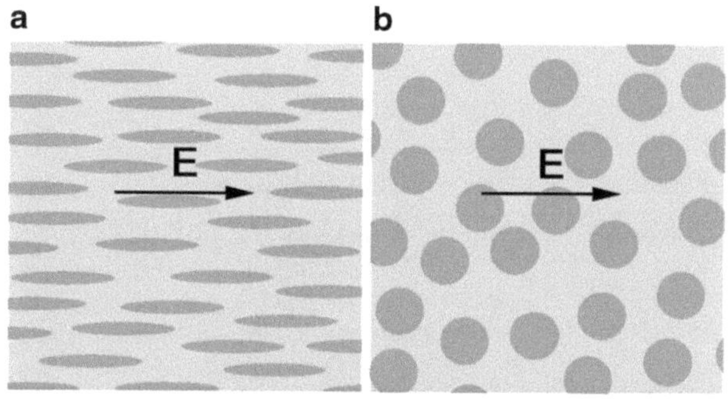

Fig. 4.2 (**a**) Artistic representation of anisotropic tissue exposed to a uniform electric field. The elongated elliptic shapes represent the cells composing the bulk tissue. In this case, the direction of the electric field vector affects the electric field induced in the cell membranes, as the projection of the electric vector onto the membrane surface tangent is dependent on the orientation of **E**. (**b**) Uniform electric field in isotropic tissue composed of spherical cells. The direction of the electric field vector is in this situation not affecting the net induced electric field in the cell membranes

A glance at the equation for transmembrane potential (see Chap. 3) reveals that the induced effect on a cell is proportional to the form factor, f (equals 1.5 for a spherical cell), and to the projection of the electric vectors onto the tangents of the cell surface, at every surface point, $E{\cdot}\cos\theta$. Therefore, the electric field "sees" different geometries from different directions in situation (a), but not in situation (b).

Interpretation of "V/m"

When characterizing the electric field of an electrode system, a common practice is to designate it by the nominal electric field strength. For instance, if we have a plate electrode with an inter-plate distance of 1 cm and voltage difference of 100 V between the plates, we assign to it the voltage-to-meter ratio of 10,000 V/m or 100 V/cm. In most cases, this is indeed a good approximation to the actual electric field strength between the plates, which can be calculated exactly as the ratio: voltage difference to inter-plate distance (valid for plate electrodes where plate dimensions (not thickness) are much larger than the distance between the plates (Fig. 4.3a1)).

If we, instead, consider an electrode unit with two pins or needles and an inter-electrode distance of 1 cm and voltage difference of 100 V between the pins (Fig. 4.3b1), we can still choose to designate the voltage-to-meter ratio of 100 V/cm to the electrode system. In this case, however, we have no idea what the actual electric field strength distribution looks like in the region between the pins, much less where "100 V/cm" is. If we, in this case, estimate the electric field strength by this fraction, we will make a big error. *The main message here is: "V/m" is a unit, not a formula!*

For some electrode systems, it is not even obvious what is meant by the fraction "V/m". If we consider the electrode in Fig. 4.3c1, we will need to define the symmetry plan and voltage encoding of the electrode arrangement before making an attempt to employ the "V/m" characteristic. "V/m" in this case is not self-explanatory.

In order to reduce the possibility of misinterpretation and drawing false conclusions regarding the electric field strength, it is recommended to instead state the nominal *voltage* of the electrodes, and provide precise and concise geometry data. Having said that, it should be mentioned that the fraction "V/m" *can* be quite handy in studies where the same electrode is used in different voltage

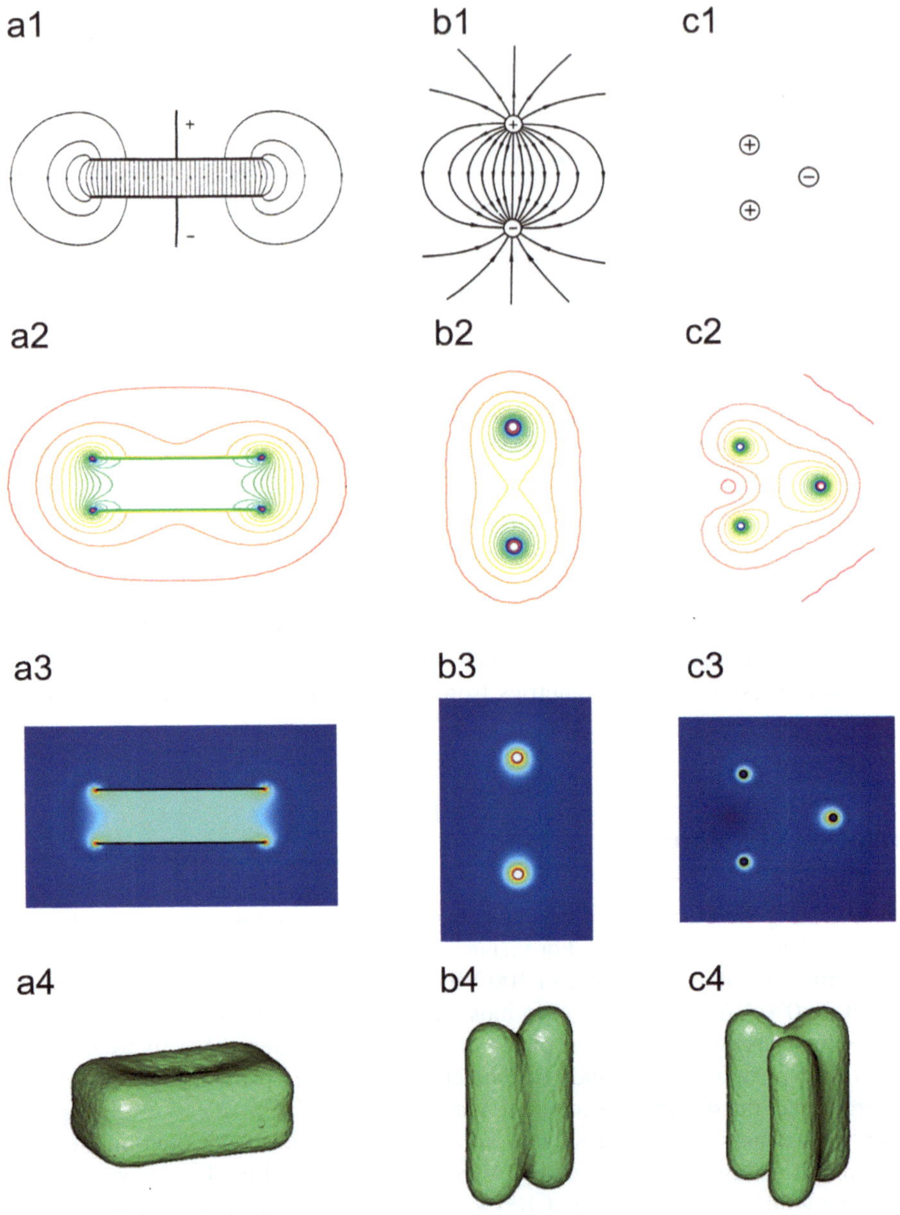

Fig. 4.3 Four types of representation of the electric fields generated by three simple electrode configurations. (a1, b1) field line plots; (a2, b2, c2) contour plots; (a3, b3, c3) slice plots; (a4, b4, c4) visualization of the electric field by 3D iso-surface plots. The graphical refinement increases downwards, whereas electrode arrangement becomes more complex from *left* to *right*. Usually, more than one type of data illustration is needed to complement the understanding of a given electric field distribution. The contour plots, slice plots, and iso-surface plots are generated by COMSOL Multiphysics ver. 3.5a (COMSOL AB, Stockholm, Sweden)

conditions. Here, it is possible to use "V/m" as comparison of the different voltages used, to make a *relative* statement about the electric field strength. This is possible due to the linear relation between the voltage amplitude and the electric field strength. In general, there is no such linearity between the electric field strength and the geometry of the electrode system.

Electric Field Parameters

The electric field can be affected by a large number of factors; therefore, the determination of it is subject to great uncertainty. Figure 4.4 gives an overview of the most critical/significant factors influencing the electropermeabilization yield. The ones that are highlighted are those responsible for altering the electric field and consequently affecting the level of induced permeability of the cell membrane.

Pulse Generator

The most well-controlled and well-understood way of influencing the electric field strength is by adjusting the applied voltage. According to the mathematical relations of electrostatics (see Section "Basic Concept and Definitions"), a change in the applied voltage will always result in a linear response of the electric field strength; that is, a doubling in the voltage amplitude yields a doubling in the electric field strength. In general,

$$E' = EU'/U,$$

where E' is the new electric field strength expressed as the old electric field strength, E, multiplied by the ratio of the new and the old applied voltage. Other adjustment options of the applied voltage pulses, such as frequency and shape, are not relevant in the discussion of the static electric field distribution; they are, however, nontrivially linked to the biological response of the cells (e.g., [3–7]).

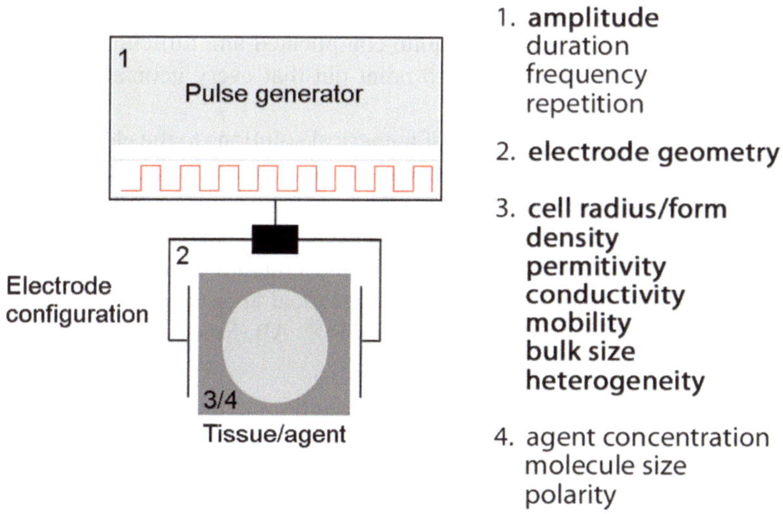

Fig. 4.4 Overview of the parameters affecting the effectiveness of electrotransfer. The parameters can be divided into four categories: *1* pulse generator, *2* electrode geometry, *3* tissue properties, and *4* agent properties. *Boldface letters* indicate factors that modify the procedure through alteration of the electric field. Besides pulse amplitude (voltage) and electrode geometry, various properties of the medium (tissue) can be mentioned as directly accountable for changes to the electric field

Electrode Geometry

From Section "Basic Concept and Definitions", it follows that charge distributions are intrinsically linked to the electric field distribution; thus, the size and shape of the electrodes are directly responsible for the electric field strength. However, the relations between geometry and electric field distribution are usually quite complicated to determine.

Even so, the laws of electromagnetics hold one simple consequence that one can benefit from when designing or redesigning an electrode configuration: Any given electrode geometry can be rescaled simply by multiplying all dimensions of the electrode configuration, including the voltage amplitude, by a factor corresponding to the required new size, and the electric field distribution can be preserved accordingly. In contrast, if an electrode system is developed from applying different scaling factors to the geometry of an existing design, the electric field of the new electrode system will have a new (relative) distribution.

As far as inter-electrode distances are concerned, we can very easily deduce the result in the case of a plate electrode. The analytical solution for the electric field between two infinite parallel plate electrodes is $E = U/d$, where U is the applied voltage and d is the distance between the electrodes. This, of course, means that the electric field strength is linked to the inter-electrode distance as

$$E' = E\, d/d',$$

where the marks indicate the new electric field strength and inter-plate distance, respectively. The result holds for most real-life plate electrodes when considering central regions of the electrode, that is, not too close to the "edges". For pin electrodes, we know that the electric field strength is inversely proportional to the distance (r) from the center of the electrode. For any interesting or clinically relevant configurations of pin electrodes, that is, with more than one pin, the principle of superposition must be applied to express the resulting electric field of all pins in any given point in space as a function of the distance to the pins. The analytical solution can be found in the literature [8].

Thickness and length of the pins of a pin electrode configuration is also related to the electric field distribution. Again, these relations are quite complicated and difficult to state as generalized formulas. Nevertheless, we mention it here to point out that every geometrical change results in changes to the electric field.

In the next section, we will give examples of numerical solutions to the electric field distributions of common electrode geometries. The use of commercial computer packages is by far the preferred way of handling electric field distributions, due to the speed and simultaneous simulation of multiple physical conditions. The reader should note, however, that handling simulation software still requires knowledge of the physics, as the outcome of the simulation is dependent on the input relations. The finite element method (FEM) is the mathematical approach employed by popular commercial packages like COMSOL Multiphysics (COMSOL AB, Stockholm, Sweden).

The Tissue

The heterogeneity and morphology of the tissue involved can have tremendous impact on the electric field in the target region (the local electric field).

On a microscopic scale, the electric field is very difficult to determine due to tissue heterogeneity. For example, local changes in cellularity causes perturbation of the local electric field, resulting in either a reduction or increase of the local field strength [3]. Cell shape, size and density affect the induced transmembrane electric field, and the relationship is often described by an approximated mathematical expression (see Chap. 3, Equation 3.1). The mobility of cells has also been investigated but has shown little relevance in clinical electroporation protocols, due to the relatively short duration of the electric field pulses compared to the rotational (and also translational) movement of the cells [6].

From a macroscopic perspective, the size of the bulk target volume and electrical resistance of the tissue types involved are important parameters. For example, if the electric conductivity of the target volume (e.g., a tumor) is higher than the conductivity of the surrounding tissue (both enclosed by the electrode system), we get a reduction of the electric field strength in the target volume, compared to a situation with equal conductivities, and vice versa [9]. Skin is a good example of a biological system that comprises of many different conductivities. The total voltage drop across the individual layers of the skin is simply distributed proportionally to the resistances of the layers, and the electric field strength can then be obtained after division by the layer thicknesses. Figure 4.5 shows the electric field distribution in a skin fold resulting from the use of a plate electrode. The potential drop across the very resistive outmost layer, the stratum corneum, is much greater than across the rest of the skin fold, even though the stratum corneum is much thinner. This results in very high electric field intensities in the stratum corneum, as compared to the remainder of the skin

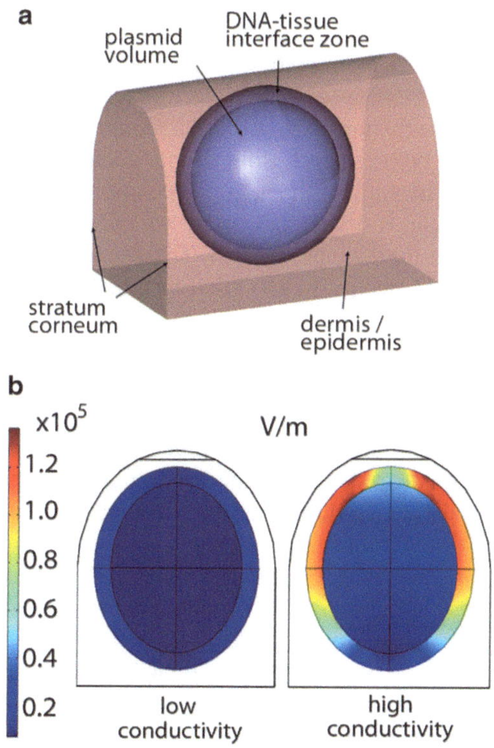

Fig. 4.5 (**a**) A simplistic model for numerical calculation of the electric field inside a skin fold containing a plasmid volume for the gene electrotransfer procedure (see Chap. 17). Plate electrodes are not modeled geometrically; instead the surface of the skin is defined by an electric potential (i.e., a boundary condition). (**b**) Central cross sections showing slice plots (see Section "Electric Field Distributions of Clinical Electrodes") of the electric field distribution in the fold. The difference in electric field distribution is clear when comparing the low and high conductivity conditions of stratum corneum, underlining the necessity of awareness when anisotropic tissue is involved (the conductivity of the stratum corneum is initially low and increases due to strong electric fields)

fold. In reality, the electric properties of skin exhibit highly nonlinear dynamics in response to the applied electric field [10]. Nevertheless, in this simplistic approach, the impact on the electric field is evident from the comparison of heterogeneous and homogeneous conditions.

For any specific tissue type, the bulk electric field generated in it is the primary parameter of concern. In treatment situations, there are many types of tissues involved, and the geometry of the tissue will often require the use of numerical computer calculations to allow for a good estimate of the electric field distributions. The calculations, however, rely on input values such as conductivities and thicknesses of various tissue types – something that is associated with large degrees of uncertainty [11]. Moreover, since biological tissue displays characteristics of both a conductor and an isolator, it must be ascribed to both an ability to be polarized (permittivity) and an ability to transport free charges (conductivity). Although sparse, data on the electric properties of tissue do exist, and one should implement as much valid information into the numerical model as possible. Even better is to sweep through different possible values of the electric parameters, to evaluate the range and sensitivity of the calculation results.

Electric Field Distributions of Clinical Electrodes

The aim of this section is to provide interested physicians and researchers with a qualitative understanding of the electric field distributions. This can be used to select appropriate electrodes for intended applications, but primarily it is to give some notion about the electric fields generated in the laboratories or treatment rooms from common electrode devices, through illustrations of the electric field distributions. In order to emphasize different features of the electric field distributions, different plotting techniques will be presented using simple geometries.

It is crucial to bear in mind the limitation of the calculations when viewing the graphics. As described previously in this chapter, if tissue parameters are not regarded, there is a risk of making very large errors in the assessment of the electric field. That is, a distinction must be made between the bulk electric field and the local electric field. Only bulk electric fields are presented.

Figure 4.3 shows four different ways of visualizing the electric field of the same electrode configurations. The method of field lines (Fig. 4.3a1, b1), despite being the most simple from a graphical point of view, holds a lot of information: (1) the arrows give the direction of the field **E**; (2) the density of lines represents strength of the field; (3) a line starts at positive charge and ends at negative charge; (4) the number of lines starting from a charge, q, is equal to q/ε_0.

The plots in Fig. 4.3a2, b2, and c2 show so-called contours of the electric field strength. Each curve represents points of equal electric field strength. This plot type is very practical for a quick overview of the field strength distributions. More details can be found in the slice plots (Fig. 4.3a3, b3, and c3), which are basically very dense contour plots. The slice plot is very useful for detailed analysis of the electric field and is the preferred 2D plot used in numerical calculations. This plot type also reveals "edge effects," which are basically very strong electric fields caused by sharp edges of electrode geometries (especially evident in Fig. 4.3a3). It is important to be aware of the edge effect, as there is a high risk of necrosis in the tissue adjacent to electrode edges (and near pins). Color legends are normally provided with slice plots for assessment of the absolute field strength distributions. 3D iso-surface plots are shown in Fig. 4.3a4, b4, and c4. They show the surfaces formed by points of equal preset electric field strengths. This visualization method is useful for evaluating the "coverage" of a predefined treatment volume, and to for example, estimate the degree of normal tissue involvement. The iso-surface plot does not, however, depicture the electric field inside the surface. Most often, a combination of two or more graphical representations is necessary to get all the information that is needed.

Treatment Planning

Which factors need to be considered to ensure that the prescribed electric field is delivered exclusively to the target volume? We will try to address this question in relation to the critical steps of the procedure. It should be noted that the intention of this description is not to provide medical guidelines for the treatment procedure (for those we would refer to Chap. 8) [12]. Rather, the idea is to put forward important factors related to the electric field distribution, in an explanatory fashion. The outline can serve as inspiration or as a checklist for physicians or researchers planning to implement this technology in their department/laboratory.

The following disposition is inspired by the treatment planning concept in radiation therapy, replacing the absorbed dose distribution with the electric field distribution.

Prescription

First, the electric field strength is prescribed according to target tissue. This can be stated both in terms of bulk electric field strength (electrode geometry and voltage amplitude) and local electric field strength (the actual electric field strength applied to target tissue), depending on what preexisting information is available in the literature, what equipment is at the disposal of the researcher, or which protocol is to be tested.

Geometrical Error

Errors can arise in the preparation stage of a treatment and include setup errors, target volume delineation errors, equipment calibration errors, calculation errors, and organ motion in the imaging scanner. Errors in the treatment delivery situation include target motion, patient, and equipment setup.

The components of the geometrical error of the electrode system should be quantified to assess the size of the necessary margin around the target tissue [13], for the following reasons: (1) the electric field can cause damage to normal tissue; (2) the target tissue must be sufficiently covered by the electric field; and (3) the uncertainty of the geometry can be considered in the evaluation of the results.

Definition of Critical Tissue

It is crucial to identify the normal tissue in close proximity to the electrodes. The risk of exposing normal tissue to the electric field should be assessed and evaluated clinically. Normal tissue (e.g., blood vessels) can skew the electric field distribution of the target volume, and thereby complicate the interpretation of the outcome.

Electrode Selection

Choosing the most appropriate electrode type normally requires advanced knowledge of electric fields and electrodes; however, clinical applicators exist with standardized numbers of electrodes and electrode configurations (as described in Chap. 5), and clinical data have been reported from their applications (as described in later chapters). Application with individually designed electrodes would normally require simulation software but generally offers a better match to a desired target volume.

Calculation of the Electric Field

Realistic calculation of the electric field distribution is only possible using simulation software where both electrode geometry and tissue properties have been modeled. Knowledge of the electric field is not always needed, if the used electrode and the involved tissue compose a standardized procedure or have been reported in the literature.

Optimization of the Electric Field

In advanced treatment planning, the electrode geometry can be improved using optimization procedures. The variables can be chosen as appropriate for the specific electropermeabilization procedure. For example, in electrochemotherapy, the following parameters can be included in the optimization: (1) the fraction of tumor volume which is exposed to an electric field strength lower than a predefined lower threshold value for reversible electroporation; (2) the fraction of tumor volume which is exposed to an electric field strength higher than a predefined upper threshold value for electroporation (beginning of irreversible electroporation); (3) the mean field strength inside the total tumor volume; (4) the standard deviation of the electric field strength; and (5) the amount of normal tissue exposed to an electric field strength above the lower and upper threshold values, respectively [14].

Conclusion

The basic concept of the static electric field can be understood through Coulomb's law and the principle of superposition. The electric potential and electric field are definitions introduced for convenience. The electric field is a vector; however, in practice it is the strength of the electric field and not the direction of the electric field that is important to know. In cases of well-defined anisotropy of the tissue, however, the directions of the electric field vector can be important. The electric field distributions are governed by the electrode configuration and amplitude of the applied voltage. In particular, the electric field strength changes linearly with the voltage applied to the electrodes. For very simple electrode geometries such as the plate electrode, we can hand calculate the bulk electric field to a good approximation. Other electrode configurations, like the pin electrode devices, require the aid of computer calculations. The tissue permeabilization is, in addition to the external electric field, influenced by a number of tissue parameters, including cell size and density. Electric field distributions can be illustrated most appropriately in contour plots or slice plot in 2D, and in iso-surface plots in 3D. To ensure correct delivery of the electric field to the target tissue, several aspects must be considered for example: the prescription of the correct electric field strength according to the target tissue, the calculation of the electric field for specialized electrode devices, required geometrical margins, and the involvement of critical normal tissue.

References

1. Schwan HP, Kay CF. The conductivity of living tissue. Ann NY Acad Sci. 1007;1957:65.
2. Feynman RP, Leighton RB, Sands M. The Feynman lectures on physics. Mainly electromagnetics and matter, vol. 2. California: Addison-Wesley Publishing Company Inc; 1964.
3. Canatella PJ, Karr JF, Petros JA, et al. Quantitative study of electroporation-mediated molecular uptake and cell viability. Biophys J. 2001;80:755–64.
4. Prausnitz MR, Lau BS, Milano CD, et al. A quantitative study of electroporation showing a plateau in net molecular transport. Biophys J. 1993;65:414–22.
5. Puc M, Kotnika T, Mir LM, et al. Quantitative model of small molecules uptake after *in vitro* cell electropermeabilization. Bioelectrochemistry. 2003;60:1–10.
6. Rols MP, Teissie J. Electropermeabilization of mammalian cells quantitative analysis of the phenomenon. Biophys J. 1990;58:1089–98.
7. Canatella PJ, Black MM, Bonnichsen DM, et al. Tissue electroporation: quantification and analysis of heterogeneous transport in multicellular environments. Biophys J. 2004;86:3260–8.
8. Dev SB, Dhar D, Krassowska W. Electric field of a six-needle array electrode used in drug and DNA delivery *in vivo*: analytical versus numerical solution. IEEE Trans Biomed Eng. 2003;50(11):1296–300.
9. Polk C, Postrow E. Handbook of biological effects of electromagnetic fields. 2nd ed. USA: CRC Press; 1996.
10. Pliquett U, Langer R, Weaver JC. Changes in the passive electrical properties of human stratum corneumdue to electroporation. Biochimica et Biophysica Acta. 1995;1239:111–21.
11. Jadoul A, Bouwstra J, Préat V. Effects of iontophoresis and electroporation on the stratum corneum. Adv Drug Deliv Rev. 1999;35:89–105.
12. Mir LM, Gehl J, Sersa G, et al. Standard operating procedures of the electrochemotherapy: instructions for the use of bleomycin or cisplatin administered either systemically or locally and electric pulses delivered by the Cliniporator™ by means of invasive or non-invasive electrodes. EJC Suppl. 2006;4:14–25.
13. ICRU Report 50, Prescribing, Recording, and Reporting Photon Beam Theray. International Commission on Radiation Units and Measurements; 1993.
14. Mahmood F, Gehl J. New clinical electrode device for electroporation of intracranial tumors - semiempirical designoptimization and geometrical tolerance assessment, Bioelectrochemistry. 2011;doi:10.1016/j.bioelechem.2010.12.002.

Chapter 5
Generators and Applicators: Equipment for Electroporation

Lasse G. Staal and Richard Gilbert

Abstract This chapter provides an introduction to the equipment available for treatments based on electroporation. The purpose is to acquaint the reader with the equipment available for the performance of electroporation-based treatments. To that end, pulse generators and applicators are presented along with details on their use. Particular features of relevance to the clinician are described, and manufacturers of the different types of equipment are introduced.

Keywords Pulse generator • Applicator • Electrode • Electrochemotherapy • Gene electrotransfer • DNA vaccination • Irreversible electroporation

Electroporation System

In general, there are three clinically related elements involved with electroporation-based treatments; the protocol, the pulse generator, and the pulse applicator. A therapeutic agent may also be involved if prescribed by the protocol. Each element has a specific role to perform. Each is as important as the others. However, it is the optimal integration of these elements that assures the best electroporation results.

Figure 5.1 shows a cartoon of the two hardware components of an electroporation system. It does not represent any specific manufacturer's equipment but does indicate what is included in any electroporation system. The pulse generator, as the name implies, generates and distributes the electric pulses that are responsible for creating the electroporation effect. It is essentially a "black box" of electronic components usually controlled by a computer. The computer provides the interface between the user and the functions provided by the electronics. In addition, data collection and data analysis options are also provided. The pulse applicator is responsible for transmitting the pulses from the pulse generator to the tissue to be treated. This cartoon version shows four electrodes shaped as needles. Other electrode shapes are available (see "Applicator options"). The number and shape of the electrodes depend on the equipment manufacturer and the treatment application. The hardware components may be combined with a therapeutic agent, and the treatment itself is governed by a protocol. A brief overview of this integration, provided in the following subsections, will help to highlight the function of the electroporation system. A more detailed description of the

R. Gilbert (✉)
Department of Chemical and Biomedical Engineering, University of South Florida, Tampa, FL, USA
e-mail: gilbert@eng.usf.edu

S.T. Kee et al. (eds.), *Clinical Aspects of Electroporation*,
DOI 10.1007/978-1-4419-8363-3_5, © Springer Science+Business Media, LLC 2011

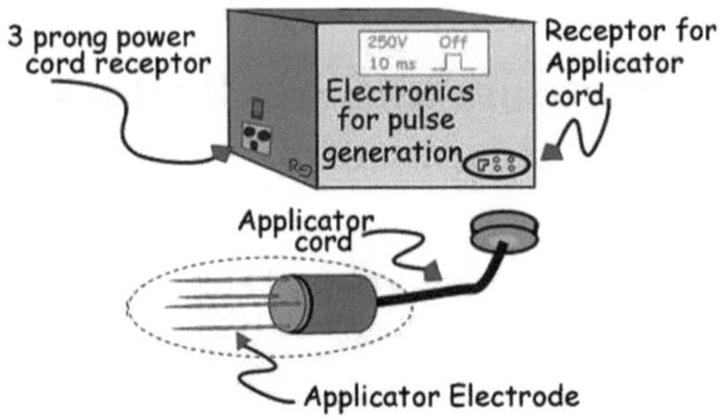

Fig. 5.1 Generic electroporation system illustrating a 4-needle applicator that can be attached to the pulse generator electronics housing. The number and shape of electrodes vary with treatment applications

electric field-mediated therapies supported by each available electroporation system is provided in Section “Vendor Information.”

Electroporation clinical applications are focused on various primary and metastatic tumor systems and infectious diseases. Two generic treatment approaches exist. In protocols based on reversible electroporation, a plasmid or a drug such as bleomycin or cisplatin may be delivered systemically or at a local treatment site. For the local situation, a typical three step protocol would call for the injection of the agent directly into the intercellular volume of the tissue to be treated, the insertion of the applicator’s electrode unit into that same region, and the use of the pulse generator to apply an electric field across the applicator’s electrodes to mediate the transport of the agent into the tissue. If an irreversible electroporation (IRE) protocol is used, the first step, the administration of a therapeutic agent, is not carried out. Instead, a very high field is applied, and the ablation action is due to the energy transfer to the treatment volume as defined by the treatment’s target position within the electric field.

In the following, please find a more in-depth discussion of the basic elements of the electroporation system, providing insight into those aspects that are deemed to be of use in the translational and clinical settings.

Pulse Generators

With the duties of the major elements of an electroporation protocol in mind, the multiple tasks that the electronics in the pulse generator are responsible for include: (1) the creation of the electrical signal shape of the pulse that is applied to the applicator’s electrodes (needles, plates, or pins), (2) the delivery of the desired energy (the amplitude of the pulse) as a function of time, and (3) the number of times that desired electrical signal waveform (pulse) is applied. A specific combination of pulse amplitudes, pulse durations, and pulse repetitions is called an electroporation signature. The delivery of this electroporation signature to an applicator with a specific number and arrangement of electrodes (needles, plates, or pins) and electrode polarities define the geometry of the electric field which, in turn, determines the actual treatment volume. Some vendors permit extensive manipulation of the pulse electrical signal wave forms and parameters while others offer precalibrated equipment tailored to specific treatments. Details on these topics are presented in the following subsections after a review of the safety factors connected with the use of pulse generators.

Safety Aspects

Safety aspects for pulse generators can be classified in terms of equipment issues and operator issues. The equipment safety issues for pulse generators are deemed to be satisfied when the equipment has received the appropriate market clearance from a relevant regulatory agency (e.g., FDA or CE Mark). Please note that it does not follow automatically that a pulse generator approved for use in the United States, an FDA-approved device, can automatically be used in the European Union, i.e., equipment with a CE Mark. Pulse generators not cleared for marketing may qualify for a clinical evaluation/investigational device exemption (IDE) status. A status as an IDE device will permit the pulse generator use in a clinical evaluation setting, since this exemption is based on the manufacturer following normal good manufacturing practices.

Safety practices are governed by the design of the pulse generator and the degree of the clinician's involvement in the protocol. If, for example, the "approved for clinical application" electroporation protocol does not allow any variations in pulse amplitude, duration, or replication, then most of the safety characteristics should be built into the generator equipment itself. This safety strategy would also include shape restraints on the input terminal plugs that accept the wire connections from the approved applicator(s) (electrode connectors). Under this scenario, the clinician would simply plug the applicator into the pulse generator the only way it can be attached and then follow the prescribed protocol. To provide additional safety against inadvertent activation, some pulse generators have foot-pad-based switches that instigate the execution of the protocol. Manufacturers also provide internal test sequences that the pulse generator executes before delivering the preprogrammed pulse wave form to the applicator terminal.

The increase in degrees of freedom an operator has with an electroporation pulse generator dramatically increases the implications of an operator error from a safety perspective. For most clinical protocol development situations, researchers want almost total control of the parameters of the electroporation signature. Pulse generators are available that allow the operator to select the number of pulses to be applied within a specified unit of time, the amplitude of all, or perhaps, each of these pulses, and the number of times this pulse application sequence is to be applied. The pulse generator may also allow the operator to assign which electrode pairs in the applicator receive the pulses as well as the polarities of the electrodes receiving these pulses. Under these conditions there may be safety constraints associated with each of the components of the electroporation signature that the operator may wish to alter, including the time between pulse applications.

Besides the built-in safety of the manufactured equipment, there are common safety expectations of pulse generators involved in both the single-specific and multiple-variations protocol applications. The pulse generator should have a series of interlocks that do not allow pulse generation if the applicator is not plugged in or the applicator's electrodes do not have proper contact with the target tissue. In addition, the nature of how the high-voltage pulses are generated requires that the generator's electronics be well grounded by means of a three-plug power cord and enclosed in a shielded case. The case will also be difficult to dismantle. It is not advisable to work with any equipment that does not have these safety features.

Pulse Types and Parameters

The vocabulary associated with electroporation is the result of the convolution of principles and practices found in physics, electrochemistry, biomedical engineering, and medical science. Thus, words and phrases in the electroporation vocabulary may take on multiple meanings. Pulse types represent one example of this mixed vocabulary in practice. Figure 5.2 illustrates three electroporation pulse types.

A pulse is typically envisioned as a signal that has a magnitude that is different from zero for a small period of time. A pulse signal may be a current or a voltage. For most electroporation pulse generators, the signal is a voltage and the magnitude of that voltage always starts out and returns to 0 volts (V). Electroporation pulse duration is not defined for a specific fixed short period of time. A square wave pulse, for instance (Fig. 5.2a), can rise very quickly to 1,000 V, remain at 1,000 V,

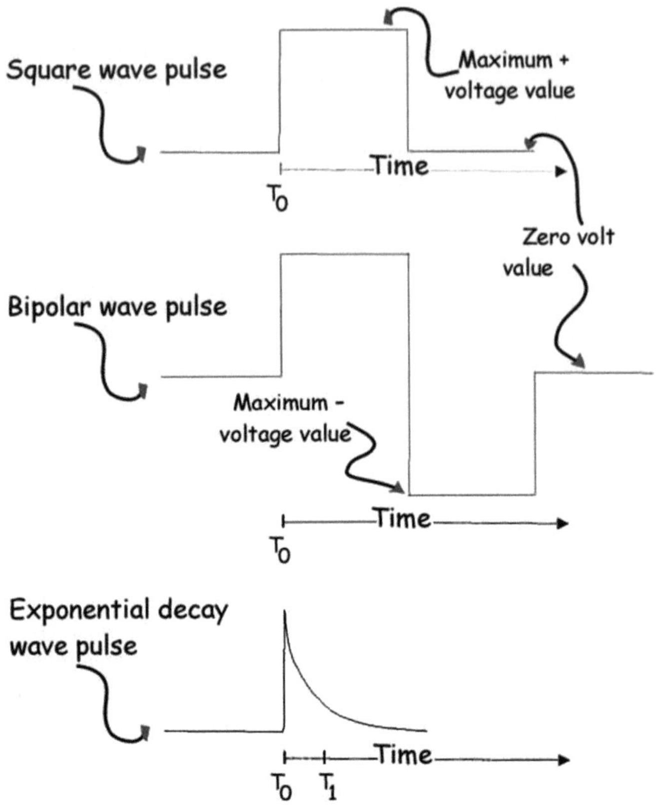

Fig. 5.2 Three common wave forms used when applying the voltage to create the electric field. The bipolar wave pulse is the only wave form that has negative voltage signals. The time mark, T_0, indicates the rise in the voltage signal in each of the three wave forms, while T_1 represents the time required for voltage value to decrease to about one-third of its maximum value

and then return to 0 V. If this entire process took 10 μs, the pulse would be labeled a 10-μs square wave pulse. During almost all of the time the pulse exists, it provides a 1,000-V signal. Thus, the square wave pulse is characterized by the pulse's total amplitude and total time, for which the examples provided are 1,000 V, 10 μs and 1,000 V, 10 ms.

An additional pulse used in electroporation is an exponential decay pulse (Fig. 5.2b). This exponential decay pulse has the same very fast rise time as the square wave, but the signal's voltage value begins to immediately decay. This exponential decay is characterized by the time constant of the signal. For convenience, the time constant is defined as the time value required for the wave to decay to approximately one-third of its maximum value. Thus, the characterization of the exponential electroporation pulse requires the maximum voltage amplitude and the time constant value.

Other wave forms are possible. If the signal begins at 0 V, rises to a positive maximum value and then falls to a negative maximum value before it returns to 0 V, the signal is known as a bipolar pulse (Fig. 5.2c). The bipolar electroporation pulse is characterized by the positive and negative maximum voltage values and the duty cycle of the pulse. The duty cycle of a bipolar pulse can be defined in one of two ways: Either as the time the pulse has a positive voltage divided by the time the pulse has a negative value or as the time the pulse has a positive voltage divided by the total time.

Classic electroporation practices were driven by whatever type of pulse could be produced by the generator. Today, square wave pulses tend to be the preferred choice. However, as the generators become more sophisticated, more complicated waveforms are possible. These individualized or mix-mode waves combine elements of square, exponential, and sine wave signals to produce an electroporation pulse for a specific application. Electroporation practitioners should expect that new electroporation pulse generators will provide some flexibility in the type of electroporation pulse the equipment can create.

Electroporation Pulse Regimes

In the current state-of-the-art use of electroporation for clinical application, electric field strength and pulse duration time are used to identify electroporation operating regimes. These characterization values are not specific to any particular treatment protocol but serve the function of a general classification tool. Current clinical treatment protocols are grouped as either high field, short duration pulse protocols or low field, long duration pulse protocols. For example, when a drug such as cisplatin or bleomycin is used, a pulse that is μs long with a field strength (see Chap. 4) of at least 800 V/cm might be used. By contrast, if a plasmid is used the pulse might have a low field strength (between 100 and 600 V/cm) and much longer pulse (ms) duration. In addition, there are protocols that combine high field pulses and low field pulses to take advantage of the electroporative effect of the high fields and the electrophoretic contribution of the low field (as described in Chap. 6).

This pulse regime classification practice becomes important if one is developing a variety of electroporation protocols. Not all electroporation pulse generator manufacturers offer generators that can produce pulses in both of the operating regimes. However, some of the newer pulse generators do provide the option of mixing high and low-voltage pulses. Specific details on various manufacturers' equipment are provided in Section "Vendor Information."

User Interface Considerations

Electroporation pulse generator interfaces are categorized by the degrees of freedom the manufacturer provides. One category of interfaces are typically PC-based and provide the user with various options to select pulse parameters, while the other interface category exemplifies a simplified operation strategy by automatically matching pulse parameters to the chosen applicator with its corresponding predetermined treatment protocol. Some manufacturers provide instrument interfaces that enable the physician to operate applicators containing many electrodes. Such interfaces assign pulses to the individual electrode pairs of an applicator. This feature may be either built into the pulse generator itself, or are provided as a plug in stand-alone unit. All manufacturers of clinical pulse generators provide software-based logs that record the basic details (the time, date, and electroporation signature) associated with each patient's electroporation session.

Electroporation Applicators

Successful electroporation requires the compatible combination of an effective protocol that may or may not include a therapeutic agent, a reliable pulse generator, and an appropriate applicator. The physical issues with the hardware combination of generator and applicator are usually straightforward, with the equipment footprint in the clinic and the ease of use being the important issues. However, the selection of the pulse generator and the appropriate applicator to represent this hardware combination does present some challenges. This section addresses the design, function, and selection options associated with the applicator.

The types of applicators a clinician has to direct attention toward depends on the goal of the electroporation effort, and there are two extremes with respect to electroporation efforts. One extreme is when the aim is to employ electroporation to treat a specific target disease, using an established protocol. In this case, there may be a "turn-key" approach available for that task and there are vendors that can supply that "turn-key" solution. The other extreme is when there is a desire to use electroporation on a target disease but there are no protocols and only initial research results to indicate that the impact of a given therapeutic agent will be magnified by an electroporative approach. Obviously, situations closer to the second rather than the first extreme demand much more attention and knowledge of applicators and applicator options. This section presents the applicator options, followed by a discussion about situations close to the first extreme, and then addresses potential applicator issues arising when the project is closer to the second extreme.

Applicator Options

A typical applicator design is shown in Fig. 5.3. The applicator comprises a power cord that is connected to the pulse generator, a handle, and an electrode unit. The use of a disposable, detachable electrode unit is meant to bring down treatment costs, and several vendors have adopted this design principle – see Section "Vendor Information" for further details.

It is convenient to identify electroporation applicators as either penetrating or nonpenetrating. The classic nonpenetrating applicator geometry consists of two thin rectangular stainless-steel pads or plates. The plates are tightened against the sides of the tissue to be treated, and the electric field is imposed from the right plate to the left plate and then imposed from the left plate to the right plate, or vice versa. To promote field uniformity in the entire tissue volume, the applicator is removed, rotated 90°, retightened against the tissue, and then the electric field application procedure is repeated.

A refinement in this plate electrode applicator design removes the treatment volume uncertainty by eliminating this physical electrode plate rotation step. These refined applicators have multiple plate electrode pairs (Fig. 5.4a) and the field is rotated within the treatment volume by the pulse generator electronically switching to different single plate pairs. In an alternative protocol, two separate groups of multiple plates are connected together to act as single plate pairs. New nonpenetrating applicator designs replace the squeezing electrode plate strategy with an applicator that has an array of beveled nubs (Fig. 5.4b). As with the rectangular pad applicators, the electroporation pulse is directed to the nub pairs by the pulse generator. The mechanical distinction between the nonpenetrating nub applicator and plate applicator designs is that the former makes contact with the top of the treatment area while the latter makes contact with the sides of the treatment volume.

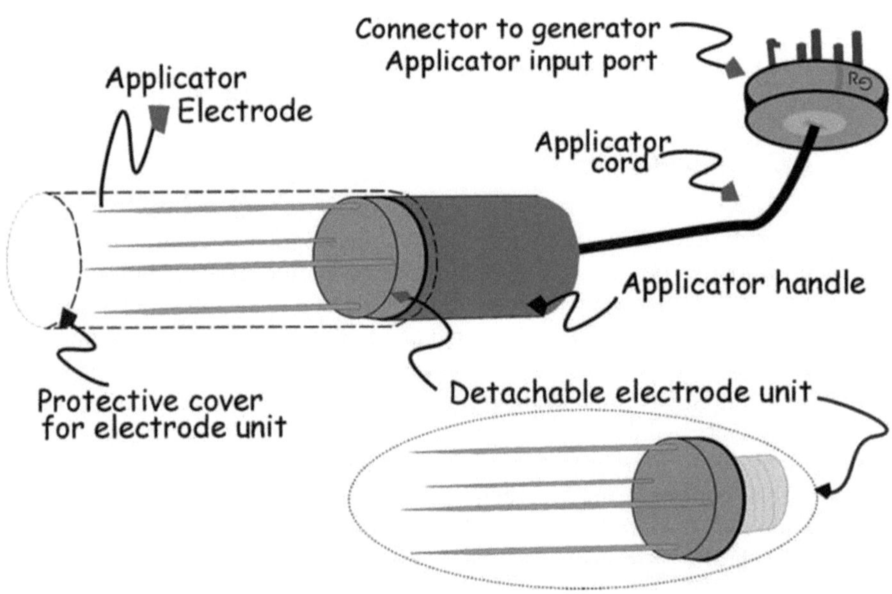

Fig. 5.3 Components of an applicator. The connection to a pulse generator may be keyed – meaning that the applicator may only be used with specific pulse generators, and the electrode(s) unit is detachable from the applicator handle. The number and shape of the covered detachable electrodes vary with treatment applications

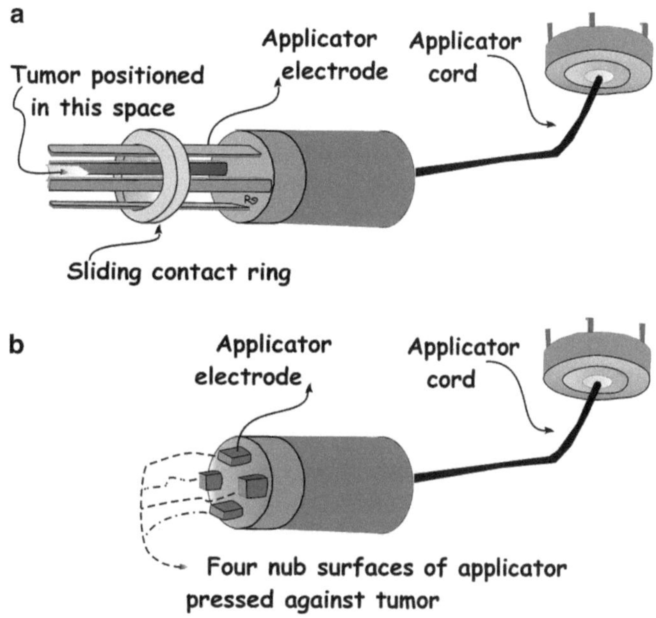

Fig. 5.4 Two nonpenetrating applicator designs. (**a**) Tumor is positioned within the space defined by the four plate electrodes. Sliding contact ring is pressed to the left to tighten electrode surfaces onto the tumor surface. (**b**) Applicator is pressed against surface of tumor so that all four nub surfaces of the applicator are in tight contact with tumor. The number and shape of nub-surfaced electrodes vary with treatment applications

Adequate electrode to tissue contact pressure in the nub applicator is accomplished by the physician pressing the applicator down on the tissue.

The electrodes of the penetrating applicator are designed to accept the electroporative pulse from the pulse generator and create the desired electric field the same way this task is accomplished with nonpenetrating electrode applicators. The penetrating electrode is usually a needle type construction with a tip designed to penetrate tissue. Penetrating applicators can consist of a single pair of electrodes or a large array of electrodes with pairs of these needle-shaped electrodes accepting the electric pulse from the pulse generator as dictated by a predetermined sequence that may be programmed into the computer memory of the pulse generator.

There are three mechanisms for acquiring electroporation applicators. Applicators can be built, leased, or purchased. The first option is the typical choice for in vitro experiments and animal studies. The second option might be the choice for the clinical trial phase of the project, while the third option is the preferred option by most equipment manufacturers, since their complete package usually includes the applicator, the pulse generator, and, when possible, a specific drug or plasmid.

Applicator Considerations for Established Electroporation Protocols

Although the option to obtain a turn-key system for use with an established protocol may be a physician's choice for the treatment of a specific cancer or infectious disease, there are still some application and applicator considerations that may influence the selection of a turn-key system or service provider. The first consideration is whether a turn-key *system* or a turn-key *service* is what is desired. The first option implies equipment ownership with a fixed and usually negotiable one-time investment cost that may or may not include maintenance of or initial training on that system. The second option typically shifts equipment performance and liability issues to the service provider but may include additional reoccurring fees connected to license agreement clauses that impose long-term time and/or system utility constraints.

In either turn-key option mentioned above, there are applicator considerations common to both. Initial factors deal with the applicator mode of use as well as questions about its source and supply. From the mode-of-use perspective, the applicator will most likely be designed for one-time use but if not, what are the number of times and criteria for reuse? From the source and supply point of view, does the pulse generator manufacturer also supply the applicator? If not, who does? Are there any and/or separate license requirements associated with the applicator? If the turn-key system includes multiple protocols, are there different applicators for separate protocols or different electrode units or both? If so, when these applicators are in storage, are they easy to identify? When the applicator is being attached to the system, is there a plug-in interlock (hardware or software) provision that prevents incorrect applicator attachment to the pulse generator?

Applicator Considerations for Translational Electroporation Protocols

The development or translation of electroporation-based treatment protocols into clinical applications imposes a completely different and more stringent initial set of complications associated with the selection of the appropriate applicator. The clinician on this research pathway does have additional degrees of freedom with respect to the applicator portion of the project; however, the ultimate objective for the applicator is the same as the applicator used in turn-key scenarios. The applicator has to be compatible with a clinically acceptable pulse generator and it must be manufactured in quantities and conditions that are appropriate for clinical use.

A review of the original clinical protocol literature published in the 1990s may lead to the tempting conclusion that the applicator selection is not critical. In most of those publications, the emphasis was on the successful field-mediating effect to improve the antitumor performance characteristics of the drug and, as such, the applicators used in those clinical trials accomplished that task and were simply identified with minimal comment. The total reality of the situation then and now is that the applicator has a major impact on the success of such electric field-mediated drug delivery protocols.

For instance, for protocols that use an agent combined with an electric field, the desired tissue response is the results of the therapeutic agent's presence inside of – not proximal to – the cells to be treated. The agent is transferred from the tissue's intercellular to intracellular environment because of the porating impact the electric field exerts on the membranes of the tissue. Thus, the desired treatment effect requires that the cells be exposed to a sufficient amount of agent shortly before, during, or shortly after the cell's exposure to the minimally required field strength. If the electrode shapes and geometric arrangement in the applicator electrode unit or the applicator's position in the tissue do not provide the minimally required field strength in the entire tissue volume, some tissue cells will not be treated. This is a particular issue in the treatment of tumors, where coverage of the entire tumor volume is critical and where great care should be taken to ensure that especially the deeper margins are treated.

The brief summary discussion of the previous paragraph suggests the crux of the applicator selection task for the translational research-focused clinician developing protocols. The proper electric field intensity, strength, and – if needed – an adequate dose of the therapeutic agent must be in near proximity of the tumor for the agent to be transported into the tumor cells. The applied electric field geometry and field strength are dependent on the geometry of the applicator's electrodes. The applicator electrode geometry is dependent on the objectives of the task, and the task changes as the investigator moves the work from its initial in vitro experimental stage through the animal studies and into the phase I, protocol safety evaluation, stage. Sometimes the animal and initial clinical trial stages may use the same applicator electrode design and arrangement, but if in vitro studies are required, the optimal applicator electrode geometry for that task seldom reaches the clinic due to the different size and insertion depth requirements.

Despite what now may seem to be a daunting challenge, there are some rules of thumb that significantly simplify applicator electrode design or selection activities. As suggested above, the guiding principle is to remember that cells within the target tissue that are not exposed to the appropriate electric field strength will not respond as intended. In addition to field strength, the field gradients are also important aspects to consider. When the electric field gradients translate into a large fraction of the voltage drop in confined regions of the tissue volume, the cells in the remaining tissue treatment volume may be exposed to field strengths below the required minimum for electroporation. Regions of high field gradients are always present near sharp edges on applicator electrodes. Fortunately, the sophistication of current modeling software allows an applicator designer to create three-dimensional computer views of the expected electric field strength and gradient profile for most electrode shapes and arrangements. In order to avoid regions of tissue that experience either subminimal or excessive field strength, the use of such software is recommended for any reader involved in the application development portion of a translational protocol effort. For more information on field strength, see Chap. 4.

This entire discussion of applicator design and selection is based on one assumption and does come with a few closing cautions. The assumption is that the investigator that needs the applicator needs it as a component of a system and/or protocol that will ultimately be used in an environment characterized by a large number of patents. The cautions deal with issues of material selection and patent infringement.

With respect to the physical electrode itself, when it comes to electroporation, not all electrodes are the same. Electroporation involves the application of voltages across electrodes that will always support electrochemical reactions at the electrode/tissue interface. Imprudent selection of electrode materials results in ions from the electrode material entering the cell cytoplasm as a result of electrochemical oxidation and reduction half-reactions. Introduction of metallic ions into an in vitro investigation could immediately contaminate the cells and complicate the experimental results.

A severe complication related to potential patent infringement is when the researcher does not realize that a patent is being infringed upon. This is particularly the case if an applicator is included in the final electroporation treatment protocol as a part of a device commercialization effort. A simple electrode system for an electroporation experiment is easy to fabricate. However, over the last 2 decades there has been a considerable amount of applicator development work conducted in the university and corporate research environments. As a result, a large number of applicator electrode geometry and electroporation method patents already exist. In most cases, applicator electrode geometry and arrangements that have been described in the electroporation research literature are already patent protected, and any transfer or modification of such applicators to support a commercial endeavor is likely to be a patent infringement. On the bright side, the wealth of information that is available from the patent literature is an important source of inspiration for aspiring applicator designers.

Vendor Information

While the concept of electroporation has been known since the 1960s, electroporation as a treatment modality is still early in its life cycle. As a result, there is a limited number of vendors that sell equipment that may be used in the clinic.

The goals of this section are as follows:

1. To inform the reader about the core focus areas of the different vendors, enabling the reader to determine which equipment may be the most appropriate for the considered treatment.
2. To inform the reader about the core features differentiating one system from another.
3. To provide the reader with an overview of the clinical experience obtained with the equipment of the different vendors.

In the following section, vendors that are providing commercially available equipment or equipment that either has been or is planned to be used in a clinical setting will be introduced in alphabetical order. It is outside the scope of this production to give directions regarding the construction of electroporation equipment. Please also note that the section will not review equipment that is only suitable for animal studies.

Angiodynamics: www.angiodynamics.com

Angiodynamics is the manufacturer of the Nanoknife™ system, which is built for treatments based on IRE (Fig. 5.5). The system is commercially available for use by physicians and has obtained market clearances in the EU, the US, Australia, and Canada for soft tissue indications.

The Nanoknife™ system is not meant to be used in combination with chemotherapy or other therapeutic substances. Instead, it is based on the concept of IRE. As explained in Chap. 19, IRE exploits the application of fields with very high field strengths to permanently permeabilize cell membranes. In order to provide increased field homogeneity and ensure best possible conformance with tumor geometry, the system provides the option of using up to six applicators that are placed either in or around the tumor. The aim is to treat lesions with a volume of up to 70 cm^3.

The Nanoknife™ pulse generator provides the user with a number of standard treatment protocols based on predefined target area configurations, but also features a software interface enabling the user to create electroporation signatures by varying pulse lengths, numbers and amplitudes, applicator geometries, and electrode placement patterns.

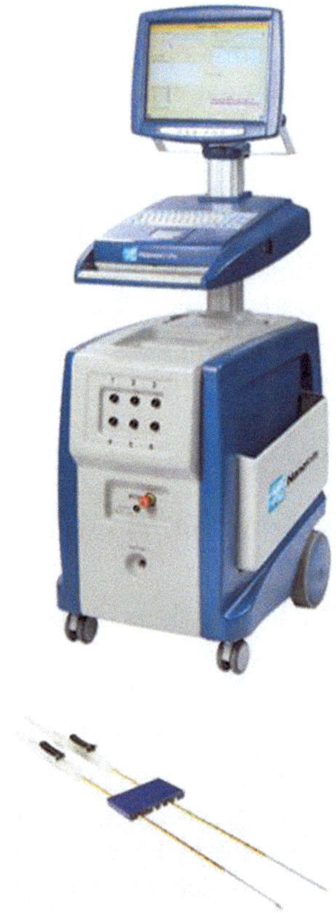

Fig. 5.5 Parameters, Nanoknife 2009 edition: Number of applicator outputs: 1–6, Number of pulses: 10–100, Pulse amplitude: 100–3,000 V, Pulse length: 20–100 μs, Max. current: 50 A

Nanoknife™ applicators are fully disposable and exclusively applicable with the Nanoknife™ pulse generator. They differ from other applicators for electroporation by being longer and thicker, enabling percutaneous insertion, and targeting of deep-seated tumors. A further difference is the option of varying the length of the electrically active area between 0 and 40 mm. This feature increases customization options and enables the user to treat small as well as larger tumors with the same type of probe.

The applicators are configured to be inserted individually or in pairs to conform to the geometry of a given lesion. As a result, the Nanoknife™ system provides the user with a high degree of freedom in tailoring the field to the tumor profile.

In use, the NanoKnife™ system allows the physician to create a patient profile and determine the appropriate placement and number of applicators according to the size and position of a given lesion. The physician also determines the appropriate protocol/pulse parameters to use, and plugs the applicators into the generator. After placement of the applicators at the site of treatment (ultrasound and/or CT may be used), the generator is activated and delivers a test pulse to determine whether treatment conditions are fulfilled. If the test is successful, the generator charges and, when triggered by the user, delivers the desired number of pulses to the treatment site. Immediately after delivery, the pulse train delivered to the patient may be read out and analyzed by means of the software interface. Treatment parameters are also stored automatically under the patient profile.

Current clinical experience involving the Nanoknife™ includes percutaneous and laparoscopic treatments of prostate, liver, lung, kidney, bone, pancreas, and lymph node [1]. A clinical trial targeting early-stage hepatocellular carcinoma was launched in February 2010.

Nanoknife™ features:

- Variable active electrode length.
- Two probe styles: single electrode applicator and bipolar applicator (two electrodes built together to form an electrode pair).
- Variable number of applicators – up to six.
- Variable applicator patterns possible.
- Automatic storage of treatment parameters, with real-time dosimetry, informing the user of the voltage and current levels delivered in a given treatment.

Cytopulse

Cytopulse was aquired by Cellectis and subsequently BTX (btxonline.com) September 2010. The paragraph below describes the products as there were at the time of acquisition.

Cytopulse was the manufacturer of the Demarvax™ and Easy Vax™ systems which are built for intradermal vaccine delivery (Fig. 5.6). Both systems were available under license for clinical evaluation purposes. The system is configured to provide delivery of DNA vaccines to the dermis.

DNA vaccination, as explained in Chap. 18, is a method for creating an immune system response by transfecting e.g. skin cells with a plasmid encoding a disease-specific antigen. The rationale behind targeting the dermis for DNA vaccination is the abundance antigen-presenting cells found in the skin. Furthermore, targeting of the skin reduces the discomfort experienced by the patient. For further information about electrotransfer to skin, please refer to chapter 17.

The Dermavax™ pulse generator software in built on Pulse Agile® waveform protocols. In a pulse agile® protocol, high-voltage short pulses and low-voltage long pulses are combined to enhance uptake of therapeutic substances. The goal is to permeabilize the target cells using high-voltage pulses, and subsequently drive the DNA vaccine into the cells using the electrophoretic forces of the longer-duration low-voltage pulses. The system automatically calibrates pulse parameters based on the configuration of the applicator selected.

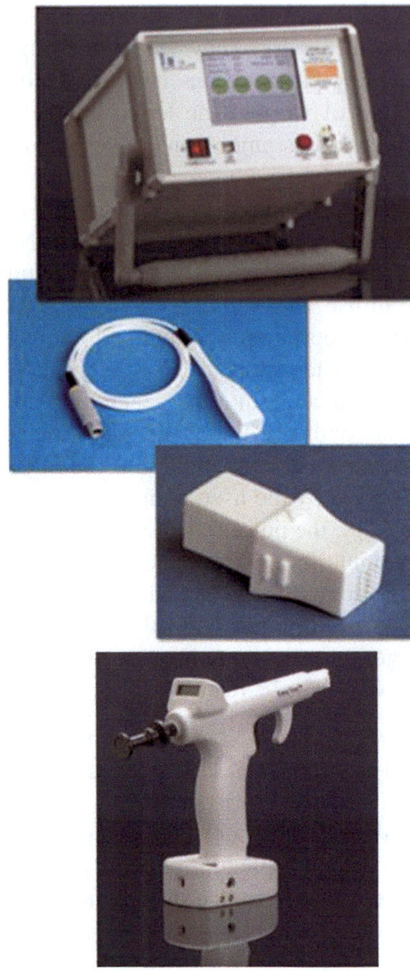

Fig. 5.6 Parameters, Dermavax/Easy Vax 2009 edition: Number of applicator outputs: 1, Pulse amplitude: 50–1,000 V/20–140 V, Pulse length: 50 μs–10 ms, Pulse interval: 200 μs–1,000 ms

The Easy Vax™ pulse generator is a handheld, battery-powered device that is configured to be portable. It is built on Pulse Agile® waveform protocols, but voltage levels are adapted to the considerably lower output of current battery technology. Calibration is fully automatic, with a smart-chip in the applicator communicating directly with the pulse generator to set parameters.

Applicators for the Dermavax™ system are exclusively applicable with the Dermavax™ pulse generator and are based on parallel needle arrays, with a selection of variable needle lengths, thicknesses, and numbers to cover applications in the dermis as well as deeper-lying tissue regions. The applicator comprises a reusable handle and a disposable single-use electrode unit featuring two parallel rows with either four or six needles in each row. The electrode unit features an electrode ID number that is used in the calibration of the Dermavax™ pulse generator.

The Easy Vax™ disposable electrode units are adapted to the lower voltage output from the Easy vax™ generator. This means that electrode needles are smaller and that the spacing between electrode rows is reduced. The electrode needles are dry-coated with the DNA vaccine, simplifying usage by eliminating the need for separate injections of therapeutic substances prior to pulsing.

In use of the Dermavax™, the physician selects an appropriate electrode unit for the planned indication. The electrode ID is entered into the Dermavax™ waveform generator, and the electrode unit is mounted in the handle. After connecting the handle and the pulse generator and injecting the intended therapeutic substance, the physician may place the electrodes in the target tissue region and trigger pulse delivery. After activation of pulse delivery to the tissue, pulse parameters are automatically stored in a digitized format on a USB key. If treating larger lesions, multiple overlapping electrode placements may be needed.

The Easy Vax™ pulse generator is automatically calibrated through insertion of an electrode unit with a smart-chip containing pulse parameter settings. The physician places the electrode unit against the skin of the patient and deploys the needles. Pulsing is triggered, and the needles are retracted to protect against needle-stick injuries. Data may be accessed through a mini USB connection.

Plans for obtaining clinical experience with the Dermavax™ include a phase I/II prostate cancer trial to investigate the safety of a xenogenic DNA vaccine delivered by the Dermavax™ intradermal electroporation system.

Furthermore, Cytopulse planned (as of October 2009) a colorectal cancer study to evaluate the delivery of a DNA vaccine which expresses Carcinoembryonic Antigen (tetwgCEA) and an HIV study to assess the safety and feasibility of administering plasmid DNA carrying multiple HIV-1 genes together with dermal electroporation.

The Easy Vax™ system has been approved for phase I testing for safety and tolerability.

Dermavax™ features:

- Pulse Agile® waveform protocols.
- Electrode units for intradermal and intratumoral applications.
- Automatic, digitized storage of pulse parameters for quality control.
- Touch-screen user interface.

Easy Vax™ features:

- Pulse Agile® waveform protocols.
- Fully handheld and portable, with rechargeable battery.
- Electrode units with dry-coated vaccines and smart-ship calibration of pulse generator.

Ichor: www.ichorms.com

Ichor is the manufacturer of the TriGrid™ system (Fig. 5.7). Devices are available for either intramuscular or intradermal DNA delivery. TriGrid™ is available under the license for clinical evaluation purposes.

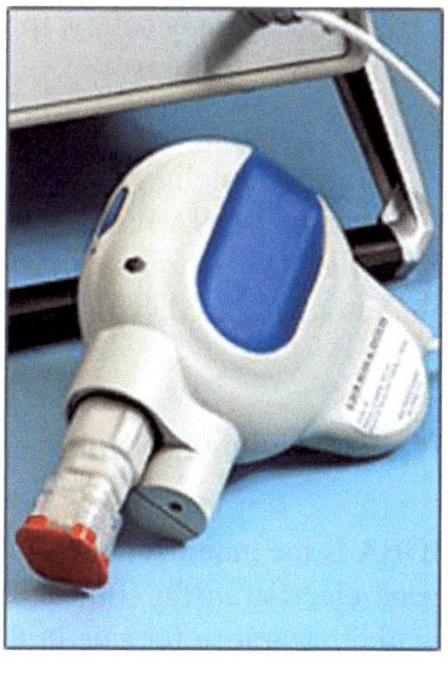

Fig. 5.7 Parameters, TriGrid 2009 edition: Number of applicator outputs: 1, Pulse amplitude: 250 V/cm, Pulse length: 40 ms, Pulse train duration: 400 ms

The Ichor pipeline is built for the delivery of plasmid DNA to muscle or skin tissue and has three focus areas:

1. Therapeutic cancer vaccines – where targeted antigens are used to enhance immune system responses, potentially along with immunostimulatory genes to increase the efficiency of the treatment.
2. Infectious diseases – where plasmid antigens delivered intramuscularly or intradermally may induce a rapid and durable antibody response to pathogens such as anthrax bacterium, HIV, and hepatitis B virus.
3. Therapeutic proteins – where a durable protein expression may be accomplished through the intramuscular delivery of plasmid DNA.

For further information about electrotransfer to tumors and muscle, please refer to Chaps. 14 and 16.

The TriGrid™ system is configured for maximum ease of use. Consequently, the pulse generator interface offers no pulse parameter customization options. The calibration of pulse parameters is based on the desired application as defined in collaboration with Ichor, and is done prior to first use of the device.

The TriGrid™ applicator is exclusively applicable with the TriGrid™ pulse generator. The TriGrid™ applicator differs from most other electroporation applicators by featuring a disposable cartridge with an integrated, centrally located injection needle in addition to the four electrode needles. The needle is connected to a DNA reservoir in the form of a syringe. According to Ichor, the arrangement of electrodes and central injection needle combined with the automated, user independent injection improves DNA placement accuracy and consistency of the procedure, and enables a full DNA administration procedure to be executed with a single push of a button. The applicator furthermore comprises all necessary mechanics for automatic deployment of electrode needles and injection needle.

In use, the TriGrid™ applicator is connected by the physician to the pulse generator and inserts a disposable cartridge in the applicator. Insertion depth is adjusted to ensure distribution of the agent within the target tissue. Upon placement of the applicator against the target region, the physician may initiate a treatment sequence by pushing a button on the applicator. Deployment of the electrode needles and the injection needle into the target tissue is done automatically, and administration of therapeutic agent as well as pulsing follows upon successful deployment. After pulsing, an automatic stick shield deploys over the sharps to prevent needle-stick injury.

Current clinical trials involving the TriGrid™ system include a phase I melanoma trial to study the safety and immunogenecity of a DNA vaccine encoding a melanosomal antigen [2], a phase I trial to study the safety and efficacy of ECT for the treatment of pancreatic cancer [3], and a phase I HIV trial to study safety, tolerability, and immunogenicity [4].

TriGrid™ features:

- Fully integrated applicator featuring injection needle as well as electrode pins.
- Automated delivery of therapeutic molecules and electric pulses in a single step.
- Integrated DNA reservoir in the form of a syringe.
- Variable insertion depth of deployable electrodes.
- Automatic needle-stick protection.

IGEA – www.igeamedical.com

IGEA is the manufacturer of the Cliniporator™ system, which is built for electrochemotherapy and gene electrotransfer (Fig. 5.8). The system is commercially available for use by physicians, with market clearance for sale in the EU (CE mark).

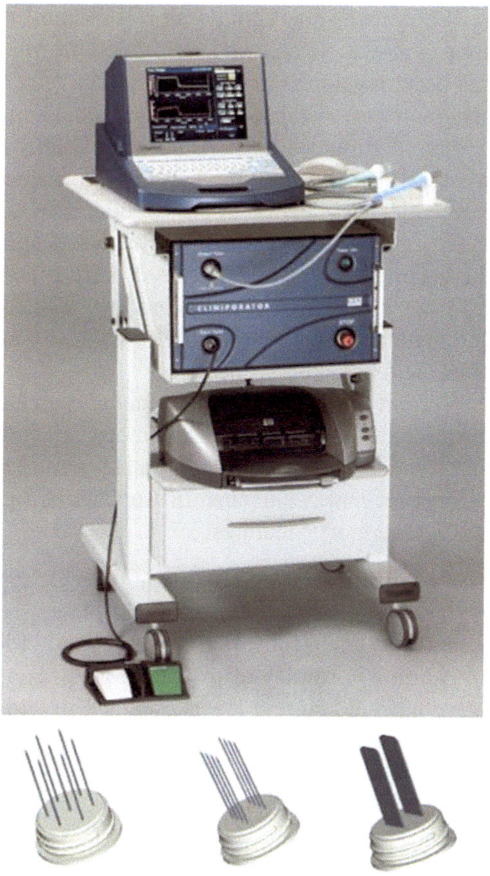

Fig. 5.8 Parameters, Cliniporator 2009 edition: Number of applicator outputs: 1, Number of pulses: 1–20, Pulse amplitude: 100–1,000 V, Pulse length: 30–5,000 μs, Max. current: 16 A

The Cliniporator™ pulse generator is built to support both electrochemotherapy and gene electrotransfer and provides a software interface for the selection between the two options.

In the electrochemotherapy mode, the pulse generator automatically sets parameters based on the geometry of the applicator chosen by the user. To shorten treatment time, the electrochemotherapy treatment mode furthermore includes the option of pulsing at 5 kHz, as opposed to the normal 1 Hz pulse frequency.

In the gene electrotransfer mode, the user has considerably more freedom to create electroporation signatures by varying pulse length, number, and amplitudes. Typically, high-voltage pulses are used for permeabilization of cells, with subsequent low-voltage pulses to promote electrophoresis. The high-voltage pulse parameters are similar to those of the electrochemotherapy mode (μs range), whereas the low-voltage pulses are characterized by being longer (ms range) and of considerably reduced amplitude. For further information about electrochemotherapy and gene electrotransfer, please refer to Chaps. 8, 9, and 13.

IGEA has focused on the treatment of skin tumor lesions, and provides a selection of applicators suited for cutaneous and subcutaneous applications. These are exclusively applicable with the Cliniporator™ pulse generator and include plate electrode units for superficial or protruding lesions with a diameter of less than 8 mm. Furthermore, needle electrodes with parallel array and hexagonal configurations are provided for deeper-lying tissues and/or larger tissue regions. Each applicator is built as a reusable handle that is connected to a disposable electrode unit featuring the electrode needles or plates.

When using the Cliniporator™ system, the physician creates a patient profile and selects an appropriate applicator and electrode unit in accordance with the standard operating procedure that has been developed in the ESOPE trial [5]. The electrode code sequence is entered into the pulse generator and the applicator cable is inserted in the pulse generator. As mentioned above, parameters are automatically set if the physician has chosen to work in the electrochemotherapy mode, whereas the gene electrotransfer mode enables customization of pulse parameters. Upon successful test sequence, injection of the intended therapeutic substance, and placement of the electrodes at the treatment site, the physician may load and charge the pulse generator. When triggered by the user, the generator delivers the desired pulse train to the target tissue, and treatment parameters may be read out and analyzed by means of the software interface. Treatment parameters are also stored automatically under the patient profile. If treating larger lesions, multiple overlapping electrode placements may be needed.

Current clinical experience includes treatment of cutaneous and subcutaneous tumors such as breast cancer, colon cancer, squamous cell carcinoma of the skin, squamous cell carcinoma of cervix, and Kaposi and leiomyosarcoma [6]. In addition, a clinical trial targeting chest wall recurrences of breast cancer was launched in August 2008 [7].

Cliniporator™ features:

- Two different modes of operation – electrochemotherapy and gene electrotransfer.
- Three different applicator types (plate, parallel array (4 × 4 electrodes), hexagon).
- 5 kHz pulsing for faster treatment and reduced discomfort.
- Automatic storage of treatment parameters, with real-time dosimetry, informing the user of the voltage and current levels obtained in a given treatment.
- Foot-pedal based activation.

Inovio – www.inovio.com

Inovio is the manufacturer of three systems for DNA vaccination and other DNA-based therapeutics (Fig. 5.9). The Medpulser® system is built for intramuscular vaccine delivery. The Elgen® system and the CELLECTRA® system are built for both intramuscular and intradermal DNA vaccine delivery. All three systems are available under the license for clinical evaluation purposes.

The Inovio pipeline is built around the delivery of DNA plasmid-based vaccines to skin and muscle tissue. The company is focusing on two specific treatment areas:

1. Therapeutic Cancer Vaccines – where targeted antigens are used to enhance immune system responses, potentially along with immunostimulatory genes to increase the efficiency of the treatment.
2. Infectious Diseases – where plasmid antigens delivered intramuscularly may induce a rapid and durable antibody response to pathogens such as HIV, hepatitis C virus, human papilloma virus, and influenza virus.

The three Inovio pulse generators offered are all optimized for DNA vaccination applications. This is reflected in the voltage levels (in the 40–250 V/cm range) and in the pulse lengths (10–60 ms). The Inovio pulse generators offer different user interfaces and levels of treatment customization:

- The Medpulser® pulse generator is remote-controlled, and treatment parameters are automatically set when the physician inserts the chosen applicator in the pulse generator.
- The Elgen® pulse generator features a flash-card-based computer interface enabling the user to customize treatment parameters including pulse and injection parameters, and to store patient and electroporation data following treatment.

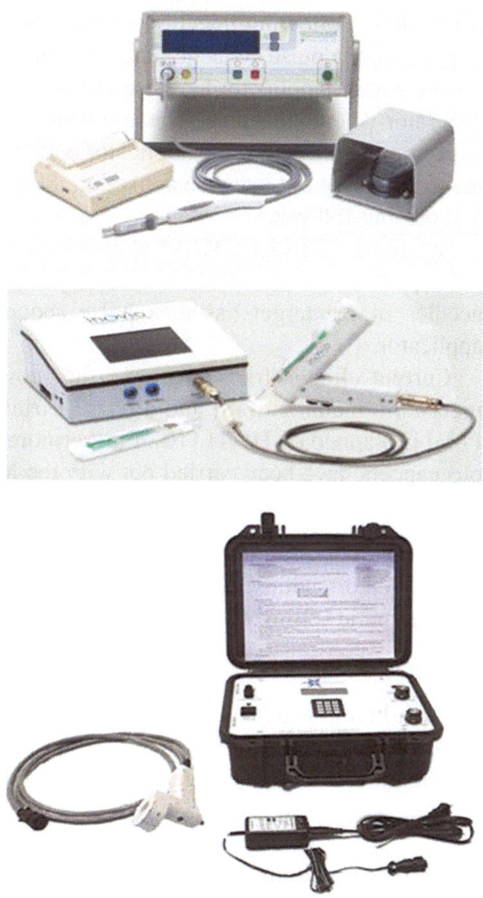

Fig. 5.9 Parameters, Medpulser/Elgen/Cellectra 2009 editions: Number of applicator outputs: 1, Pulse amplitude: 50–250/50–250/40–200 V, Pulse length: 60/10–60/52

- The CELLECTRA® pulse generator provides the option of customizing depth of insertion, voltage levels, timing between injection and pulsing, pulse duration, and injection volume. Treatment parameters are stored, and may be downloaded and analyzed after treatment. The battery-operated pulse generator is built for field assignments, and is encased in a water-resistant, shock-proof carrier.

Inovio offers a number of different needle applicators that are exclusively applicable with the respective Inovio pulse generators:

- The Medpulser® system features an applicator comprising a four-needle array with variable insertion depth. The array comes in different sizes, with each applicator having a unique built-in electronic identifier that automatically calibrates pulse generator parameters to conform to the applicator geometry.
- The Elgen® system features an applicator comprising a two-needle array with built-in syringes. The needles serve as delivery channels for the DNA vaccine, ensuring colocalization of the vaccine and the needles. The applicator furthermore serves as a device controller, and features a push button that is used to activate the pulse controller.
- The CELLECTRA® system features two applicators, one for intradermal and one for intramuscular applications. The intramuscular applicator also facilitates colocalization of the vaccine within the volume enclosed by the needle array. Both applicators feature push buttons that are used to activate the pulse controller.

In use, the Medpulser® applicator is connected to the Medpulser® pulse generator to set treatment parameters. Following injection of the DNA vaccine and insertion of the applicator needles in the target tissue, a pulse sequence may be initiated with a remote control.

The Elgen® applicator likewise features an electronic identifier that communicates with the pulse generator when connected. The applicator comprises built-in syringes containing the DNA vaccine to be administered, and the applicator is furthermore configured to deploy the electrode needles into the target tissue upon device activation. Following insertion, the vaccine is automatically dispensed, and pulsing follows.

In use, the CELLECTRA® applicator is connected to the CELLECTRA® pulse generator and pulse parameters are set. Following injection of the DNA vaccine and insertion of the applicator needles in the target tissue, a pulse sequence may be initiated by pushing the button on the applicator.

Current clinical trials involving the Inovio electroporation systems include a phase I trial on metastatic melanoma [8] and a phase I trial on Human Papilloma Virus [9]. In addition, a phase I trial is planned on HIV-1 [10]. Furthermore, several ECT trials targeting cutaneous and subcutaneous cancers have been carried out with the MedPulser equipment [11–15].

Medpulser® features:

- Remote-controlled operation.
- Applicators with variable needle length for intramuscular delivery.
- Automatic setting of pulse parameters based on applicator geometry.

Elgen® features:

- Push-button activated, fully automated deployment, injection, and pulsing.
- Applicators for intramuscular and intradermal delivery.
- Integrated DNA reservoir in the form of twin syringes.

CELLECTRA® features:

- Automatic, continuous measurements of tissue resistance.
- Applicators for intramuscular and intradermal delivery with push-button activation.
- Enhanced portability through enclosed, chargeable battery and water-resistant, shock-proof casing.

Sonion – www.sonion.com

Sonion is the manufacturer of the Ellisphere system which is built for the treatment of deeper-lying tissue regions (Fig. 5.10). The system is scheduled for its first clinical evaluation in 2011.

The Ellisphere system is configured to enable the less-invasive application of electroporation to deeper-lying tissues. To enable access to such deeper-lying tissues, the Ellisphere disposable applicator differs from other applicators by featuring electrode needles that may be deployed from a thin introducer shaft to cover a larger treatment region. Thus, it is possible to treat lesions with diameters up to 30 mm with a single insertion of an applicator with a 5-mm shaft.

The applicator is primarily intended for use in the brain, but other indications in deeper-lying organs are considered. It is mounted on a stereotactic head frame by means of a reusable guide system that is built to stabilize the applicator during insertion and to provide control of insertion depth. For further information about electrochemotherapy in the brain, please refer to Chap. 11.

When using the Ellisphere system, the physician prepares the patient, programs the pulse generator with the desired pulse parameters, and injects the intended therapeutic substance. The guide system and the applicator are mounted on the head frame, the applicator is inserted to

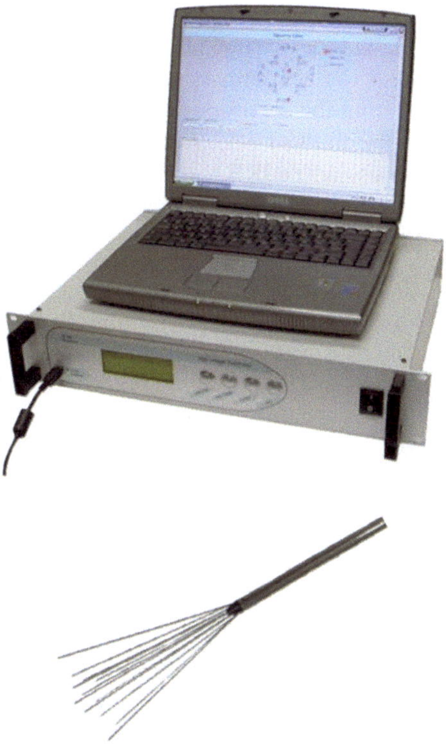

Fig. 5.10 Ellisphere 2009 edition

the desired position and the electrode needles are deployed (proper positioning may be verified by e.g., intraoperative CT). Activation of pulsing and postoperative data handling depends on the pulse generator chosen.

A clinical trial is being prepared to test safety and efficacy of electrochemotherapy, primarily against brain metastases.

Ellisphere features:

- Introducer with deployable electrodes enabling the treatment of large lesions through a small incision.
- Multicompatible pulse controller.

Perspectives

While electroporation is still a young and evolving field of medicine, it is evident from the above that a lot of efforts have been invested in advancing this promising treatment modality.

In the field of *electrochemotherapy*, standard operating procedures are now available to help practitioners new to the field prepare for the treatment of patients. Standardized equipment is commercially available to doctors in the EU, and the first study on the pharmacoeconomics and cost efficiency [16] has been published to show that electrochemotherapy is a cost-efficient alternative to conventional treatments of a number of cancers.

In the field of *gene electrotransfer*, several companies and a substantial number of research institutions are currently in the process of validating the potential of DNA vaccination as a means to prevent and alleviate a number of debilitating and life-threatening diseases. As it is apparent from the vendor section, a number of different approaches to gene electrotransfer are currently being tested, with dry-coated electrodes and integrated syringes offering colocalization of drug and field, emerging as alternatives to the traditional approach of separating the injection of the therapeutic agent from the electroporation procedure.

In the field of *IRE*, equipment is now commercially available in the US, the EU, and other countries. While IRE is the most recent addition to the armamentarium of the physician, a number of trials have been initiated to validate this treatment.

In terms of future device development on the equipment side, the next stages of pulse generator development will likely result in:

- More advanced interface options, with enhanced simulation environments that may eventually feature image fusion to enable the correlation of pre- and postoperative imaging with field properties. Thus, physicians may experience better treatment planning as well as the option of altering treatment parameters in real-time to reflect changing tissue conditions.
- More advanced pulse modulation options, with new pulse patterns and sequences emerging as a result of better understanding of tissue responses to field application.
- Better real-time surveillance of tissue conditions during treatment, potentially enabling the pulse generator itself to adapt voltage levels and durations to tissue conditions in the microenvironment encountered between individual electrode pairs.

Regarding the development of applicators, we see the coming period offering:

- More specialized applicators, enabling access to tissue regions currently outside the reach of treatments.
- Further integration of applicators and drugs, with integrated drug delivery systems and new coating technologies enhancing uptake and treatment precision.
- Further integration with other fields of medicine, with sonoporation, photoporation, and plasma-based treatments serving as further enhancements. The potential of electroporation as a supplementary treatment will also require validation, with the preoperative treatment of tumor margins following resection being the likely first target.

When looking at the electroporation industry as a whole – and taking into consideration the likely proliferation of new technologies and treatment modalities – we note that the absence of industry standards may eventually become a hindrance. History shows that industries grow beyond the constraints imposed by the capabilities of individual companies when standards emerge, to the benefit of the entire industry. At the present stage, a number of different approaches are being validated and some will eventually emerge as more successful. We entertain the (perhaps naïve) hope that increasing convergence will result from this validation, enabling crossovers between equipment made by different vendors and increasing the freedom of the individual physician to tailor treatments to the patient without undue equipment constraints.

In concluding this chapter, we find substantial reasons for excitement. A number of important breakthroughs have been made in the last decade, and judging from the rapidly increasing pace of development, more will follow in the near future. But already today, we have safe, reliable equipment and well-tested protocols that are helping us treat patients who would otherwise have few or no alternatives.

References

1. http://investors.angiodynamics.com/releasedetail.cfm?ReleaseID=434361. 2010.
2. Safety and Immunogenicity of a Melanoma DNA Vaccine Delivered by Electroporation, NCT00471133, http://clinicaltrials.gov. 2009.

3. Electroporation Therapy With Bleomycin in Treating Patients With Pancreatic Cancer, NCT00027521, http://clinicaltrials.gov. 2009.
4. Study of a Potential Preventive Vaccine Against HIV in Healthy Volunteers (ADVAX-EP), NCT00545987, http://clinicaltrials.gov. 2009.
5. Mir LM, Gehl J, Sersa G, Collins CG, Garbay JR, Billard V, et al. Standard operating procedures of the electrochemotherapy: Instructions for the use of bleomycin or cisplatin administered either systemically or locally and electric pulses delivered by the Cliniporator (TM) by means of invasive or non-invasive electrodes. Ejc Supplements. 2006;4(11):14–25.
6. Marty M, Sersa G, Garbay JR, Gehl J, Collins CG, Snoj M, et al. Electrochemotherapy – an easy, highly effective and safe treatment of cutaneous and subcutaneous metastases: results of ESOPE (European Standard Operating Procedures of Electrochemotherapy) study. Ejc Supplements. 2006;4(11): 3–13.
7. Electrochemotherapy for Chest Wall Recurrence af Breast Cancer: Present Challenges and Future Prospects, NCT00744653, http://clinicaltrials.gov. 2009.
8. A Trial to Evaluate the Safety of Intratumoral VCL-IM01 Followed by Electroporation in Metastatic Melanoma, NCT00223899, http://clinicaltrials.gov. 2008.
9. Phase I of Human Papillomavirus (HPV) DNA Plasmid (VGX-3100) + Electroporation for CIN 2 or 3, NCT00685412, http://clinicaltrials.gov. 2009.
10. Study of PENNVAX™-B (Gag, Pol, Env) + Electroporation in HIV-1 Infected Adult Participants (HIV-001), NCT01082692, http://clinicaltrials.gov. 2010.
11. Study Using the MedPulser Electroporation System With Bleomycin to Treat Cutaneous and Subcutaneous Cancer, NCT00198276, http://clinicaltrials.gov. 2007.
12. Study Using the Medpulser Electroporation System With Bleomycin to Treat Head and Neck Cancer, NCT00198263, http://clinicaltrials.gov. 2007.
13. Medpulser Electroporation With Bleomycin Study to Treat Anterior Head and Neck Squamous Cell Carcinoma, NCT00198315, http://clinicaltrials.gov. 2007.
14. Medpulser Electroporation With Bleomycin Study to Treat Posterior Head and Neck Squamous Cell Carcinoma, NCT00198328, http://clinicaltrials.gov. 2007.
15. Bleomycin With or Without Electroporation Therapy in Treating Patients With Stage III or Stage IV Melanoma, NCT00006035, http://clinicaltrials.gov. 2009.
16. Colombo GL, Matteo SD, Mir LM. Cost-effectiveness analysis of electrochemotherapy with the Cliniporatortrade mark vs. other methods for the control and treatment of cutaneous and subcutaneous tumors. Ther Clin Risk Manag. 2008;4(2): 541–8.

Part II
Electrochemotherapy

Chapter 6
Cell Electropermeabilization and Cellular Uptake of Small Molecules: The Electrochemotherapy Concept

Aude Silve and Lluis M. Mir

Abstract The cell membrane is an impassable barrier for small hydrophilic molecules, termed nonpermeant, that are too hydrophilic for diffusing through the plasma membrane, and moreover are not recognized and internalized by a transporter, channel, or receptor system. Reversible cell electropermeabilization allows the cellular uptake of these nonpermeant small molecules. Studies demonstrating that bleomycin is a nonpermeant anticancer drug possessing a very high intrinsic cytotoxicity (the toxicity displayed when the drug has no biological barrier separating it from its target) have lead to the development of the electrochemotherapy concept. Indeed, cell electropermeabilization can increase bleomycin toxicity several thousand-fold in vitro and about thousand-fold in vivo. At the dosages used, bleomycin selectively kills the dividing cells by a mitotic cell death process. The physico-chemical bases reported in this chapter give light to the interesting aspects of the electrochemotherapy revealed and/or confirmed by the clinical trials, in particular, its efficacy and safety.

Keywords Electrochemotherapy • Bleomycin • Cisplatin • Electroporation • Electropermeabilization • Nonpermeant molecules • Low-permeant molecules • Intrinsic activity • Vascular lock • Molecular transport across membranes • Mitotic cell death • Cell death • Antitumor treatment • Electropermeabilization monitoring • Drug vectorization • Targeting

Introduction

In pharmacology, most of the current drugs are molecules that act on receptors or on molecules located at the cell surface. However, in the specific case of anticancer pharmacology, the classical cytotoxic drugs have their targets located inside cells.

The control of transport across the plasma membrane is of the highest importance in cell physiology and homeostasis. On the one hand, internalization of metabolites necessary for cell function (e.g., sugars, amino acids, cofactors, ions) is mediated and precisely controlled by membrane transporters or channels. On the other hand, there is no mechanism for a controlled crossing of the cell

L.M. Mir (✉)
Univ Paris-Sud, Unité Mixte de Recherche (UMR) 8203, Institut Gustave-Roussy, 114 rue E. Vaillant, 94805 Villejuif, France
and
Centre Nationale de la Recherche Scientifique (CNRS), Unité Mixte de Recherche (UMR) 8203, Institut Gustave-Roussy, 114 rue E. Vaillant, 94805 Villejuif, France
e-mail: luismir@igr.fr

S.T. Kee et al. (eds.), *Clinical Aspects of Electroporation*,
DOI 10.1007/978-1-4419-8363-3_6, © Springer Science+Business Media, LLC 2011

membrane in the case of macromolecules and small xenobiotic molecules like most of the anticancer cytotoxic drugs. Using this knowledge, important factors to consider are:

- Only plasma membrane crossing, either at the cell surface or in structures like the caveolae, results in direct access to the cell cytosol and the nucleosol; that is, to the "true" inside of the cell where replication, transcription, and transduction take place.
- Endocytosis, in most forms, gives access to the vesicles of the cell via the generation of endosomes, and therefore, the endocytosed molecules do not directly reach the cytosol even though they are inside the cell.
- The nuclear envelope is not a physical barrier for the small molecules that already reached the cytosol, because such molecules are able to freely cross the nuclear pores (up to a molecular weight of about 30,000 Da).

As will be detailed in Section "Penetration of Small Molecules into the Cell Interior," the small xenobiotic molecules fall into three categories: (1) the first category comprises "foreign" molecules that easily enter the cells and reach the cytosol because they take the place of physiological molecules on membrane transporters that mediate the uptake of their substrates into the cell interior (e.g., the anticancer drugs melphalan and methothrexate); (2) the second category includes most of the xenobiotic active molecules: these molecules are lipophilic or amphiphilic (possessing both hydrophilic and lipophilic properties) compounds that also easily enter the cells because the plasma membrane is not a barrier (these molecules, like actinomycin D and many other anticancer drugs, diffuse through the lipid bilayer and accumulate inside the cells); (3) the last category corresponds to a very small group of xenobiotic molecules, termed *nonpermeant* molecules, that do not easily enter the cells (this concept will be described in detail in Section "Penetration of small molecules into the cell interior"). If a nonpermeant molecule, which rarely reaches the cell interior (e.g., bleomycin), is physiologically (i.e., therapeutically) active, it is because the presence of very few of these molecules inside the cell is sufficient to provoke the physiological effect at the cell level. This means that such molecules possess a very high *intrinsic* activity (an activity fully revealed when the molecules can really reach the cell interior). The molecules belonging to this last category are those that fully benefit from their combination with membrane-permeabilizing procedures.

In this chapter, we will review the physico-chemical properties of the small molecules to show why some of them can become much more efficient through their combination with membrane-permeabilizing procedures, in particular with electric pulses able to transiently and reversibly permeabilize the cells. The concept of electrochemotherapy will thus be defined and the basics of this treatment reviewed. Subsequently, procedures for the detection, follow-up, and quantification of cell electropermeabilization, in vitro and in vivo, will be described in order to give the basis for a rational use of small molecules in combination with reversible electropermeabilization. Finally, the differences existing between in vitro and in vivo situations, in terms of the uptake of small molecules by cells or tissues exposed to permeabilizing electric pulses, will be discussed to understand how effects detected in vitro can be easily translated for use in an in vivo situation.

Penetration of Small Molecules into the Cell Interior

Whereas it is obvious that very large molecules may not freely cross the plasma membrane of the cell, the plasma membrane is also an effective barrier for certain small molecules. Indeed, the ease with which molecules enter a cell depends both on their physico-chemical properties and their biological characteristics. For example, molecules are taken up actively by cells when they participate in cell metabolism and are essential elements of cell life (e.g., amino acids, glucose). The penetration of all these categories of molecules through the plasma membrane is modified by cell electropermeabilization [1]. The purpose of the following paragraphs is to review how the normal mechanisms of transport across the cell membrane can be affected by the exposure of cells to electric pulses reversibly permeabilizing the cell membrane.

Hydrophobic and Amphiphilic Molecules (With and Without Electropermeabilization)

The plasma membrane is not an impassable barrier for hydrophobic and amphiphilic molecules, at least provided the size (and thus the molecular weight) of these molecules does not exceed certain limits [1]. It is difficult to give a value for these limits, as many parameters influence them, such as the three-dimensional conformation of the molecules, the number and position of the polar groups in the molecule, and the substances (e.g., DMSO, ethanol) in which these molecules, which can be poorly soluble in water, are dissolved before their dilution in physiological (water-based) media. Most of the classical molecules of the chemotherapy armamentarium (thus not considering, e.g., the new classes of antibodies against specific receptors at the tumor cells surface) are molecules falling in this physico-chemical category. Therefore, the activity of these molecules (e.g., Actinomycin D, Adriamycin, Doxorubicin) is based on their capacity to enter and eventually accumulate in the cells. As a matter of fact, these molecules can indeed accumulate inside cells up to a point in which their internal concentration is higher than their external concentration, because they often have an elevated affinity for their corresponding intracellular targets, for example, DNA, tubulin protein (either free or assembled in microtubules), etc. Often, the intrinsic cytotoxicity of these molecules (i.e., the actual cytotoxic potential of one of these molecules inside the cell) is low; the molecules are in fact therapeutically active because they accumulate in very large numbers inside the cell – a process facilitated by the ability of these molecules to easily enter the cell. The transport mechanism involved is simple passive diffusion through the plasma membrane, which implies that the molecule is able to enter the membrane (in other words to "dissolve" in the plasma membrane, transiently staying inside it). This transport mechanism is clearly permitted by the physico-chemical properties of both the molecules and the cell membrane.

As expected from the consequences of the physico-chemical properties of hydrophobic and amphiphilic molecules on their potential activity, cell electropermeabilization does not greatly modify their activity profile. In very early studies, it was shown that the cytotoxicity of molecules like Actinomycin D or *N*-methyl-9-hydroxy-ellipticium [1, 2] can be increased in vitro by a maximum of 2–4-fold (under optimal electropermeabilization conditions and for very short durations of cell exposure to these drugs). This can be attributed to a corresponding increase in the amount of internalized molecules, as the same factor of sensitization to Actinomycin D as was seen in sensitive cells was also found in a partially resistant cell line derived from the sensitive cells. This is in agreement with the fact that resistance to Actinomycin D is mainly due to a multidrug resistance mechanism based on the activity of pumps that expel the drug from the cell interior. Obviously, the difference in drug efficacy between the electropermeabilized cells and the control cells will rapidly decrease with an increase in the duration of the contact between the cells and the drugs, as drugs can continuously enter the nonpermeabilized cells. This is why, in several other reports, no effect of cell electropermeabilization was found in the case of drugs such as Adriamycin, Doxorubicin, or Paclitaxel (see also Table 6.1).

Table 6.1 Increase of drug cytotoxicity by electroporation

Drugs tested	Potentiation
Bleomycin (nonpermeant molecule)	100–5,000-fold
Cisplatin (low-permeant molecule)	3–80-fold
Carboplatin (low-permeant molecule)	10–13-fold
Methotrexate, Melphalan, Mithramycin, Actinomycin D, Adriamycin, Cyclophosphamide, Mitomycin C, Doxorubicin, 5-fluorouracil, Vinblastine, Vincristine, Paclitaxel, Taxotere	None

Small Hydrophilic Molecules (With and Without Electropermeabilization)

Two sorts of molecules must be considered here: those that mimic physiological molecules, and those that do not show any structural similarity with the substrates of permeases (that allow for facilitated transport) or of membrane-bound active transporters (often ATPases).

Small molecules of the first category enter cells because they are able to occupy the binding site of physiological molecules on the transporters (e.g., anticancer drugs such as melphalan or methotrexate, which are internalized by leucine transporters or reduced folate transporters, respectively). Even in such cases, it is possible to detect an effect of cell electropermeabilization. For example, transport, and thus cytotoxicity, of melphalan is regulated by the external concentration of leucine. Indeed, as melphalan is conveyed by the leucine transporters, the presence of high leucine concentrations outside the cell reduces the capability of melphalan transport, whereas the absence of leucine will exacerbate melphalan toxicity. Under a given set of electropermeabilization conditions and concentration of external leucine, it was found that the toxicity of melphalan on electropermeabilized cells (EC_{50} = 3.5 × 10^{-5} M) was similar to the toxicity on nonelectropermeabilized cells (EC_{50} = (5.5 ± 1.0) × 10^{-5} M). The toxicity on the nonelectropermeabilized cells increased nearly twofold in the absence of external leucine and decreased to an equal extent in the presence of 1.8 mM leucine (in contrast to 0.3 mM in the usual electroporation medium) [2]. Conversely, the toxicity on the electropermeabilized cells was not dependent on the external leucine concentration; a finding that corresponds with the fact that the diffusion across the membrane (permitted by cell electropermeabilization) is not a saturable transport mechanism. Even though the toxicities were similar with or without electric pulses at a concentration of 0.3 mM external leucine, the differences in the toxicity dependency on the concentration of external leucine reveal the change in uptake mechanism [2].

The second type of small hydrophilic molecules are those that cannot penetrate the cells in the absence of any type of cell permeabilization treatment or chemical modification of the molecular structure altering their hydrophilic characteristics, for instance, bleomycin. Bleomycin is a natural substance produced by *Streptomyces verticillis* [3]. It has antibiotic and cytotoxic properties and is an anticancer drug that has been used to treat patients since the middle of the 1970s. This molecule is not considered particularly active. However, since it is almost devoid of side effects (except for lung fibrosis after the administration of a cumulated dose of 300 mg/m^2, and some skin reactions), bleomycin is still used for specific cancer treatments or in combination with other drugs. Bleomycin is hydrophilic and does not diffuse through the plasma membrane [4]. It tightly binds to specific (still unidentified) membrane molecules [5]; however, these surface molecules do not mediate the direct transfer of the drug through the plasma membrane in the way that leucine transporters can do with melphalan [6]. Instead, Bleomycin uptake is linked to the number of binding sites at the cell surface and the endocytosis rate, which corresponds to the flux of molecules of bleomycin conveyed by the binding sites [7]. Since the cytotoxic effects of bleomycin are due to the generation of double-strand DNA breaks (DSBs) (one DSB per molecule of bleomycin on the average), the number of molecules entering the cell per unit of time must be large enough to compensate for the capability of the cell to repair the DSBs during the same time period. This is the reason why many cell types can withstand very large external concentrations of bleomycin. At the same time, there is a lot of bleomycin entering the cell by pinocytosis, which is not responsible for bleomycin toxicity, as these molecules will remain in the endosomal compartments [4, 7]. In certain ways, the mechanism of internalization of the bleomycin molecules responsible for their cytotoxicity shares some features with those of vegetal and fungal toxins, in particular ricin, for which the internalization by receptor-mediated endocytosis is well documented [8–10]. Chain B in the entire ricin binds to any galactose residue exposed at the cell surface, that is, about 1–2 × 10^7 binding sites per cell [8], whereas the catalytic chain A of ricin binds to the mannose specific receptor present at the surface of certain cells (1.5–2.0 × 10^5 sites per cell), for example, macrophages and the Kupffer cells of the liver.

The ricin molecules internalized through this specific receptor are the most cytotoxic [8]. Since bleomycin can specifically bind a specific membrane protein, its uptake mechanism appears to resemble the second ricin uptake pathway.

In a more general way (i.e., including large molecules like some proteins and nucleic acids), what we call nonpermeant molecules are those molecules that are devoid of any cellular internalization mechanism. This means molecules that are either too hydrophilic or too large for diffusing through the plasma membrane, and that moreover are not recognized and transported by a transporter or receptor system. In the cases in which those molecules have a pharmacological interest because of their intracellular targets or intracellular mode of action (essentially, small molecules like cancer drugs or large molecules like DNA or proteins), it is desirable to develop appropriate techniques aimed at their penetration into the cytosol. This is also true for some other, low-permeant molecules (oligonucleotides and certain cytotoxic drugs like the cisplatinum derivatives) which have only a very limited cellular internalization capability, due to a slow and limited diffusion across the plasma membrane or to a low-efficiency transporter- or receptor-mediated mechanism of translocation across the membrane.

Large Hydrophilic Molecules (With and Without Electropermeabilization)

Even though large hydrophilic molecules are outside the strict scope of this chapter, it is interesting to discuss their case. Nucleic acids and proteins may fall in this category, and techniques such as those presented in this book (e.g., electrochemotherapy) can be extended to these large molecules. Indeed, electric-pulse-mediated gene transfer is also gaining momentum. From preclinical studies (published 10 years ago) showing its efficacy, particularly for the transfer of plasmids to skeletal muscle [11–13], and from ulterior studies describing the mechanisms of gene electrotransfer [14, 15], this approach is now under clinical trials [16]. The first of such trials was recently published and shows that this approach can be applied on humans [17]. It is important to mention that these molecules do not easily enter the cells even after optimal membrane permeabilization. In the case of proteins, very large external concentrations are necessary, as the larger the molecule the lower its diffusion rate through the permeabilized membrane. In the case of plasmid molecules, with an extremely high molecular weight (a plasmid of 6-kbp has an approximate molecular weight of 6×648 kDa/kbp = 3,700 kDa), the permeabilization of the cell membrane is insufficient in several tissues: the DNA must additionally be pushed towards the cell membrane [18]. Long electric pulses or combinations of short high-voltage pulses and of long low-voltage pulses are necessary, as the long pulses introduce an electrophoretic component that effectively pushes the nucleic acids (which are highly charged molecules that move easily under the electric fields) [12, 15]. Therefore, the issues for these molecules is not only the absence and presence of electropermeabilization, but also the type of electric pulses used holds great significance.

Electrochemotherapy

Electrochemotherapy Concept

The concept of electrochemotherapy was based on the analysis by Dr. Mir and colleagues of the behavior of bleomycin on cells exposed to permeabilizing electric pulses. Bleomycin behavior is a classic example of the nonpermeant category of hydrophilic molecules described above (Fig. 6.1). The concept was later extended by Prof. Sersa and colleagues to cisplatin, a typical low-permeant

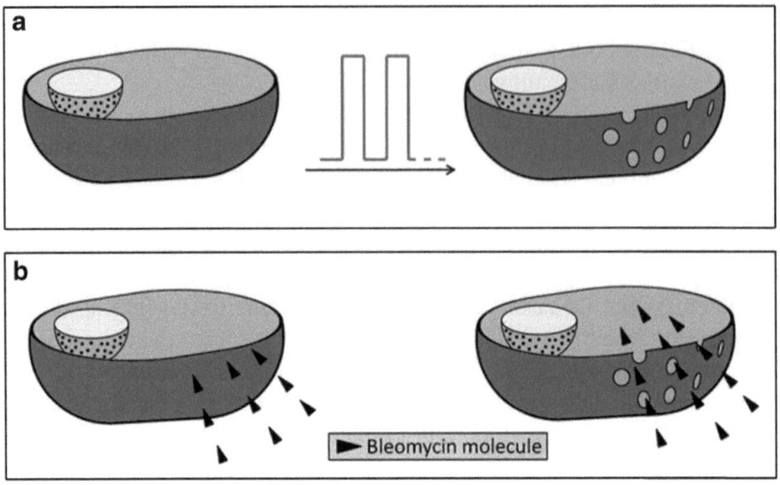

Fig. 6.1 The electrochemotherapy concept. (**a**) Permeabilization of the cell membrane by application of electric pulses. (**b**) Penetration of bleomycin into an electropermeabilized.cell

molecule (part of its uptake occurs by diffusion while part of it is mediated by other mechanisms yet to be fully elucidated; therefore, membrane crossing is also a limiting step in cisplatin efficacy). Bleomycin holds great interest for therapeutic use because it possesses a very high intrinsic cytotoxicity: 500 molecules in the cell cytosol entering at the time of cell electropermeabilization are sufficient to kill the cell through the generation of DSBs. Because the nonpermeant molecules can only enter the cell when the membrane is permeable (i.e., for a few minutes only: after delivery of the electric pulses and before resealing of the membrane), there is no time for extensive accumulation of drug inside the cell to occur. Thus, the therapeutic nonpermeant molecules must be very active when they are in the cell cytosol, which, as mentioned, is the case with bleomycin.

The concept of electrochemotherapy can also be extended to molecules other than the classical anticancer drugs, and even to large molecules. An example was provided by the Pokeweed Antiviral Protein (PAP) [2]. This molecule is a member of the vegetal and fungal cytotoxic proteins. Like some of the other members of this family of proteins, PAP kills the cells by the catalytic inactivation of one of the ribosomal RNAs, resulting in total arrest of protein synthesis. A single molecule in the cytosol is able to kill the cell. Contrary to the other members of this family of proteins, PAP does not possess any cell-binding domain, and therefore the catalytic chain is a nonpermeant natural substance with a very high intrinsic toxicity. Interestingly, it was possible to show that cell electropermeabilization results in an increase of PAP cytotoxicity of 200,000 times [2]. This result proved (1) that a huge increase in the cytotoxicity of nonpermeant molecules can be achieved by cell electropermeabilization (the basic concept of electrochemotherapy) and (2) that cell electropermeabilization gives direct access to the cell cytosol, where the target of PAP was strictly located. These data show potential perspectives for the future development of this new pharmacological approach.

Electrochemotherapy Definition

Electrochemotherapy is the local potentiation, by means of *permeabilizing* electric pulses, of the antitumor activity of a *nonpermeant* anticancer drug possessing a high intrinsic cytotoxicity (e.g., bleomycin) or of a *low-permeant* anticancer drug (e.g., cisplatin) already possessing a good level of cytotoxicity on the unpermeabilized cells. The electric pulses are locally delivered to the tumors.

Vectorization and Targeting

In the previous section, we emphasized that the action of a drug on its targets (i.e., the tumor cells) can be ameliorated by either the vectorization of the molecule or the specific targeting of the tissues of interest. Actually, in electrochemotherapy, the electric fields do both:

- *Vectorization*: The electric field has a real role in facilitating drug uptake and thus in increasing drug efficiency, because, in the volume affected by the electric pulses, the consequences on the cells of the electric field application is the permeabilization of the cell membrane.
- *Targeting*: Because the electric field is locally delivered, targeting is achieved by the electric field distribution in the body. This implies the ability to correctly choose the electrode geometry and the applied voltage-to-distance ratio (V/cm) as these parameters must fit the tumor geometry (size and shape).

Cancer Agents in Electrochemotherapy

Several research groups have examined the potential increase of the toxicity of anticancer drugs by means of cell electropermeabilization with very coherent results, in spite of differences in the cell types used, conditions of electroporation, duration of the incubations, etc. [2, 19] (Table 6.1). As expected, delivery of electric pulses does not improve the cytotoxic activity of molecules that are already permeant.

Basis of Electrochemotherapy Efficacy

The principal basis of electrochemotherapy efficacy is the combined, complementary, and synergistic use of permeabilizing electric pulses and nonpermeant (bleomycin) or low-permeant cytotoxic drugs (cisplatin). The combined effects of these physical and chemical agents are completed by the biological mechanisms listed below.

Type of Cell Death

It is very important to highlight that cell death is not caused by the electric pulses when reversible electroporation parameters are used. Cells reseal, and thus, after some time, they can restore their internal ionic levels (as described in Chap. 2). Therefore, the necrosis associated with the loss of homeostasis is not the main mechanism of cell death. Acting directly on the DNA molecule (whatever the type of genes expressed), cisplatin and bleomycin induce the formation of DNA adducts or DNA single- and double-strand breaks, respectively. When bleomycin is administered intravenously at a classical therapeutic dose (15,000 IU/m^2), as in the case of electrochemotherapy, the bleomycin concentration in the interstitial fluids of the tissues is very low due to bleomycin dilution in the whole body. Still, as mentioned earlier, the low number of DSBs caused by bleomycin even at very low concentrations are toxic [20]. Moreover, with a small number of these breaks, the cell will still be metabolically active but unable to divide, as, at the next mitosis, the chromosomes will be fragmented and the formation of the daughter cells completely impaired, resulting in cell death. This mitotic cell death pathway is very important, as it introduces an intrinsic targeting in electrochemotherapy that under these conditions results in the selective and efficient killing of the dividing tumor cells, while the nondividing normal cells also exposed to the electric pulses (and thus permeabilized as well) will survive. Such a mechanism may explain the very good cosmetic effects often reported after the treatment of superficial lesions [21]. It also allows for the preventive treatment of the tissues located just around tumors that frequently show local recurrences.

Induction of Vascular Lock

The delivery of permeabilizing electric pulses to tissues provokes an arrest of the blood flow in the tissue. If a drug is injected intratumorally, this *vascular lock* phenomenon prevents the washing of the drug from the tumor by the blood flow. In the case of the low-permeant cisplatin, this retention effect could be very important, as cisplatin will enter the cells not only during the time the cells are permeabilized but also after the cells are resealed. If bleomycin is injected intravenously, the effect of the vascular lock makes it essential that injection precede the delivery of electric pulses. The vascular lock can also contribute to the electrochemotherapy efficacy due to the long-term reduction in blood flow greatly reducing glucose and oxygen supply to the tumor.

The vascular lock is a general reaction of the tissues. In the case of normal tissues like skeletal muscle, the blood stops flowing for less than 2 min and the mechanism is partly based on a histamine-dependent reaction [22]. In this case, the duration of the blood flow interruption is insufficient to generate hypoxia or any other deleterious consequences. In tumors, the irregular vasculature results in a much longer duration of the blood flow interruption. Moreover, the endothelial cells in tumor tissues are dividing cells that constantly generate new vessels. Therefore, these dividing cells are sensitive to the drugs used in electrochemotherapy, which results in a long-term reduction of the blood flow in the tumor, greatly contributing to the electrochemotherapy efficacy.

Host Immune Response

Since the initial preclinical experiments, it has been shown that there are differences in the response to electrochemotherapy of tumors as a function of the animal immune system status. While complete regression was achieved in both the cases of immunocompetent and immune-deficient animals, a curative effect was achieved only in the former case while tumors reappeared after some time in the latter case [23]. The addition of various types of immunomodulating molecules has demonstrated the implication of the host immune system in cure achievement. Depletion in T lymphocyte numbers dramatically reduced the curative rate in mice [23], while the addition of interleukin-2 (which activates the helper and the killer T lymphocytes) [23, 24] or of Toll-like receptor ligands (which activate the dendritic cells, i.e., the antigen-presenting cells responsible for the recruitment and activation of T cells) [25] increased the curative rate of the treated tumors. Moreover, these molecules also induced the achievement of systemic antitumor effects either on an untreated secondary transplanted tumor (that mimics a large metastasis) [24, 25] or on the appearance of visceral [26] or pulmonary metastases [27]. The first clinical trial combining electrochemotherapy and several local injections of low amounts of interleukin-2 showed an increase in the T cell response [28]. Further clinical trials should analyse the potential of this type of combination of electrochemotherapy and molecules regulating the activity of the host immune system.

Monitoring Cell and Tissue Electropermeabilization Using Small Molecules

Because cell electropermeabilization is one of the two principal bases of electrochemotherapy, assessment of cell electropermeabilization in vivo has been fundamental, both for establishing that electrochemotherapy mechanisms are actually based on cell electropermeabilization, and, later on, for optimizing the treatment; that is, for validating models of electric field distribution (and thus electric-field-mediated permeabilization). This allows for the definition and validation of optimal electrode geometry and optimal voltages to apply to the electrodes as a function of electrode geometry and tissue characteristics. Nowadays, clinical procedures can be validated and there is no further need to repeat the type of experiments described in the following sections, unless new types of electrodes are designed and tested. There are basically two types of assessment methods, based on chemical and physical approaches. Because this chapter deals with the uptake of small molecules, only the chemical methods using small molecules are described here.

Biological Effects of Bleomycin

At low bleomycin concentrations, only the electropermeabilized cells will be killed owing to the huge increase in drug toxicity resulting from cell electropermeabilization [29]. Thus, the toxic effects of bleomycin can be used as a marker for cell electropermeabilization, both in vitro, ex vivo, and in vivo [29]. However, in essence, this is only valid for dividing cells (that is, for tissues like tumors). It is important to mention that in the presence of high concentrations of bleomycin, the morphology of all the electropermeabilized cells changes drastically just a few minutes after pulse delivery. One such change entails the nucleus becoming apoptotic in appearance (accordingly, bleomycin has also been termed an apoptosis-mimetic drug) [30]. Therefore, histology performed on tissues collected a few minutes after treatment with electric pulses and high doses of bleomycin can show the areas affected by the treatment and, thus, the field distribution in the tissue, even in the case of tissues composed of nondividing cells (e.g., the liver) [31].

Other Bleomycin-Based Methods

Because of the truly nonpermeant characteristic of the bleomycin molecule, bleomycin-based radioactive compounds have been designed in order to analyze tissue electropermeabilization.

^{57}Cobalt and bleomycin form an extremely stable complex. Moreover, the ^{57}Co-bleomycin complex not only possesses a high specific radioactivity, but it is also nontoxic: the cells will not be killed by the internalized ^{57}Co-bleomycin. It is therefore a highly useful molecule for studying electropermeabilization even though time-consuming washes may be necessary to remove the ^{57}Co-bleomycin that did not enter the cell [32]. It has been extensively used in vitro [4]. In vivo, its use is limited because of the low renal clearance of the complex (resulting in slow washing of the tissues), the need to maintain the animals for 3 days in metabolic cages, and the problem of the radioactive waste (^{57}Co half-life is 270 days) [29].

^{118}In, on the contrary, has a very short half-life. ^{118}In-bleomycin (Persson et al., personal communication) has a very high specific radioactivity allowing for the use of gamma cameras to visualize the electropermeabilized tissues. The use of this complex could also reduce the radioactive waste problem.

Non-Bleomycin-Based Markers

A large number of fluorescent or radioactive small molecules have been used to detect electropermeabilization in tissues, such as propidium iodide [33], lucifer yellow [34], calcium-green in calcium-rich medium, FluxOR™ in thallium-enriched medium, (99m)Tc-DTPA [35, 36], and ^{51}Cr-EDTA [37, 38]. In vivo, ^{51}Cr-EDTA is the most interesting molecule. ^{51}Cr has a short half-life (15 days) and also a very rapid renal clearance, which means that the complex is very rapidly washed from the tissues. This greatly facilitates experimental protocols. In skeletal muscle, the difference between permeabilized and nonpermeabilized muscle cells is already detectable 1 h after pulse and ^{51}Cr-EDTA delivery. However, in this short time, the washing of complex that has not been captured by the reversibly eletropermeabilized cells is not yet complete. Therefore, determination of the amount of ^{51}Cr-EDTA internalized into the electropermeabilized cells requires measurement of the radioactivity still present in a control tissue, for example, the contralateral muscle [38]. After 24 h, washing is complete, and there is no remaining radioactivity in the control tissue, and thus, uptake corresponds to the net radioactivity in the pulsed tissues. It is important to remember that in the case of an excessive (irreversible) electropermeabilization, uptake decreases as the radioactive molecules that entered the cells will leak. The quantitative ^{51}Cr-EDTA test for evaluation of the in vivo electropermeabilization level has allowed researchers (1) to determine the reversible and irreversible electroporation thresholds in various tissues, (2) to show differences in the voltage-to-distance ratios to apply when using either internal or external electrodes, (3) to show differences between pulses of different durations, when pulses are applied to a given tissue using given electrode type and geometry, (4) to show similarities between the same tissue in different species, and (5) to show differences between different tissues [37–40].

Differences Between In Vitro and In Vivo Situations

After having shown the principles of transport of small molecules into cells, as well as the changes caused by cell membrane electropermeabilization and the tests to determine cell permeabilization in vitro and in vivo, we will next discuss the differences that exist between in vitro and in vivo situations. Indeed, the points that are described below may largely interfere with the expected potential results from the working hypothesis, particularly when moving from bench experiments in vitro to preclinical trials in vivo.

Tissue Heterogeneity

The first thing to consider is that in vitro, the cells exposed to electric pulses usually come from cell cultures, thus consisting of a single cell type. In vivo, even in the case of a homogeneous tissue (e.g., a liver lobe), the cell composition is much more complex, as many cell types associate to form a tissue. Tissues will mainly contain a single tissue-specific cell type (e.g., the muscle fibers in skeletal muscle), even though some tissues contain various specific cell types (e.g., the hepatocytes and Kupfer cells in the liver). Aside from the cells conferring the specificity to the tissue, most tissues contain endothelial vascular cells, smooth muscle fibers, blood cells, nerve cells (or at least the part of the axons located in the tissue), fibroblasts, and also, as shown a few years ago, stem cells. As the different cells in a tissue have different shapes and different sizes, their electropermeabilization thresholds can differ greatly. Therefore, an overall analysis of the permeabilization level of a tissue is not precise enough. It is necessary to analyze which cell types have been electroporated and thus electromanipulated (particularly in the case of the use of electroporation to transfer genes into specific cells in the tissue, in order to ensure that the transfected cells are indeed the targeted ones).

In the case of electrochemotherapy, this is not a real problem since, in addition to the permeabilization of the tumor cells, the electropermeabilization of the endothelial cells leads to antiangiogenic effects (see section "Induction of vascular lock") that can contribute to electrochemotherapy efficacy. Moreover, the nerves will not be affected, because the axon diameter is much smaller than the cell diameter (thus, the transmembrane potential induced is not sufficient to affect the membrane structure), and even if some amount of cytotoxic agent could enter the axon and be transported to the cell nucleus, nerves are absolutely postmitotic cells and would not be killed by low amounts of drug.

Geometrical Considerations

Another significant difference between in vitro and in vivo situations lies with simple geometrical considerations. In vitro, usually 1–2 × 10^6 cells are treated in a volume of 50–200 μl, meaning that less than 1–2% of the volume is occupied by the cells, and that 98–99% of the volume is just medium. Thus, under the usual conditions, permeabilization of one cell may have no influence on the permeabilization of the neighboring cells. Cell permeabilization can be considered as independent events [41], except in extremely dense cell suspensions [42].

On the contrary, in vivo, at least 10%, and up to 80%, of the volume is occupied by cells. In such cases, the permeabilization of one cell introduces changes in the local conductivity of the tissue and, thus, in the electric field distribution. As a consequence, permeabilization of neighboring cells are interdependent events. This is the reason why models for electric field distribution and cell permeabilization in tissues are necessary.

The geometrical and structural differences also have direct consequences on the ways in which drugs, permeabilization markers, or any other molecule of interest can be brought in contact with cells. In vitro, contact is very easy as there is a lot of medium surrounding the cells. Thus, molecules are introduced into the medium, and subsequently there are no other obstacles for them to pass in order to enter the cells once electropermeabilization is achieved. On the contrary, in vivo, or even ex vivo (tissues or pieces of tissues), there are other cells and membranes surrounding the cells (e.g., fascia in muscles). As an obvious consequence, the distribution of permeabilization markers or drugs around the cells is difficult and heterogeneous.

Direct injection in the tissue is possible (meaning that a relatively homogeneous distribution of the injected substance is achievable) only if tissue is enclosed by a membrane (e.g., muscle), or if, in large animals, the volume of interest is artificially limited by injections of vasoconstricting molecules (e.g., lidocaine). Otherwise, a uniform distribution is almost unachievable. Molecules must be injected in a large volume of liquid compared to the tissue volume even though this procedure can be painful in some tissues. Intravascular (intravenous or intraarterial) injections are possible (meaning that some efficacy can be achieved) only if the molecule of interest can be largely diluted and still have biological effects (like bleomycin).

Drug Access and Washing

Drug access and washing is very different between in vitro and in vivo situations. In particular, it is very important to consider the timing of when to inject the drugs or permeabilization markers in vivo for treatments in combination with permeabilizing electric pulses, as well as how the drugs or the markers are washed from the tissues after treatment. Indeed, among the differences between in vitro and in vivo situations, it is necessary to highlight the vascular lock phenomenon. While in vitro markers can be added before or after pulse delivery (up to a certain extent, depending on the temperature and on the permeabilization level achieved), in vivo markers can only be injected before pulse delivery, at least if the marker is injected intravenously. Of course, local injections can also be performed after pulse delivery, as cells remain permeable for several minutes in vivo. However, better uptake is generally obtained when markers are injected before pulse delivery.

For bleomycin, experiments in mice have shown that, if injected intravenously, the drug must be administered 3 or 4 min before pulse delivery; in rats, 4 min before; while in humans, it is necessary to wait 8 min before applying pulses to the nodule(s) to be treated. In humans, pulses can be delivered for at least 20 min (that is, up to 28 min after the bolus injection) with maximal efficacy, but pulses can also be delivered for some more minutes with excellent antitumor effects [43]. The reader should note that in all cases, bleomycin must be rapidly injected to reach the highest possible levels first in the blood plasma and then in the tissues. In humans, the bolus injection must be performed in 30–45 s. The times provided above correspond to the delay necessary to reach the intratissue peak concentration after the bolus injection.

Conclusion and Perspectives

The permeabilization of cells, either in vitro or in vivo, opens the way to use potentially interesting drugs acting specifically on intracellular targets. Several physical and chemical means for cell permeabilization have been used in vitro. Not all of these methods can be easily used in vivo, in particular the chemical ones. The cell electroporation technique, also termed cell electropermeabilization, that uses electric pulses of 100 μs duration and field amplitudes in the range of a few hundred V/cm, is nowadays clinically used routinely in electrochemotherapy, as effectively displayed in this book, in particular in Chaps. 8 and 9.

Moreover, the concept of electrochemotherapy with anticancer drugs is extending. New promising therapies based on specific modifications of gene expression may employ relatively small nonpermeant molecules (natural or modified oligonucleotides, in antisense or antigene strategies), or even large nonpermeant molecules like coding DNAs or RNAs which may benefit from cell electropermeabilization to facilitate entry into the cells, as already described in Section "Penetration of Small Molecules into the Cell Interior" of this chapter. This nonviral procedure, termed nucleic acid electrotransfer (or DNA electrotransfer, gene electrotransfer, or electrogenetherapy) is very useful, as it extends the concept of electrochemotherapy, not only to other molecules but also to treatment of diseases other than benign or malign tumors.

References

1. Orlowski S, Mir LM. Cell electropermeabilization: a new tool for biochemical and pharmacological studies. Biochim Biophys Acta. 1993;1154(1):51–63.
2. Orlowski S, Belehradek Jr J, Paoletti C, Mir LM. Transient electropermeabilization of cells in culture. Increase of the cytotoxicity of anticancer drugs. Biochem Pharmacol. 1988;37(24):4727–33.
3. Umezawa H, Maeda K, Takeuchi T, Okami Y. New antibiotics, bleomycin A and B. J Antibiot. 1966;19(5):200–9.
4. Poddevin B, Orlowski S, Belehradek Jr J, Mir LM. Very high cytotoxicity of bleomycin introduced into the cytosol of cells in culture. Biochem Pharmacol. 1991;42(Suppl):S67–75.
5. Pron G, Belehradek Jr J, Mir LM. Identification of a plasma membrane protein that specifically binds bleomycin. Biochem Biophys Res Commun. 1993;194(1):333–7.
6. Pron G, Belehradek Jr J, Orlowski S, Mir LM. Involvement of membrane bleomycin-binding sites in bleomycin cytotoxicity. Biochem Pharmacol. 1994;48(2):301–10.
7. Pron G, Mahrour N, Orlowski S, et al. Internalisation of the bleomycin molecules responsible for bleomycin toxicity: a receptor-mediated endocytosis mechanism. Biochem Pharmacol. 1999;57(1):45–56.

8. van Deurs B, Sandvig K, Petersen OW, Olsnes S, Simons K, Griffiths G. Estimation of the amount of internalized ricin that reaches the trans-Golgi network. J Cell Biol. 1988;106(2):253–67.
9. Simmons BM, Stahl PD, Russell JH. Mannose receptor-mediated uptake of ricin toxin and ricin A chain by macrophages. Multiple intracellular pathways for a chain translocation. J Biol Chem. 1986;261(17):7912–20.
10. van Deurs B, Pedersen LR, Sundan A, Olsnes S, Sandvig K. Receptor-mediated endocytosis of a ricin-colloidal gold conjugate in vero cells. Intracellular routing to vacuolar and tubulo-vesicular portions of the endosomal system. Exp Cell Res. 1985;159(2):287–304.
11. Mir LM, Bureau MF, Gehl J, et al. High-efficiency gene transfer into skeletal muscle mediated by electric pulses. Proc Natl Acad Sci USA. 1999;96(8):4262–7.
12. Andre F, Gehl J, Sersa G, et al. Efficiency of high and low voltage pulse combinations for gene electrotransfer in muscle, liver, tumor and skin. Hum Gene Ther. 2008;19:1261–71.
13. Hojman P, Gissel H, Andre F, et al. Physiological effects of high and low voltage pulse combinations for gene electrotransfer in muscle. Hum Gene Ther. 2008;19:1249–60.
14. Satkauskas S, Bureau MF, Puc M, et al. Mechanisms of *in vivo* DNA electrotransfer: respective contributions of cell electropermeabilization and DNA electrophoresis. Mol Ther. 2002;5(2):133–40.
15. Satkauskas S, Andre F, Bureau MF, Scherman D, Miklavcic D, Mir LM. Electrophoretic component of electric pulses determines the efficacy of *in vivo* DNA electrotransfer. Hum Gene Ther. 2005;16:1194–201.
16. Heller LC, Heller R. *In vivo* electroporation for gene therapy. Hum Gene Ther. 2006;17(9):890–7.
17. Daud AI, DeConti RC, Andrews S, et al. Phase I trial of interleukin-12 plasmid electroporation in patients with metastatic melanoma. J Clin Oncol. 2008;26(36):5896–903.
18. Villemejane J, Mir LM. Physical methods of nucleic acid transfer: general concepts and applications. Br J Pharmacol. 2009;157:207–19.
19. Gehl J, Skovsgaard T, Mir LM. Enhancement of cytotoxicity by electropermeabilization: an improved method for screening drugs. Anticancer Drugs. 1998;9(4):319–25.
20. Tounekti O, Kenani A, Foray N, Orlowski S, Mir LM. The ratio of single- to double-strand DNA breaks and their absolute values determine cell death pathway. Br J Cancer. 2001;84(9):1272–9.
21. Marty M, Sersa G, Garbay JR, et al. Electrochemotherapy – an easy, highly effective and safe treatment of cutaneous and subcutaneous metastases: results of the ESOPE (European Standard Operating Procedures of Electrochemotherapy) study. Eur J Cancer Suppl. 2006;4(11):3–13.
22. Gehl J, Skovsgaard T, Mir LM. Vascular reactions to *in vivo* electroporation: characterization and consequences for drug and gene delivery. Biochim Biophys Acta. 2002;1569(1–3):51–8.
23. Mir LM, Orlowski S, Poddevin B, Belehradek Jr J. Electrochemotherapy tumor treatment is improved by interleukin-2 stimulation of the host's defenses. Eur Cytokine Netw. 1992;3(3):331–4.
24. Mir LM, Roth C, Orlowski S, et al. Systemic antitumor effects of electrochemotherapy combined with histoincompatible cells secreting interleukin-2. J Immunother Emphasis Tumor Immunol. 1995;17(1):30–8.
25. Roux S, Bernat C, Al-Sakere B, et al. Tumor destruction using electrochemotherapy followed by CpG oligodeoxynucleotide injection induces distant tumor responses. Cancer Immunol Immunother. 2008;57(9):1291–300.
26. Ramirez LH, Orlowski S, An D, et al. Electrochemotherapy on liver tumours in rabbits. Br J Cancer. 1998;77(12):2104–11.
27. Orlowski S, An D, Belehradek Jr J, Mir LM. Antimetastatic effects of electrochemotherapy and of histoincompatible interleukin-2-secreting cells in the murine Lewis lung tumor. Anticancer Drugs. 1998;9(6):551–6.
28. Andersen MH, Gehl J, Reker S, et al. Dynamic changes of specific T cell responses to melanoma correlate with IL-2 administration. Semin Cancer Biol. 2003;13(6):449–59.
29. Belehradek Jr J, Orlowski S, Ramirez LH, Pron G, Poddevin B, Mir LM. Electropermeabilization of cells in tissues assessed by the qualitative and quantitative electroloading of bleomycin. Biochim Biophys Acta. 1994;1190(1):155–63.
30. Tounekti O, Pron G, Belehradek Jr J, Mir LM. Bleomycin, an apoptosis-mimetic drug that induces two types of cell death depending on the number of molecules internalized. Cancer Res. 1993;53(22):5462–9.
31. Miklavcic D, Semrov D, Mekid H, Mir LM. A validated model of *in vivo* electric field distribution in tissues for electrochemotherapy and for DNA electrotransfer for gene therapy. Biochim Biophys Acta. 2000;1523(1):73–83.
32. Poddevin B, Belehradek Jr J, Mir LM. Stable [57Co]-bleomycin complex with a very high specific radioactivity for use at very low concentrations. Biochem Biophys Res Commun. 1990;173(1):259–64.
33. Rols MP, Delteil C, Golzio M, Dumond P, Cros S, Teissie J. *In vivo* electrically mediated protein and gene transfer in murine melanoma. Nat Biotechnol. 1998;16(2):168–71.
34. Mir LM, Banoun H, Paoletti C. Introduction of definite amounts of nonpermeant molecules into living cells after electropermeabilization: direct access to the cytosol. Exp Cell Res. 1988;175(1):15–25.
35. Engstrom PE, Persson BR, Salford LG. Studies of *in vivo* electropermeabilization by gamma camera measurements of (99m)Tc-DTPA. Biochim Biophys Acta. 1999;1473(2–3):321–8.

36. Grafstrom G, Engstrom P, Salford LG, Persson BR. 99mTc-DTPA uptake and electrical impedance measurements in verification of in vivo electropermeabilization efficiency in rat muscle. Cancer Biother Radiopharm. 2006;21(6):623–35.
37. Gehl J, Mir LM. Determination of optimal parameters for *in vivo* gene transfer by electroporation, using a rapid in vivo test for cell permeabilization. Biochem Biophys Res Commun. 1999;261(2):377–80.
38. Gehl J, Sorensen TH, Nielsen K, et al. *In vivo* electroporation of skeletal muscle: threshold, efficacy and relation to electric field distribution. Biochim Biophys Acta. 1999;1428(2–3):233–40.
39. Batiuskaite D, Cukjati D, Mir LM. Comparison of *in vivo* electropermeabilization of normal and malignant tissue using the 51Cr-EDTA uptake test. Biologija. 2003;2:45–7.
40. Cukjati D, Batiuskaite D, Andre F, Miklavcic D, Mir LM. Real time electroporation control for accurate and safe *in vivo* non-viral gene therapy. Bioelectrochemistry. 2007;70(2):501–7.
41. Susil R, Semrov D, Miklavcic D. Electric field induced transmembrane potential depends on cell density and organization. Electro Magnetobiol. 1998;17:391–9.
42. Pucihar G, Kotnik T, Teissie J, Miklavcic D. Electropermeabilization of dense cell suspensions. Eur Biophys J. 2007;36(3):173–85.
43. Domenge C, Orlowski S, Luboinski B, et al. Antitumor electrochemotherapy: new advances in the clinical protocol. Cancer. 1996;77(5):956–63.

Chapter 7
Vascular-Disrupting Action of Electrochemotherapy: Mode of Action and Therapeutic Implications

Gregor Sersa and Maja Cemazar

Abstract Besides having a direct cytotoxic effect on tumor cells, electrochemotherapy also has a vascular-disrupting effect. Application of electric pulses to the tumor induces transitory, but profound, reduction in tumor perfusion and oxygenation of tumors. When bleomycin or cisplatin are present at the time of tissue electroporation, endothelial cells in tumor blood vessels are also affected, leading to their apoptotic death. As a consequence, blood flow in the treated tumor is reduced, leading to extensive tumor cell necrosis and regression. Therefore, electrochemotherapy can be beneficially used in the treatment of bleeding metastases, as demonstrated in several reported cases. A model of vascular changes after application of electric pulses to the tumor and a model of vascular changes after electrochemotherapy are proposed.

Keywords Electrochemotherapy • Vascular-disrupting effect • Electroporation • Bleomycin • Cisplatin

Introduction

A functioning vascular supply is essential for solid tumor growth and metastasis. It is known that in the absence of angiogenesis, tumors are not able to develop beyond a few millimeters and therefore remain dormant. The angiogenic switch enables neovascularization of tumors and consequently rapid tumor growth, metastasis, and tumor progression [1]. The newly developed vessels have specific physiological and biological features that distinguish them from normal vessels. These differences include a relative lack of vascular smooth muscle cells, abnormal and chaotic branching patterns, and the absence of innervation. Endothelial cells in neovascularized tumors differ from those in normal tissue; they have distinct molecular markers, and their proliferation is much faster. Therefore, tumor vasculature, due to its physiological and molecular specificity, is a specific target for tumor treatment [2].

There are two concepts of *vascular-targeted agents* as cancer therapeutics that act on tumor blood vessels; those inhibiting the formation of new blood vessels (*antiangiogenic agents*), and those that act on the established blood vessels (*vascular-disrupting agents*). Antiangiogenic agents

G. Sersa (✉)
Department of Experimental Oncology, Institute of Oncology Ljubljana,
Zaloska c. 2, SI-1000 Ljubljana, Slovenia
e-mail: gsersa@onko-i.si

S.T. Kee et al. (eds.), *Clinical Aspects of Electroporation*,
DOI 10.1007/978-1-4419-8363-3_7, © Springer Science+Business Media, LLC 2011

are considered cytostatic in nature, in contrast to vascular-disrupting agents, which are thought to be cytotoxic. The antiangiogenic agents exert their effect within days and require chronic dosing, oral or intravenous, whereas vascular-disrupting agents are effective within minutes and require acute dosing, mostly intravenously [3].

Both categories of vascular-targeted therapies are clinically available, the prominent antiangiogenic agent being bevacizumab (avastin), whilst combretastatin A4-P is the major vascular-disrupting agent. Although they are distinguished by their mode of action, there is some overlap between the two groups, with agents classified according to their primary site of action [4–6].

Electrochemotherapy

Electrochemotherapy consists of chemotherapy followed by local application of electric pulses to the tumor to increase drug delivery into cells. Drug uptake can be increased by electroporation only for those drugs whose transport through the plasma membrane is normally impeded [7]. Among many drugs which have been tested so far, only bleomycin and cisplatin have transitioned from preclinical testing to clinical trials. In vitro studies demonstrated a several-fold increase in their cytotoxicity after electroporation of cells. In vivo, electroporation of tumors after local or systemic administration of either of the drugs, that is, electrochemotherapy, proved to be an effective antitumor treatment. In preclinical studies on several tumor models, electrochemotherapy with either bleomycin or cisplatin was assessed in detail, and parameters for effective local tumor control were determined [8, 9]. Several clinical studies were performed demonstrating that electrochemotherapy is effective in local tumor control of cutaneous and subcutaneous tumor nodules of different histology. So far, predominantly melanoma skin metastases have been treated, with ~70% long-lasting complete responses of the treated nodules [10–12].

Besides membrane electroporation, which facilitates drug transport and its accumulation in the cell, other mechanisms that are involved in antitumor effectiveness of electrochemotherapy have been described [8, 9].

Modifying Effect of Electric Pulses on Tumor Blood Flow

The application of electric pulses to tissues induces a transient but reversible reduction in blood flow. Several studies have investigated changes in blood volume, perfusion, and oxygenation in tumors and normal tissue after application of electric pulses. The first study, using albumin-(Gd-DTPA) contrast-enhanced magnetic resonance imaging (MRI), has demonstrated that 30 min after application of electric pulses to SA-1 tumors, tumor blood volume is reduced from 20% in untreated tumors to 0% in electroporated tumors [13]. A pharmacological study with ^{86}RbCl extraction technique in the same tumor model was also done, exploring time dependence of the perfusion changes. A significant reduction of tumor perfusion (~30% of control) was observed within 1 h following the application of electric pulses to the tumors. Thereafter, tumor blood flow slowly recovered, almost reaching the pretreatment level within 24 h. No change in perfusion was induced in untreated contralateral normal leg muscle. A similar pattern of blood flow reduction was induced when a second set of electric pulses was applied to the tumor following a 24-h interval. The degree of tumor blood flow reduction was dependent upon the number of electric pulses applied; a smaller effect was observed if less than eight pulses were applied. Furthermore, the degree of blood flow reduction was also dependent on the amplitude of electric pulses applied; electric pulses with an amplitude higher than 600 V induced reduction in tumor blood flow [14]. In subsequent studies, it was demonstrated that the results obtained with the ^{86}RbCl extraction technique correlated with the Patent Blue staining technique, which is a much more simple method for measuring tissue perfusion [15].

The changes in tumor perfusion were shown to correlate with changes in tumor oxygenation, as measured by the electron paramagnetic resonance (EPR) technique. The maximal reduction in partial oxygen pressure (pO_2) level was observed 2 h after application of electric pulses to the tumor (~40% of control), with recovery to the pretreatment level within 10 h after application [16]. This study also demonstrated that changes in the tumor blood flow are instantaneous, occurring during the application of electric pulses, as demonstrated by laser Doppler flowmetry [17].

In vitro studies have shown that application of electric pulses to a monolayer of endothelial cells results in a profound disruption of microfilament and microtubule cytoskeletal networks, loss of contractility, and loss of cadherin-formed cell-to-cell junctions in the vascular endothelial lining immediately after electroporation, which recovered within 60 min after electroporation, without any significant loss of cell viability. The cytoskeletal effects of electroporation were paralleled by a rapid increase in endothelial monolayer permeability, giving an indication of putative mechanisms responsible for the observed increase in permeability and cessation of blood flow in vivo [18].

A tumor is a heterogeneous tissue consisting of tumor stromal cells and a capillary network. When a tumor mass is exposed to an electric field that is used for electrochemotherapy, all cells in the tissue are exposed [19, 20]. In a mathematical model, it was validated that endothelial cells in the lining of small tumor blood vessels are exposed to an electric field that can increase their permeability. The model predicted that endothelial cells lining the tumor blood vessels are exposed to a ~40% higher electric field than the surrounding tumor cells. This indicates that tumor endothelial cells are a valid target for electroporation [17].

A histological study of tumors exposed to electric pulse application examined blood vessel changes. Changes in endothelial cell shape were observed 1 h after application of electric pulses. Endothelial cells turned spherical in shape and became swollen, and the lumen of blood vessels was narrowed (Fig. 7.1) [17].

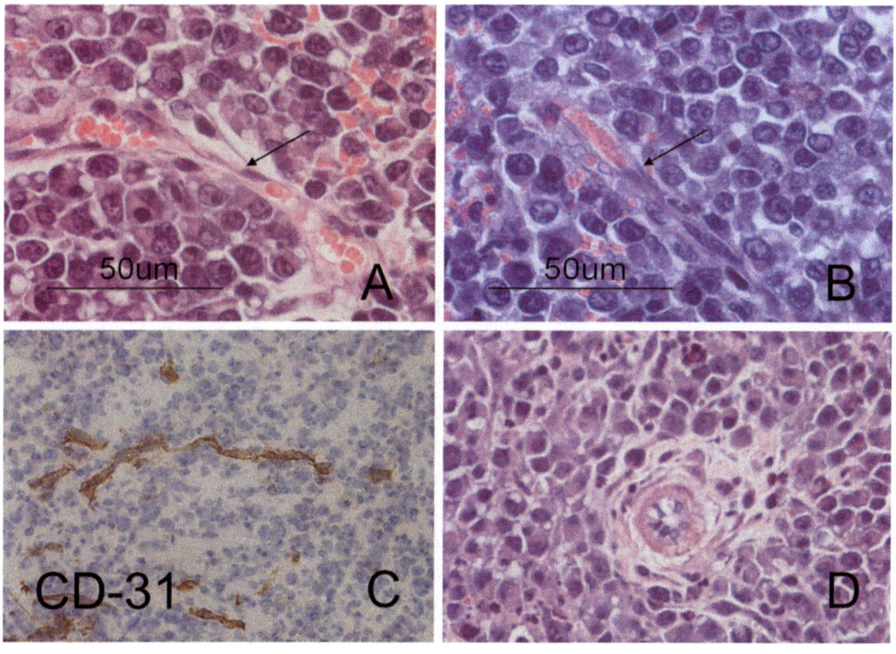

Fig. 7.1 Morphological changes in tumor blood vessels after electroporation. Swollen endothelial cells (**a**, **b**) and narrowed lumens (**c**, **d**). Tumor tissue specimens were formalin-fixed and paraffin-embedded. Two consecutive 5 μm thick sections were cut from each paraffin block and stained with hematoxylin eosin or immunohistochemically using anti-CD31 antibody to visualize blood vessels

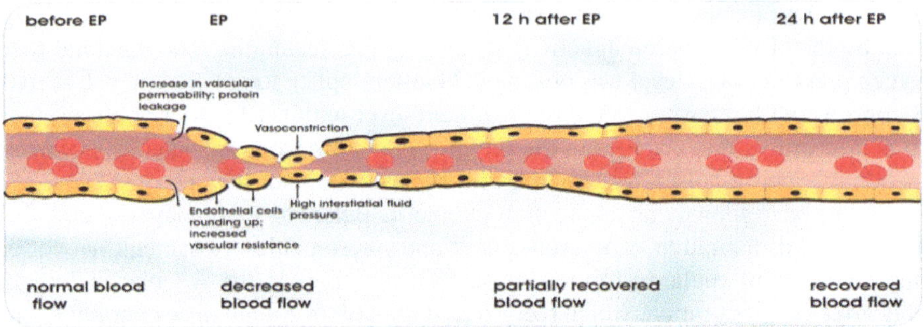

Fig. 7.2 Model of vascular changes in tumor blood vessels exposed to high intensity electric pulses as used in electrochemotherapy. *EP* electroporation

The observed effects of tumor blood flow modification after application of electric pulses were also observed in normal muscle tissue in mice. Similar effects on leg perfusion, measured by Patent Blue, were observed in mice, with a wide variety of electric pulse amplitudes and pulse durations (10–20,000 μs and 0.1–1.6 kV/cm) [21].

Based on all the gathered information on vascular effects of electric pulses in the tumor, a model of the sequence of changes is proposed (Fig. 7.2):

1. Disruption of cytoskeletal networks causing endothelial cells to turn spherical in shape.
2. Increased leakage of plasma into the interstitial space.
3. Increased interstitial fluid pressure and vascular resistance leading to a narrowed vascular lumen and reduced blood flow.
4. Restoration of tumor blood flow within 24–48 h due to the effect on endothelial cells and vascular permeability being reversible.

The studies indicate that vascular reactions induced by application of electric pulses to the tissue are important for the kinetics of drug delivery used in electrochemotherapy or plasmid delivery in gene electrotransfer. The vascular lock causes drug entrapment by temporary cessation of tissue perfusion induced by electric pulses, leading to a prolonged exposure of the tissue to the previously injected drug, plasmid DNA, or other nucleic acid molecules, as demonstrated in the case of electrochemotherapy with cisplatin [8, 21, 22].

Modifying Effect of Electrochemotherapy on Tumor Blood Flow

Modifying effects of electrochemotherapy on tumor blood flow, measured by tumor perfusion and oxygenation as well as histological changes, were studied and compared to vascular changes observed after application of electric pulses without the accompanying injection of a drug [17]. Studies on electrochemotherapy with bleomycin as well as with cisplatin have demonstrated that changes, within 2 h in tumor perfusion and oxygenation, are identical to those observed after the application of electric pulses alone. Immediately after treatment, tumor perfusion was maximally reduced. Approximately 30 min later, the tumors started to reperfuse in both groups; in the tumors treated by electrochemotherapy, the reperfusion leveled after ~1 h and stayed at 20% up to 48 h after the treatment, whereas the tumors treated with application of electric pulses alone continued to reperfuse. The changes in tumor perfusion were demonstrated to be similar when using electrochemotherapy with either bleomycin or cisplatin. The degree of changes was demonstrated to be dependent on the drug dosage used in electrochemotherapy. For example, a lower bleomycin dose

(1 mg/kg) resulted in less reduction of tumor perfusion than a higher dose (4 mg/kg). The low dose also resulted in gradual reperfusion of the tumors, which was in all cases significantly delayed compared to perfusion changes after application of electric pulses alone, whereas the higher dose of bleomycin resulted in complete shutdown of tumor perfusion and a high percentage of tumor cures (70%) [15–17].

The changes in perfusion following electrochemotherapy correlated with tumor oxygenation. EPR oxymetry demonstrated that electrochemotherapy induced an instantaneous reduction in pO_2 levels to ~25% of the pretreatment level, which is a more profound effect than the one caused by application of electric pulses alone. Tumor oxygenation subsequently correlated with changes observed after application of electric pulses for up to 2 h post-treatment; however, the recovery of tumor oxygenation was much slower, returning to the pretreatment level with a delay as long as 2 days [16, 17]. Short- and long-term perfusion changes were confirmed by power Doppler ultrasonography of tumors, as well as by determination of the hypoxic area in the tumors by staining of cells with pimonidazole, a marker of tumor hypoxia [17, 23]. Furthermore, it was demonstrated that electroporation of human endothelial HMEC-1 cells, even after short-term drug exposure, significantly enhanced the cytotoxicity of bleomycin and cisplatin [24].

All these data indicate that in vivo electrochemotherapy, especially with bleomycin, may directly damage the vascular endothelium, accounting for its vascular-disrupting effect. Detailed histological analyses of tumors after electrochemotherapy demonstrated that the same morphological changes in endothelial cells occurred as after application of electric pulses to the tumors; endothelial cells turned spherical in shape and became swollen, and the lumen of blood vessels was narrowed. However, apoptotic morphological characteristics were found in some vessels 8 h after electrochemotherapy. Furthermore, blood vessels were stacked with erythrocytes and extravasation of erythrocytes was also observed. Apoptotic endothelial cells were not observed in the control group or in tumors treated with either electric pulses or bleomycin alone (Fig. 7.3) [17].

Based on all the gathered information on vascular effects of electrochemotherapy with bleomycin or cisplatin, a model of the sequence of changes is proposed (Fig. 7.4), which shares details with the model proposed for the application of electric pulses and includes further changes due to the presence of the chemotherapeutic drug:

1. Disruption of cytoskeletal networks causing endothelial cells to turn spherical in shape.
2. Increased leakage of plasma into the interstitial space.
3. Increased interstitial fluid pressure and vascular resistance leading to a narrowed vascular lumen and reduced blood flow.
4. Apoptosis of endothelial cells due to the presence of an increased amount of the chemotherapeutic drug.
5. No or significantly delayed vascular reperfusion, depending on the degree of vascular disruption.

Clinical Application

As hemorrhaging cutaneous metastases are a common clinical problem, some reports on successful treatment with electrochemotherapy have already been described. Gehl et al. described two cases of successful management of bleeding melanoma skin metastases [25, 26]. The first case established the effectiveness of electrochemotherapy in the treatment of nine bleeding, ulcerated nodules on the chest wall, with immediate cessation of bleeding after administration of electric pulses and complete regression of all nodules [25]. The second case demonstrated a palliative effect of electrochemotherapy in dealing with eight metastases on the head and scalp, with complete regression of all but one of the metastases (87%) [26]. An even bigger skin metastasis (3.5 × 3 cm in diameter)

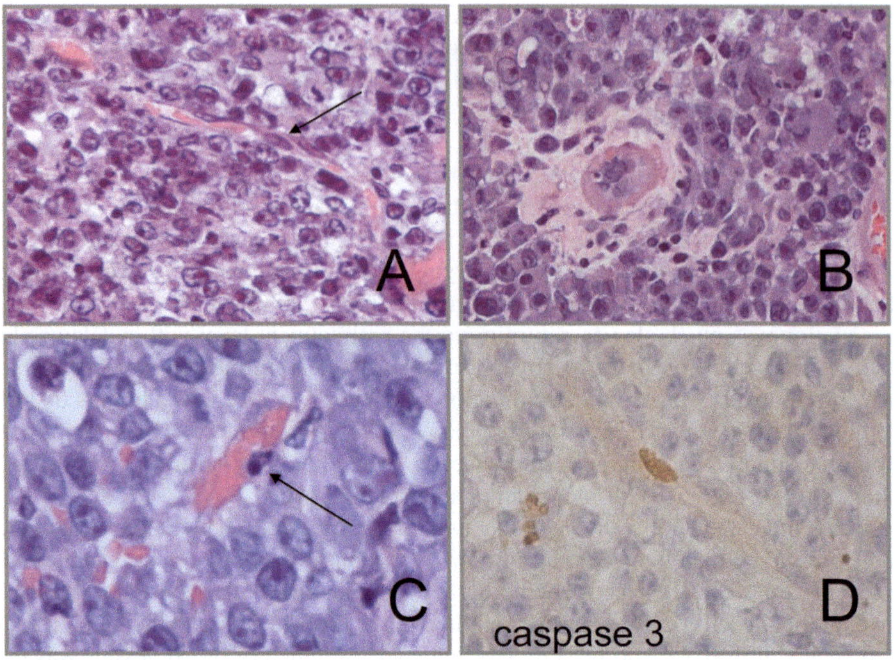

Fig. 7.3 Morphological changes in tumor blood vessels after electrochemotherapy with bleomycin. Swollen endothelial cells turned spherical in shape (**a**), increased vascular resistance to tumor blood flow (**b**), and apoptotic endothelial cells (**c, d**). Tumor tissue specimens were formalin-fixed and paraffin-embedded. Two consecutive 5 μm thick sections were cut from each paraffin block and stained with hematoxylin eosin or immunohistochemically using ant-caspase 3 antibody to visualize apoptotic cells

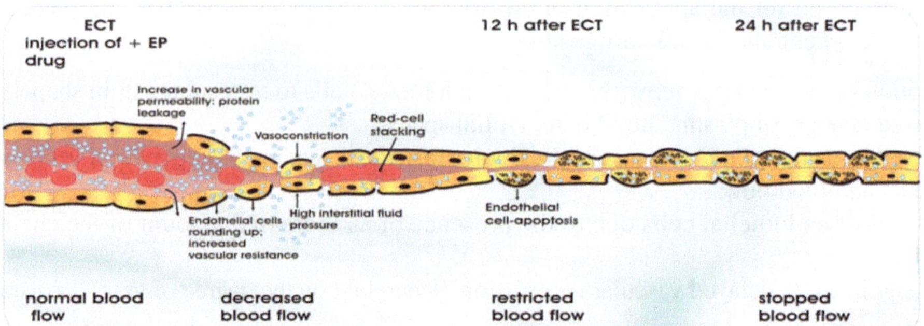

Fig. 7.4 Model of vascular-disrupting action of electrochemotherapy. *EP* electroporation; *ECT* electrochemotherapy

was treated by electrochemotherapy at our Institute of Oncology Ljubljana [27]. The bleeding metastasis was located on the leg and amputation of the leg was initially considered as a definitive cure. However, electrochemotherapy with bleomycin given intravenously was performed, and immediately after delivery of the electric pulses, the bleeding stopped and did not recur. The lesion developed a crust and decreased in size in a matter of weeks. At the end of the 3-week observation period, the lesion was in partial response (Fig. 7.5).

These reports show that electrochemotherapy represents a novel approach in the palliation of bleeding metastases. Surgery can be suitable for management of small bleeding lesions, but with

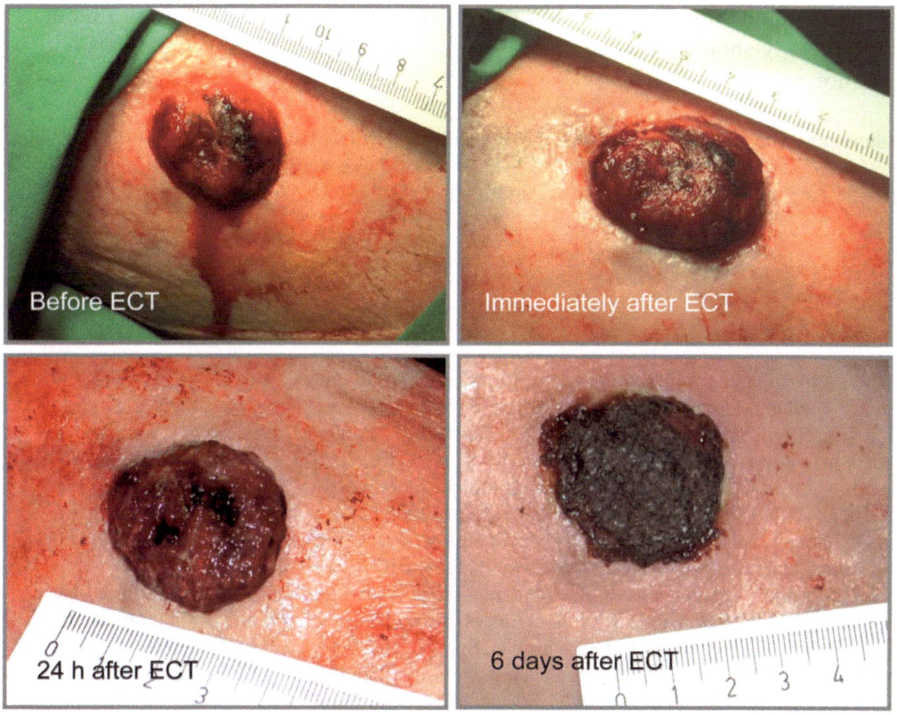

Fig. 7.5 Response of bleeding melanoma metastasis to electrochemotherapy with bleomycin. During the following week, a crust formed and fell off within 3 weeks. *ECT* electrochemotherapy

larger or multiple lesions, amputation is the only possible surgical approach [28]. Furthermore, no studies have been performed so far to establish the palliative effect of radiotherapy on bleeding melanoma nodules. On the other hand, in a study by Fraker et al., an isolated limb perfusion with melphalan and tumor necrosis factor-alpha proved to be an effective palliative treatment of advanced bleeding melanoma. Symptomatic improvement was achieved in 5 of 6 patients with bleeding or ulcerated nodules [29]. In addition, several other studies report on the limb-sparing effect of isolated limb perfusion. Noorda et al. reported on a series of 21 patients with recurrent or persistent melanoma who underwent repeated isolated limb perfusion with tumor necrosis factor alpha and melphalan, with a median follow-up of 18 months and 95% limb salvage rate [30]. In a study by Grunhagen et al., limb salvage was achieved in 36 out of 37 patients, one patient undergoing amputation due to treatment toxicity [31]. However, according to Sasso et al., intra-arterial embolization is a treatment of choice in the management of bleeding melanoma [32].

Conclusion

A comparison between isolated limb perfusion for bleeding metastases and electrochemotherapy points to the many advantages of the latter. Patients are often in overall poor physical condition and electrochemotherapy offers an excellent alternative due to its once-only treatment strategy, high probability of immediate relief, as well as the modest degree of patient discomfort experienced. Currently, its main clinical application remains restricted to palliative treatment of cutaneous and subcutaneous tumor nodules refractory to conventional treatment. However, electrochemotherapy should also be considered as a treatment modality in patients with refractory bleeding tumor nodules.

Acknowledgments The authors acknowledge the financial support from the state budget of the Slovenian Research Agency (P3-0003). The authors acknowledge the help of Prof. Marko Snoj, Prof. Andrej Coer, Dr. Simona Kranjc, and Dr. Mireille Treeby in preparation of the manuscript.

References

1. Folkman J. Anti-angiogenesis: new concept for therapy of solid tumors. Ann Surg. 1972;175:409–16.
2. Folkman J. Angiogenesis: an organizing principle for drug discovery. Nat Rev. 2007;6:273–86.
3. Siemann DW, Bibby MC, Dark GG, Dicker AP, Eskens F, Horsman MR, et al. Differentiation and definition of vascular-targeted therapies. Clin Cancer Res. 2005;11:416–20.
4. Tozer GM, Kanthou C, Baguley BC. Disrupting tumour blood vessels. Nat Rev. 2005;5:423–35.
5. Neri D, Bicknell R. Tumor vascular targeting. Nat Rev. 2005;5:436–46.
6. Hinnen P, Eskens F. Vascular disrupting agents in clinical development. Br J Cancer. 2007;96:1159–65.
7. Mir LM. Bases and rationale of the electrochemotherapy. EJC Suppl. 2006;4:38–44.
8. Mir LM, Orlowski S. Mechanisms of electrochemotherapy. Adv Drug Del Rev. 1999;35:107–18.
9. Sersa G, Cemazar M, Miklavcic D, Rudolf Z. Electrochemotherapy of tumours. Radiol Oncol. 2006;40:163–74.
10. Marty M, Sersa G, Garbay JR, Gehl J, Collins CG, Snoj M, et al. Electrochemotherapy – an easy, highly effective and safe treatment of cutaneous and subcutaneous metastases: Results of ESOPE (European Standard Operating Procedures of Electrochemotherapy) study. EJC Suppl. 2006;4:3–13.
11. Quaglino P, Montera C, Osella-Abate S, Barberis M, Illengo M, Rissone M, et al. Electrochemotherapy with intravenous bleomycin in the local treatment of skin melanoma mestastases. Ann Surg Oncol. 2008;15:2215–22.
12. Sersa G, Miklavcic D, Cemazar M, Rudolf Z, Pucihar G, Snoj M. Electrochemotherapy in treatment of tumors. EJSO. 2008;34:232–40.
13. Sersa G, Beravs K, Cemazar M, Miklavcic D, Demsar F. Contrast enhanced MRI assessment of tumor blood volume after application of electric pulses. Electro Magnetobiol. 1998;17:299–306.
14. Sersa G, Cemazar M, Parkins CS, Chaplin DJ. Tumour blood flow changes induced by application of electric pulses. Eur J Cancer. 1999;35:672–7.
15. Sersa G, Cemazar M, Miklavcic D, Chaplin DJ. Tumor blood modifying effect of electrochemotherapy with bleomycin. Anticancer Res. 1999;19:4017–22.
16. Sersa G, Krzic M, Sentjurc M, Ivanusa T, Beravs K, Kotnik V, et al. Reduced blood flow and oxygenation in SA-1 tumours after electrochemotherapy with cisplatin. Br J Cancer. 2002;87:1047–54.
17. Sersa G, Jarm T, Kotnik T, Coer A, Podkrajsek M, Sentjurc M, et al. Vascular disrupting action of electroporation and electrochemotherapy with bleomycin in murine sarcoma. Br J Cancer. 2008;98:388–98.
18. Kanthou C, Kranjc S, Sersa G, Tozer G, Zupanic A, Cemazar M. The endothelial cytoskeleton as a target of electroporation based therapies. Mol Cancer Ther. 2006;5:3145–52.
19. Miklavcic D, Corovic S, Pucihar G, Pavselj N. Importance of tumour coverage by sufficiently high local electric field for effective electrochemotherapy. EJC Suppl. 2006;4:45–51.
20. Pavselj N, Miklavcic D. Numerical modeling in electroporation-based biomedical applications. Radiol Oncol. 2008;42:159–68.
21. Gehl J, Skovsgaard T, Mir LM. Vascular reactions to *in vivo* electroporation: characterization and concequences for drug and gene delivery. Biochim Biophys Acta. 2002;1569:51–8.
22. Cemazar M, Miklavcic D, Scancar J, Dolzan V, Golouh R, Sersa G. Increased platinum accumulation in SA-1 tumor cells after *in vivo* electrochemotherapy with cisplatin. Br J Cancer. 1999;79:1386–91.
23. Coer A, Cemazar M, Plazar N, Sersa G. Comparison between hypoxic markers pimonidazole and glucose transporter 1 (Glut-1) in murine fibrosarcoma tumours alter electrochemotherapy. Radiol Oncol. 2009;43:195–202.
24. Cemazar M, Parkins CS, Chaplin DJ, Tozer GM, Sersa G. Electroporation of human microvascular endothelial cells: evidence of an anti-vascular mechanism of electrochemotherapy. Br J Cancer. 2001;84:565–70.
25. Gehl J, Geertsen PF. Efficient palliation of haemorrhaging malignant melanoma skin metastases by electrochemotherapy. Melanoma Res. 2000;10:585–9.
26. Gehl J, Geertsen PF. Palliation of haemorrhaging and ulcerated malignant cutaneous tumors using electrochemotherapy. EJC Suppl. 2006;4:35–7.

27. Snoj M, Cemazar M, Srnovrsnik T, Paulin Kosir S, Sersa G. Limb sparing treatment of blooding melanoma recurrence by electrochemotherapy. Tumori. 2009;95:398–402.
28. Fletcher WS, Pommier RF, Lum S, Wilmarth TJ. Surgical treatment of metastatic melanoma. Am J Surg. 1998;175:413–7.
29. Fraker DL, Alexander HR, Andrich M, Rosenberg SA. Palliation of regional symptoms of advanced extremity melanoma by isolated limb perfusion with melphalan and high-dose tumor necrosis factor. Cancer J Sci Am. 1995;1:104–5.
30. Noorda EM, Vrouenraets BC, Nieweg OE, van Geel AN, Eggermont AM, Kroon BB. Repeat isolated limb perfusion with TNFalpha and melphalan for recurrent limb melanoma after failure of previous perfusion. Eur J Surg Oncol. 2006;32:318–24.
31. Grunhagen DJ, de Wilt JH, Graveland WJ, van Geel AN, Eggermont AM. The palliative value of tumor necrosis factor alpha-based isolated limb perfusion in patients with metastatic sarcoma and melanoma. Cancer. 2006;106:156–62.
32. Sasso CM, Hubner C, Wall S. Intraarterial embolization of bleeding melanoma. J Vasc Nurs. 1995;13:27–8.

Chapter 8
Electrochemotherapy of Small Tumors; The Experience from the ESOPE (European Standard Operating Procedures for Electrochemotherapy) Group

Gregor Sersa, Julie Gehl, Jean-Remy Garbay, Declan M. Soden, Gerald C. O'Sullivan, Louise W. Matthiessen, Marko Snoj, and Lluis M. Mir

Abstract Electrochemotherapy, utilizing bleomycin and cisplatin as chemotherapeutic drugs along with electric pulses locally delivered to the treated tumors, plays an important role in the local control of cancers. The treatment is easy to perform, on an outpatient basis, for the treatment of skin melanoma, breast cancer, or other tumor skin metastases. An objective response rate of 80% or more is reported on the treated nodules, mostly with a long-lasting response. The treatment procedure is fully described in the published European Standard Operating Procedures for electrochemotherapy study. Currently, electrochemotherapy is used as a treatment that improves the quality of life for patients with progressive disease. Furthermore, it is ideally suited to the treatment of tumors refractory to conventional treatments like radiotherapy or surgery, or those that cannot be surgically excised due to their number and location. In addition, it can be effectively employed as a cytoreductive treatment before surgical resection in an organ-sparing procedure as well as in the treatment of bleeding skin metastases.

Keywords Electrochemotherapy • Electroporation • Bleomycin • Cisplatin • Cutaneous tumors • Melanoma

Introduction

A multimodal approach is usually employed in the treatment of cancer. However, local tumor control is a critically important part of the treatment of malignant solid tumors as it relieves symptoms, forestalls complications, facilitates responsiveness to systemic therapies, and is often curative. Despite the advances made in cancer treatment, many tumors at the time of presentation are untreatable with standard treatment approaches, local or systemic. This situation is often due to the resistance of tumor cells to chemotherapy and radiation therapy, the anatomical location of the cancer that can preclude complex excision or ablation by radiotherapy, and the presence of concurrent illnesses which either limit the application or adversely alter the risk and benefit of a standard treatment.

Locally recurrent disease, particularly after optimal treatment of for example, malignant melanoma, head and neck carcinoma, or breast cancer, is difficult to manage. The patients are often faced

G. Sersa (✉)
Institute of Oncology Ljubljana, Slovenia, Department of Experimental Oncology,
Institute of Oncology Ljubljana, Zaloska c. 2, SI-1000 Ljubljana
e-mail: gsersa@onko-i.si

S.T. Kee et al. (eds.), *Clinical Aspects of Electroporation*,
DOI 10.1007/978-1-4419-8363-3_8, © Springer Science+Business Media, LLC 2011

with obviously progressing painful, bleeding, and malodorous tumors. These patients have a poor quality of life, while their valuable remaining time may not benefit from often questionably suitable invasive treatment approaches. Therefore, the ideal treatment for cancer should be minimally invasive, targeted, and effective against a diversity of tumor types and anatomical locations. Ultimately, it should be minimally intrusive, improve the patient's quality of life, and increase life expectancy through local control or cure.

Electrochemotherapy

Electrochemotherapy is an anticancer therapeutic approach that enhances the effectiveness of a chemotherapeutic drug due to increased uptake of the drug by applying electric pulses to tumor tissue. Short intense electric pulses cause transient and reversible permeabilization of the cell membranes, therefore increasing intracellular access of otherwise nonpermeant or poorly permeant drugs [1, 2], as is also described in Chap. 6. Various chemotherapeutic drugs have been tested, but bleomycin and cisplatin were found to be the most suitable for clinical use in electrochemotherapy based on numerous in vitro and in vivo studies [3, 4]. Extensive in vivo studies were performed on different animal tumor types, either transplantable or spontaneous. High antitumor effectiveness of electrochemotherapy was demonstrated on fibrosarcomas, melanomas, and carcinomas in mice, rats, and rabbits; good clinical results were also obtained in veterinary oncology on cats, dogs, and horses [5, 6]. The mechanisms involved in electrochemotherapy are multiple. The basic mechanism is membrane electroporation which facilitates drug transport into the cells in tumors. A 2–4-fold increase in DNA binding of cisplatin was demonstrated after tumor electroporation compared to drug administration alone [7, 8]. In the case of bleomycin, a more than 300-fold increase in the cytotoxic effect may be achieved, and one internalized bleomycin molecule may cause 10–15 DNA strand breaks [9, 10]. Additional mechanisms of electrochemotherapy include drug entrapment in the tumor tissue after application of electric pulses to the tumors due to the vascular lock that is induced by the electric pulses (see Chap. 7) [11–13]. Furthermore, electrochemotherapy also has a supplementary vascular-disrupting effect of electrochemotherapy that is due to the electroporative effect of electric pulses on endothelial cells and their apoptosis after drug exposure [11, 14]. An immune response is also involved, as massive destruction of tumor cells may release tumor antigens systemically, which in turn can elicit an immune response that can contribute to the overall treatment response of electrochemotherapy [15–17].

Clinical Studies of Electrochemotherapy

A number of clinical trials have been performed on electrochemotherapy applied to different types of tumors. The first clinical trial was published in 1991 in head and neck cancer patients, which demonstrated encouraging results [18]. Thereafter, several clinical studies reported excellent results on electrochemotherapy with bleomycin or cisplatin, predominantly on melanoma [19–27], basal cell carcinoma [21–24, 28, 29], head and neck squamous carcinoma [18, 30–34], and mammary carcinoma metastases [21, 22, 24, 32]. Several case reports on electrochemotherapy treatment effectiveness in skin metastases of hypernephroma [35], ovarian cancer [36], Kaposi's sarcoma [23], urogenital carcinoma [37], and Merkel cell cancer [38] were also reported.

The history of electrochemotherapy can be divided into the periods before and after the European Standard Operating Procedures on electrochemotherapy (ESOPE) study published in 2006 [39], which represents a landmark in the translation of electrochemotherapy into a broader clinical application. Before the ESOPE study, various studies involving electrochemotherapy utilized a variety of protocols with different doses of chemotherapy, pulse parameters, and pulse generators in conjunction with different electrode types [40]. In an attempt to rectify this, the ESOPE study was launched with the aim of standardizing the technique involved in the clinical application of electrochemotherapy by the preparation of Standard Operating Procedures (SOP), based on the experience of leading European cancer centers on electrochemotherapy (Institute Gustave Roussy, Villejuif; Institute of Oncology, Ljubljana; Cork Cancer Research Center, Cork; and Herlev Hospital, Copenhagen). This was made possible by the existence of the electric pulse generator Cliniporator™ (IGEA, Carpi, Italy) which had been developed in a preceding European project. Based on the prepared SOP, the treatment response after electrochemotherapy was investigated according to the tumor type, drug used, route of administration, and type of electrodes.

Before the ESOPE study, reports of 247 patients undergoing clinical trials had been published; 655 nodules from 202 patients were treated by electrochemotherapy with bleomycin and 354 nodules from 45 patients by electrochemotherapy with cisplatin. Objective responses (ORs) of various histological types of tumor nodules were reported in 80% of cases. The majority of cases treated were skin metastases of melanoma, where 45 and 77% complete responses (CRs) were obtained when bleomycin was administered intratumorally or systemically, respectively. Correspondingly, 67 and 48% CRs were obtained when cisplatin was administered intratumorally or systemically, respectively. The treatment responses in the studies have been reviewed earlier [9, 40].

The ESOPE study was a 2-year-long, prospective, non-randomized, multi-institutional study on 41 patients evaluable for response to treatment, and 61 evaluable for toxicity [41]. Treatment response after different electrochemotherapy regimes was evaluated, with variables including the drug used (bleomycin or cisplatin) and administration route (intratumoral or intravenous (i.v.)). The type of electrodes (plate, needle) was evaluated in the treatment of melanoma or nonmelanoma nodules. After electrochemotherapy, an OR was obtained in 145 of the treated nodules (84.8%), with 11.1% being partial responses and 73.7% CRs after a single treatment. Only in a very small number of cases was a negative response observed, with either no response in 10.5% or progressive disease in 4.7% of cases.

The study showed no statistical difference in local tumor control at 150 days after the treatment (median follow-up was 133 days and range 60–380 days) between bleomycin given i.v. (88% OR) or intratumorally (73% OR), or cisplatin given intratumorally (75% OR). In some previous studies [23], an intratumoral dose of bleomycin five times higher than the one used in the ESOPE study was administered. As the intratumoral dose of bleomycin used in the ESOPE study was equally as efficient as in the previous studies, it seems that the lower dose is effective and may lead to better normal tissue tolerance and a lower total injected dose.

No statistical difference in the response of melanoma versus nonmelanoma nodules was observed, although there was a trend toward a higher OR for the nonmelanoma nodules (90%) compared to the melanoma nodules (80%), supported by a higher level of CRs (83.6 versus 66.3%).

The importance of the results of the ESOPE study is in demonstrating that, with an appropriate protocol for treatment of cutaneous metastases of different tumor types, a success rate in excess of 80% can be achieved, which is comparable to the success rate that was reported in the studies before the ESOPE study [42].

Owing to the results of the ESOPE study, this treatment approach has been adopted by several new cancer centers throughout Europe. Since the ESOPE study, electrochemotherapy is being used for the treatment of cutaneous and subcutaneous tumor nodules of different histology in a number of cancer centers. Some of the centers have already reported their experience with electrochemotherapy. Most of the studies have obtained results similar to the ones of the ESOPE study, predominantly on melanoma nodules [43, 44] but also on breast carcinoma metastases [45, 46], metastatic basal cell carcinoma [47], Kaposis's sarcoma [48], and head and neck cancer [49].

The melanoma studies demonstrated that even tumor nodules greater than 3 cm in diameter can be successfully treated by electrochemotherapy by use of repeated electrochemotherapy sessions (as described in Chap. 9).

The quality of life of the treated patients was followed in two studies [41, 43]. In the first, the ESOPE study [41], it was demonstrated that side effects of electrochemotherapy were minor and acceptable, as reported by the patients. In fact, 93% reported that they would be willing to accept another treatment if indicated. In the second study by Campana et al. [43], a more in-depth evaluation of patients' quality of life was done through a survey assessing wound healing and bleeding, esthetic impairment, daily activities, social relations, pain, treatment satisfaction, and acceptance of retreatment. Most patients reported a benefit in local-disease-related complaints and in activity of daily living (ADL).

All these studies have proved that electrochemotherapy is safe and effective in a palliative setting in all tumors treated, and useful in preserving patients' quality of life.

Summary of Treatment Advantages and Clinical Uses

Electrochemotherapy is used for the treatment of cutaneous and subcutaneous tumor nodules of different malignancies. The treatment advantages and clinical uses for electrochemotherapy can be summarized as follows:

- Easy and effective treatment of tumors of any histology in the cutaneous and subcutaneous tissue. Single nodules of sizes up to 7–8 cm in diameter can be treated in multiple electrochemotherapy sessions, and smaller nodules less than 3 cm in diameter in a single session. Multiple nodules can also be treated, 30 or more in a single session, with the possibility to retreat the remaining, previously untreated nodules in further session(s). In some cases, long-term remissions up to several years can be obtained (Fig. 8.1) [50].
- This treatment improves the quality of life of patients with progressive disease. Electrochemotherapy is currently used in a palliative intent, providing benefit to patients treated on an outpatient basis [41, 43].
- Electrochemotherapy may be used as the treatment of choice for tumors refractory to conventional treatments like radiotherapy or surgery when they cannot be surgically excised due to their number or location [41, 51]. Furthermore, electrochemotherapy can be performed on patients using local anesthesia.

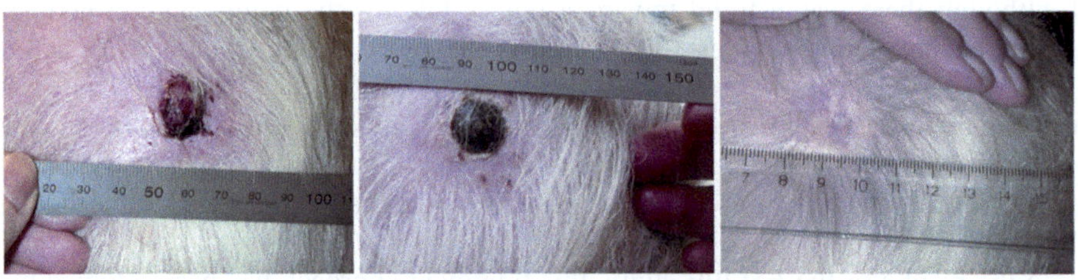

Fig. 8.1 Course of treatment for a patient with malignant melanoma metastases treated with i.v. bleomycin and type III (*hexagonal*) electrodes under general anesthesia. One of the eight treated metastases is shown. Before treatment, the metastasis was ulcerated and caused hemorrhage, pain, and discomfort. One month after treatment, the lesion was covered by a crust. Needle marks in normal tissue are visible around the crust, since both the tumor and a margin of normal tissue were covered. The normal tissue was largely unaffected, whereas the tumor area became necrotic, indicating a therapeutic window. Six months after treatment, the treated nodule was in CR. The crust fell off after 10 weeks, revealing normal skin that had healed underneath the nodule (from Gehl, Ugeskrift for laeger, 2005, with permission)

- In some cases, the benefit of electrochemotherapy has been demonstrated as a cytoreductive treatment before surgical resection in an organ-sparing treatment attempt. It has been used in such a setting before sphincter-sparing resection of anal melanoma [52, 53], digital chondrosarcoma [54], rescuing the finger from amputation, or to reduce the extent of surgery in a case of Kaposi's sarcoma of the penis [48].
- Bleeding skin melanoma metastases present a problem that is common but difficult to manage. Electrochemotherapy provides an effective way of treating them; the vascular-disrupting action of electrochemotherapy immediately stops bleeding and provides good antitumor effectiveness and symptom relief [19, 55].

How to Treat the Patients: SOP

Electric Pulse Generator

In Chap. 5, various pulse generators are discussed. The Cliniporator™ is the generator that has been used in most studies to date and was also used in the ESOPE study. Therefore, the published SOP is adjusted to use of the Cliniporator™. The generator produces square wave electric pulses of variable amplitude with two options for electric pulse frequency (1 or 5,000 Hz). In addition, it is possible to verify and document the treatment parameters, since the amplitude and electric current delivered are displayed on the screen after each set of pulses and can be stored in the electronic memory of the machine.

Drugs and Dosage

It is required that, when the electric pulses are applied, the drugs are present in a pharmacological peak at the tumor site. There are several options for drug injection, depending on the clinical situation. Bleomycin can be delivered intratumorally or systemically, whereas cisplatin must be injected intratumorally to achieve the best results. When bleomycin is delivered systemically, previous data indicate an optimal treatment time window of pulses to be delivered between 8 and 28 min after the bolus injection of the drug, likely corresponding to the pharmacokinetic half-life of bleomycin [9, 39]. Pulses may be delivered after this time; however, the effect of later pulse delivery on efficacy is not yet quantified. For intratumoral application, however, the pulses need to be delivered between 1 and 10 min after the drug injection. The standard dose for i.v. bleomycin injection is 15,000 IU/m^2, while for intratumoral injection, the dose of bleomycin is approximately 500 IU/cm^3 and of cisplatin is approximately 1 mg/cm^3, depending on the tumor volume (i.e., smaller tumors should be treated with a higher dose due to risk of wash-out to systemic circulation) [39]. Please note that bleomycin is dosed in international units (IU), units (U), or mg, respectively, depending on national preference [9].

Anesthesia

The decision to administer electrochemotherapy under general or local anesthesia is dependent upon a number of factors, that is, the site, size, and number of lesions to be treated, as well as the general medical condition of the patient. Large tumors on sensitive locations as well as multiple

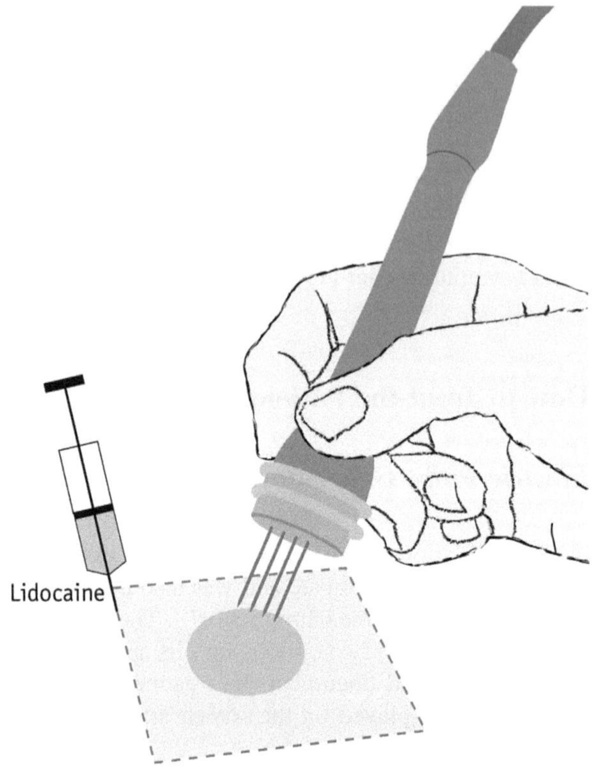

Fig. 8.2 When treating in local anesthesia, a rectangular infiltration of local anesthetic (Lidocaine, 2%, with epinephrine, 0.5%) should be laid around the area to be treated, by injection along 4 lines, so that the nodule is "fenced in" by local anesthetic. It should be ensured that an even amount of anesthetic is injected along all four sides of the rectangle, so that pain transmission is completely blocked

nodules are treated under general anesthesia. When smaller, discrete nodules are involved, for example, chest wall or limb metastases from breast adenocarcinoma or melanoma, the treatment can be carried out using local anesthesia (Fig. 8.2) [39].

Electrodes and Electric Pulse Application

Electric pulses can be applied by means of different types of electrodes (see Chap. 5). In the ESOPE study, three kinds of electrode devices were used. Type I devices consist of plate electrodes with different gap distances between them (4, 6, or 8 mm). Small superficial tumor nodules are treated using these. For treatment of thicker and/or deeper-seated tumor nodules, needle electrodes are more suitable. Type II devices consist of needle electrodes with a 4 mm gap between them and are used for the treatment of small nodules, typically in combination with local anesthesia, as the applied voltage is smaller than for the larger type III device. Type III devices consist of needle electrodes distributed in a hexagonal array and are aimed for the treatment of bigger tumor nodules (>1 cm in diameter). General anesthesia or good loco-regional anesthesia is recommended when this type of electrode is used. The application of a train of 8 electric pulses can be performed using 1 or 5,000 Hz repetition frequency. While both have the same antitumor effectiveness, as was demonstrated in the clinical study [41], the higher repetition frequency enables quicker delivery of pulses and also induces only a single muscle contraction – an effect associated with the delivery of each train of electric pulses [56].

When the tumors are bigger than the size of the electrodes, the entire tumor can be efficiently treated by moving and placing electrodes adjacently for each consecutive electric pulse application. Safety margins can and should be included in the procedure. In comparison to thermal ablation methods and other tissue-destructive methods of ablation, the benefit of electrochemotherapy is that application to the margins is greatly facilitated due to the fact that healthy tissue is less responsive to electrochemotherapy than tumor, thus facilitating a more rapid response with wider margins. Needle electrodes need to be inserted all the way through to the bottom margin of the treated tumor in order to provide adequate electric field distribution throughout the tumor [42, 57].

Selection of the Drug, Its Delivery Route, and Electrodes

Selection of the drug used in electrochemotherapy is based on the number and size of the nodules to be treated. For large or multiple tumor nodules, bleomycin injected i.v. is most appropriate. The choice of electrodes is dependent on the shape and location of the nodules. Smaller nodules in numbers up to 7 can be treated by intratumoral injection of bleomycin or cisplatin. The choice of electrodes is again dependent on the shape and location of the nodules, but predominantly Type I and II devices can be used.

The SOP describes all the treatment parameters in detail, thus giving the yet inexperienced physician in electrochemotherapy detailed guidelines for treatment [39]. The treatment procedure can be mastered in a couple of electrochemotherapy sessions; assistance in training can be sought also in cancer centers that are performing electrochemotherapy. When treating the patient, one should keep in mind that sufficient drug concentration and proper electric field distribution for coverage of the whole tumor mass are required [57] in order to ensure a high efficacy of the treatment.

Treatment Response

After electrochemotherapy, the patients can be discharged from the hospital within a few hours. No specific care of the treated nodules is required. In a few weeks [2, 3], a superficial scab forms on the nodule, which falls off after 4–12 weeks, with a longer healing time after treatment of larger nodules or previously irradiated areas. Once the scab falls off, the treatment effectiveness is visible. If the treated nodule is not completely eradicated, retreatment can be performed, usually with equally effective responsiveness (no drug resistance has been observed). De-pigmentation or scarring may occur, depending on the depth of infiltration of the cancerous lesion [36].

Conclusion

Electrochemotherapy is a feasible and safe method for the palliative treatment of metastatic melanoma and other tumors. Immediate clinical benefit is provided for patients with multiple localized cutaneous and subcutaneous metastases that are unsuitable for surgery or radiotherapy. Due to the low incidence of complications, electrochemotherapy can be repeated several times in order to maintain local control of the disease.

References

1. Mir LM. Therapeutic perspectives of *in vivo* cell electropermeabilization. Bioelectrochemistry. 2001;53(1):1–10.
2. Gehl J. Electroporation: theory and methods, perspectives for drug delivery, gene therapy and research. Acta Physiol Scand. 2003;177(4):437–47.
3. Gehl J, Skovsgaard T, Mir LM. Enhancement of cytotoxicity by electropermeabilization: an improved method for screening drugs. Anticancer Drugs. 1998;9(4):319–25.
4. Sersa G, Cemazar M, Rudolf Z. Electrochemotherapy: advantages and drawbacks in treatment of cancer patients. Cancer Therapy. 2003;1:133–42.
5. Jaroszeski MJ, Heller R, Gilbert R. Electrochemotherapy, electrogenetherapy, and transdermal drug delivery: electrically mediated delivery of molecules to cells. Totowa: Humana; 2000.
6. Cemazar M, Tamzali Y, Sersa G, Tozon N, Mir LM, Miklavcic D, et al. Electrochemotherapy in veterinary oncology. J Vet Intern Med. 2008;22(4):826–31.
7. Sersa G, Cemazar M, Miklavcic D. Antitumor effectiveness of electrochemotherapy with cis-diamminedichloroplatinum(II) in mice. Cancer Res. 1995;55(15):3450–5.
8. Cemazar M, Miklavcic D, Scancar J, Dolzan V, Golouh R, Sersa G. Increased platinum accumulation in SA-1 tumour cells after *in vivo* electrochemotherapy with cisplatin. Br J Cancer. 1999;79(9–10):1386–91.
9. Gothelf A, Mir LM, Gehl J. Electrochemotherapy: results of cancer treatment using enhanced delivery of bleomycin by electroporation. Cancer Treat Rev. 2003;29(5):371–87.
10. Tounekti O, Pron G, Belehradek Jr J, Mir LM. Bleomycin, an apoptosis-mimetic drug that induces two types of cell death depending on the number of molecules internalized. Cancer Res. 1993;53(22):5462–9.
11. Cemazar M, Parkins CS, Holder AL, Chaplin DJ, Tozer GM, Sersa G. Electroporation of human microvascular endothelial cells: evidence for an anti-vascular mechanism of electrochemotherapy. Br J Cancer. 2001;84(4):565–70.
12. Sersa G, Cemazar M, Miklavcic D, Chaplin DJ. Tumor blood flow modifying effect of electrochemotherapy with bleomycin. Anticancer Res. 1999;19(5B):4017–22.
13. Sersa G, Cemazar M, Parkins CS, Chaplin DJ. Tumour blood flow changes induced by application of electric pulses. Eur J Cancer. 1999;35(4):672–7.
14. Sersa G, Jarm T, Kotnik T, Coer A, Podkrajsek M, Sentjurc M, et al. Vascular disrupting action of electroporation and electrochemotherapy with bleomycin in murine sarcoma. Br J Cancer. 2008;98(2):388–98.
15. Mir LM, Orlowski S, Poddevin B, Belehradek Jr J. Electrochemotherapy tumor treatment is improved by interleukin-2 stimulation of the host's defenses. Eur Cytokine Netw. 1992;3(3):331–4.
16. Mir LM, Roth C, Orlowski S, Quintin-Colonna F, Fradelizi D, Belehradek Jr J, et al. Systemic antitumor effects of electrochemotherapy combined with histoincompatible cells secreting interleukin-2. J Immunother Emphasis Tumor Immunol. 1995;17(1):30–8.
17. Andersen MH, Gehl J, Reker S, Pedersen LO, Becker JC, Geertsen P, et al. Dynamic changes of specific T cell responses to melanoma correlate with IL-2 administration. Semin Cancer Biol. 2003;13(6):449–59.
18. Mir LM, Belehradek M, Domenge C, Orlowski S, Poddevin B, Belehradek Jr J, et al. Electrochemotherapy, a new antitumor treatment: first clinical trial. C R Acad Sci III. 1991;313(13):613–8.
19. Gehl J, Geertsen PF. Efficient palliation of haemorrhaging malignant melanoma skin metastases by electrochemotherapy. Melanoma Res. 2000;10(6):585–9.
20. Glass LF, Pepine ML, Fenske NA, Jaroszeski M, Reintgen DS, Heller R. Bleomycin-mediated electrochemotherapy of metastatic melanoma. Arch Dermatol. 1996;132(11):1353–7.
21. Heller R. Treatment of cutaneous nodules using electrochemotherapy. J Fla Med Assoc. 1995;82(2):147–50.
22. Heller R, Jaroszeski MJ, Glass LF, Messina JL, Rapaport DP, DeConti RC, et al. Phase I/II trial for the treatment of cutaneous and subcutaneous tumors using electrochemotherapy. Cancer. 1996;77(5):964–71.
23. Heller R, Jaroszeski MJ, Reintgen DS, Puleo CA, DeConti RC, Gilbert RA, et al. Treatment of cutaneous and subcutaneous tumors with electrochemotherapy using intralesional bleomycin. Cancer. 1998;83(1):148–57.
24. Rodriguez-Cuevas S, Barroso-Bravo S, Manza-Estrada J, Cristobal-Martinez L, Gonzalez-Rodriguez E. Electrochemotherapy in primary and metastatic skin tumors: phase II trial using intralesional bleomycin. Arch Med Res. 2001;32(4):273–6.
25. Rols MP, Bachaud JM, Giraud P, Chevreau C, Roche H, Teissie J. Electrochemotherapy of cutaneous metastases in malignant melanoma. Melanoma Res. 2000;10(5):468–74.
26. Byrne CM, Thompson JF, Johnston H, Hersey P, Quinn MJ, Michael HT, et al. Treatment of metastatic melanoma using electroporation therapy with bleomycin (electrochemotherapy). Melanoma Res. 2005;15(1):45–51.
27. Sersa G, Stabuc B, Cemazar M, Miklavcic D, Rudolf Z. Electrochemotherapy with cisplatin: clinical experience in malignant melanoma patients. Clin Cancer Res. 2000;6(3):863–7.

28. Glass LF, Fenske NA, Jaroszeski M, Perrott R, Harvey DT, Reintgen DS, et al. Bleomycin-mediated electrochemotherapy of basal cell carcinoma. J Am Acad Dermatol. 1996; 34(1):82–6.
29. Glass LF, Jaroszeski M, Gilbert R, Reintgen DS, Heller R. Intralesional bleomycin-mediated electrochemotherapy in 20 patients with basal cell carcinoma. J Am Acad Dermatol. 1997;37(4):596–9.
30. Allegretti JP, Panje WR. Electroporation therapy for head and neck cancer including carotid artery involvement. Laryngoscope. 2001;111(1):52–6.
31. Belehradek M, Domenge C, Luboinski B, Orlowski S, Belehradek Jr J, Mir LM. Electrochemotherapy, a new antitumor treatment. First clinical phase I-II trial. Cancer. 1993;72(12):3694–700.
32. Domenge C, Orlowski S, Luboinski B, De BT, Schwaab G, Belehradek Jr J, et al. Antitumor electrochemotherapy: new advances in the clinical protocol. Cancer. 1996;77(5):956–63.
33. Panje WR, Hier MP, Garman GR, Harrell E, Goldman A, Bloch I. Electroporation therapy of head and neck cancer. Ann Otol Rhinol Laryngol. 1998;107(9 Pt 1):779–85.
34. Burian M, Formanek M, Regele H. Electroporation therapy in head and neck cancer. Acta Otolaryngol. 2003;123(2):264–8.
35. Sersa G, Cufer T, Cemazar M, Rebersek M, Zvonimir R. Electrochemotherapy with bleomycin in the treatment of hypernephroma metastasis: case report and literature review. Tumori. 2000;86(2):163–5.
36. Sersa G, Stabuc B, Cemazar M, Jancar B, Miklavcic D, Rudolf Z. Electrochemotherapy with cisplatin: potentiation of local cisplatin antitumour effectiveness by application of electric pulses in cancer patients. Eur J Cancer. 1998;34(8):1213–8.
37. Kubota Y, Mir LM, Nakada T, Sasagawa I, Suzuki H, Aoyama N. Successful treatment of metastatic skin lesions with electrochemotherapy. J Urol. 1998;160(4):1426.
38. Curatolo P, Mancini M, Clerico R, Ruggiero A, Frascione P, Di MP, et al. Remission of extensive merkel cell carcinoma after electrochemotherapy. Arch Dermatol. 2009;145(4):494–5.
39. Mir LM, Gehl J, Sersa G, Collins CG, Garbay JR, Billard V, et al. Standard operating procedures of the electrochemotherapy: Instructions for the use of bleomycin or cisplatin administered either systemically or locally and electric pulses delivered by the Cliniporator™ by means of invasive or non-invasive electrodes. EJC Suppl. 2006;4(11):14–25.
40. Sersa G. The state-of-the-art of electrochemotherapy before the ESOPE study; advantages and clinical uses. EJC Suppl. 2006;4(11):52–9.
41. Marty M, Sersa G, Garbay JR, Gehl J, Collins CG, Snoj M, et al. Electrochemotherapy, An easy, highly effective and safe treatment of cutaneous and subcutaneous metastases: results of ESOPE (European Standard Operating Procedures of Electrochemotherapy) study. EJC Suppl. 2006;4(11):3–13.
42. Sersa G, Miklavcic D, Cemazar M, Rudolf Z, Pucihar G, Snoj M. Electrochemotherapy in treatment of tumours. Eur J Surg Oncol. 2008;34(2):232–40.
43. Campana LG, Mocellin S, Basso M, Puccetti O, De Salvo GL, Chiarion-Sileni V, et al. Bleomycin-based electrochemotherapy: clinical outcome from a single institution's experience with 52 patients. Ann Surg Oncol. 2009;16(1):191–9.
44. Quaglino P, Mortera C, Osella-Abate S, Barberis M, Illengo M, Rissone M, et al. Electrochemotherapy with intravenous bleomycin in the local treatment of skin melanoma metastases. Ann Surg Oncol. 2008;15(8):2215–22.
45. Rebersek M, Cufer T, Cemazar M, Kranjc S, Sersa G. Electrochemotherapy with cisplatin of cutaneous tumor lesions in breast cancer. Anticancer Drugs. 2004;15(6):593–7.
46. Larkin JO, Collins CG, Aarons S, Tangney M, Whelan M, O'Reily S, et al. Electrochemotherapy: aspects of preclinical development and early clinical experience. Ann Surg. 2007;245(3):469–79.
47. Fantini F, Gualdi G, Cimitan A, Giannetti A. Metastatic basal cell carcinoma with squamous differentiation: report of a case with response of cutaneous metastases to electrochemotherapy. Arch Dermatol. 2008;144(9):1186–8.
48. Curatolo P, Mancini M, Ruggiero A, Clerico R, Di MP, Calvieri S. Successful treatment of penile Kaposi's sarcoma with electrochemotherapy. Dermatol Surg. 2008;34(6):839–42.
49. Tijink BM, De BR, Van Dongen GA, Leemans CR. How we do it: chemo-electroporation in the head and neck for otherwise untreatable patients. Clin Otolaryngol. 2006; 31(5):447–51.
50. Snoj M, Cemazar M, Slekovec KB, Sersa G. Effective treatment of multiple unresectable skin melanoma metastases by electrochemotherapy. Croat Med J. 2007;48(3):391–5.
51. Testori A, Rutkowski P, Marsden J, Bastholt L, Chiarion-Sileni V, Hauschild A, et al. Surgery and radiotherapy in the treatment of cutaneous melanoma. Ann Oncol. 2009;20 Suppl 6:vi22–9.
52. Kubota Y, Tomita Y, Tsukigi M, Kurachi H, Motoyama T, Mir LM. A case of perineal malignant melanoma successfully treated with electrochemotherapy. Melanoma Res. 2005; 15(2):133–4.
53. Snoj M, Rudolf Z, Cemazar M, Jancar B, Sersa G. Successful sphincter-saving treatment of anorectal malignant melanoma with electrochemotherapy, local excision and adjuvant brachytherapy. Anticancer Drugs. 2005;16(3):345–8.

54. Shimizu T, Nikaido T, Gomyo H, Yoshimura Y, Horiuchi A, Isobe K, et al. Electrochemotherapy for digital chondrosarcoma. J Orthop Sci. 2003;8(2):248–51.
55. Snoj M, Cemazar M, Srnovrsnik T, Kosir SP, Sersa G. Limb sparing treatment of bleeding melanoma recurrence by electrochemotherapy. Tumori. 2009;95(3):398–402.
56. Zupanic A, Ribaric S, Miklavcic D. Increasing the repetition frequency of electric pulse delivery reduces unpleasant sensations that occur in electrochemotherapy. Neoplasma. 2007;54(3):246–50.
57. Miklavcic D, Beravs K, Semrov D, Cemazar M, Demsar F, Sersa G. The importance of electric field distribution for effective *in vivo* electroporation of tissues. Biophys J. 1998;74(5):2152–8.

Chapter 9
Electrochemotherapy for Larger Malignant Tumors

Louise W. Matthiessen, Tobian Muir, and Julie Gehl

Abstract Cutaneous metastases can present themselves in many ways and adversely affect self-esteem and body image. Management and palliative treatment of cutaneous metastases remain as clinically challenging problems. Electrochemotherapy as a palliative treatment for smaller metastases (size < 3 cm) is well investigated, whereas experience with electrochemotherapy for larger metastases (size >3 cm) mostly relies on case reports and small clinical studies.

The present chapter focuses on the knowledge obtained from case reports, clinical studies, and authors' experience. Tumor depth and the ability to cover the whole area, evaluation and benefit for the patient, repeated treatment, and penetration of the skin are some of the challenges that will be discussed.

In conclusion, electrochemotherapy for larger malignant tumors seems promising as a palliative treatment and could be a good supplement to surgery, but further investigation is needed in order to make evident indications and guidelines for such treatment.

Keywords Electrochemotherapy • Clinical • Metastases • Large tumors • Bleomycin

Introduction

Electrochemotherapy for small (less than 3 cm in diameter) cutaneous and subcutaneous metastases from different cancers is a proven, efficient, and well-documented palliative treatment, as described in Chap. 8. The efficacy and safety of electrochemotherapy in larger cutaneous metastases are much less well-documented. In the present chapter, we aim to shed light on this issue based on our own experience from an ongoing study with electrochemotherapy for chest wall recurrence of breast cancer as well as from case reports on other tumor types in various locations such as the limbs and trunk.

Cutaneous Metastases from Primary Cancer

Cutaneous metastases from solid primary tumors are uncommon, accounting for 0.7–9.0% with melanoma and breast cancer being the most common origin. The presence of a cutaneous metastasis

L.W. Matthiessen (✉)
Center for Experimental Drug and Gene Electrotransfer (C*EDGE), Department of Oncology, Copenhagen University Hospital Herlev, Herlev Ringvej 75, 2730 Herlev, Denmark
e-mail: lowima01@heh.regionh.dk

S.T. Kee et al. (eds.), *Clinical Aspects of Electroporation*,
DOI 10.1007/978-1-4419-8363-3_9, © Springer Science+Business Media, LLC 2011

is usually a grave prognostic sign [1]. Metastases to the skin are spread by either haematogenous spread, lymphatic spread, or direct extension from a primary tumor.

Cutaneous metastases can present themselves in many ways, from the fibrotic metastatic process characterized by diffuse morphea-like indurations of the skin, to multiple nodules or papules, or the ulcerated or fungating wounds that are associated with odor, exudate, and bleeding. They may adversely affect self-esteem and body image, thereby causing the patients to isolate themselves at a time when social support is needed. Treatment of these metastases is often a challenge for both the patient and the clinical caretakers. The main focus should be on controlling infection and odor, managing exudate, minimizing bleeding, protecting surrounding skin, reducing pain, and optimizing the emotional welfare of the patient.

Many non-traditional treatment approaches have been tried, for example, hyperthermia and cryotherapy; however, if surgery and radiotherapy are not options, there is no approach that has become standard treatment for cutaneous metastases in the oncological setting. In the ESOPE study (described in Chap. 8), good results were obtained when treating small cutaneous and subcutaneous metastases smaller than 3 cm with electrochemotherapy, with a complete response (CR) rate of 73% and a PR rate of 11% after a single treatment [2]. Treatment of larger cutaneous metastases with electrochemotherapy has mostly been reported in case studies and has not yet been subject to a systematic clinical investigation. Tumor depth and the ability to cover the tumor area, evaluation and benefit for the patient, retreatment, and penetration of the skin are problems that need to be addressed when applying electrochemotherapy for large nodules.

Clinical Studies of Electrochemotherapy for Larger Cutaneous Metastases

Previous Studies

One of the first reports on treatment of larger cutaneous metastases came from Domenge et al. [3]. Seven patients with either head and neck cancer or breast carcinoma were treated. The lesion sizes ranged from 1.0 × 1.0 to 8.0 × 20.0 cm, and cutaneous infiltration with permeation was seen in some of the lesions. All lesions were treated with plate electrodes, and partial, but no complete, responses were observed. Pulses could safely be delivered more than 100 times in a single treatment, and retreatment was administrated safely up to three times. Since 1996, there have been reports of successful treatment of large head and neck skin metastases [4], breast cancer recurrence [5], Kaposi Sarcoma [6], malignant melanoma [7], and Merkel Cell tumor [8].

Larkin et al. [9] treated cutaneous metastases from different primary tumors in 30 patients with electrochemotherapy. Metastases larger than 3 cm were found to be less likely to respond than smaller ones, having an objective response (OR) rate of 38% (8 of 21) compared to a total OR rate of 82%.

Campana et al. [10] treated 208 cutaneous metastases from different primary tumors in 52 patients in a nonrandomized clinical phase II trial. Of the 208 nodules, 55 were larger than 3 cm (up to 5.7 cm in diameter) and 1 was a confluent mass of small metastases. The researchers noticed an inverse correlation between CR and the maximum diameter of the target lesion. The response rates were 28% for lesions larger than 3 cm and 66% for those smaller than 1.5 cm. The larger nodules presented more problems with penetration of the skin and had lower response rates than seen in the treatment of smaller nodules.

Quaglino et al. [11] likewise observed the inverse correlation between response rate and size of the metastases. Although all treated nodules were below 3 cm in diameter, tumors less than 1 cm^2 had an OR rate of 99% in contrast to those larger than 1 cm^2 (83%). The differences in response rate were even higher when CR rates were compared: 72% in metastases smaller than 1 cm^2 versus 28% in metastases larger than 1 cm^2.

Experience from Ongoing Studies

In ongoing (as of 2009) trials at the Department of Oncology, Copenhagen University Hospital, Herlev, Denmark, we have experience with treating larger cutaneous metastases from different primary tumors.

With tumors larger than 10 cm in diameter, it can be difficult to treat the whole area in one session, and also, depending on the depth of the tumor, it can be difficult to reach the bottom of the tumor during the first treatment round (Fig. 9.1).

Ulcerated metastases have responded well to electrochemotherapy (Fig. 9.2). Although it was not possible to cover the whole of the metastasis areas, most patients obtained good symptomatic relief with less odor and exudate after one treatment. This can be due to both the easy penetration of the needles in the ulcerated area and the immediate antivascular effect of electrochemotherapy, which stops the exudate and bleeding [12–14].

Some issues pertaining to electrochemotherapy of larger cutaneous metastases are presented in the following sections.

Repeated Treatments

Retreatment may be performed in order to sequentially reduce the tumor mass from the top down. When the metastases are deep, it is not possible to reach the inner portion of the tumor tissue, and therefore only partial responses (PRs) have been obtained. The part of the tumor that is not reached in the first treatment may progress between treatments. In order to avoid extensive progression, plans for retreatment must be made on an individual basis.

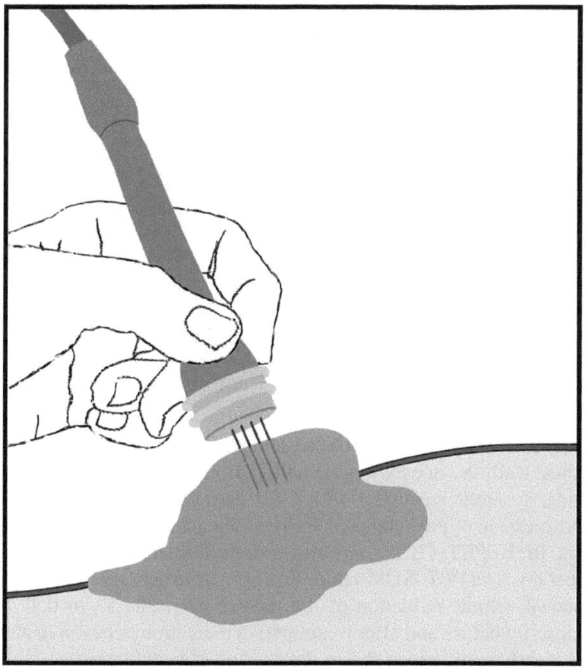

Fig. 9.1 This figure illustrates how the inner portion of a large tumor can be difficult to reach with needle electrodes during the first treatment round. If tumor mass is reduced in the first treatment, deeper parts of the tumor can be reached when treatment is repeated

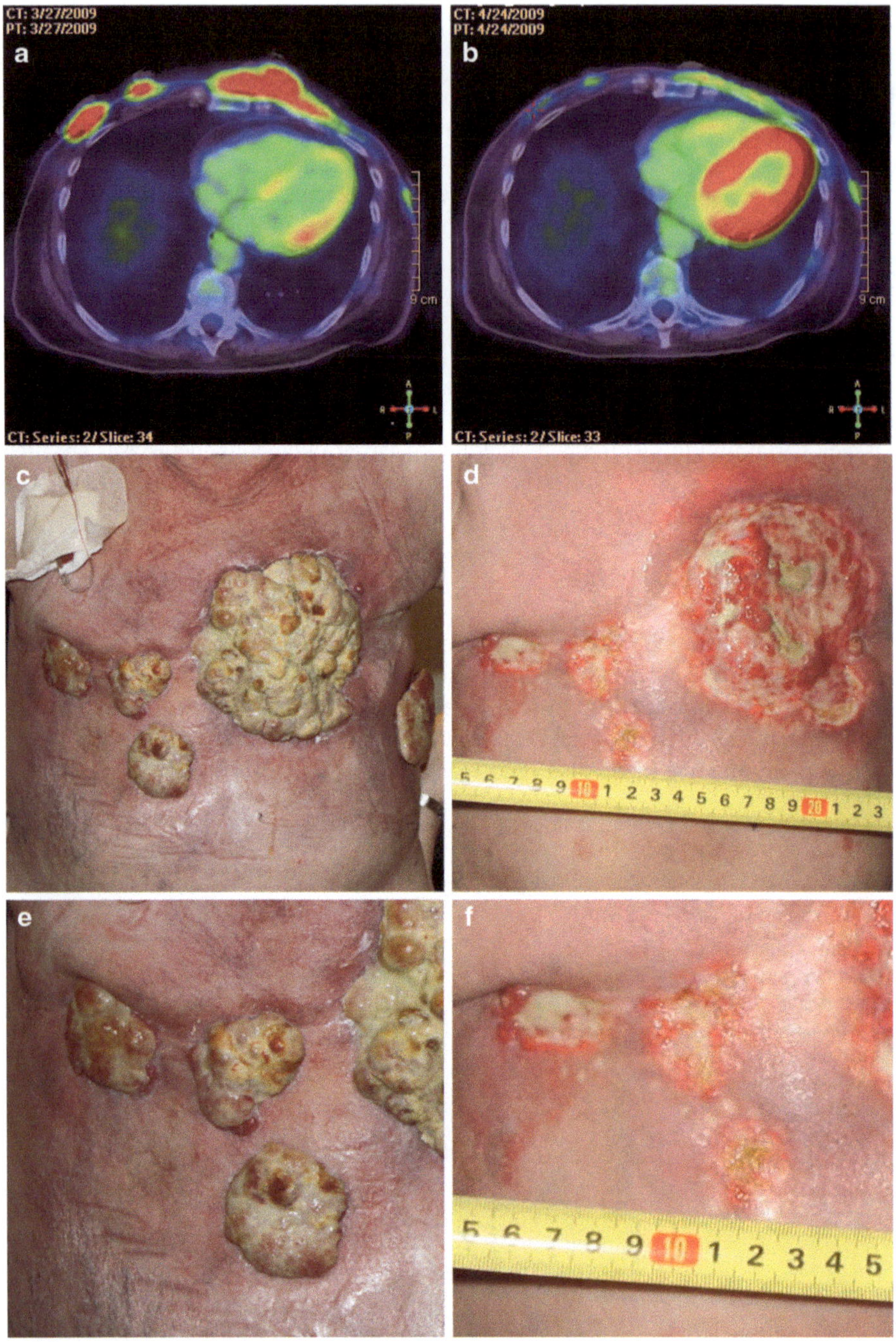

Fig. 9.2 Sixty-four-year-old patient with bilateral receptor-negative, HER2-negative breast cancer recurrence on the chest wall. Previously treated with radiotherapy 2 Gy × 24 in both sides and reirradiated with 3 Gy × 10 on the left side, systemic treatment with CEF, Taxotere, Gemcitabine, Vinorelbine, and Xeloda, but despite that continuous progression of the cutaneous lesions. The patient was treated two times with electrochemotherapy in general anesthesia. (**a**, **b**) PET–CT scan of lesions before treatment (**a**) and 1 month after second treatment (**b**) with electrochemotherapy. The PET–SUV values decrease from average 10.7 to an average of 2.9 indicating less tumor activity. CT scan shows volume reduction of the tumors from 287.58 to 0.47 cm^3. (**c**) Before treatment, (**d**) after treatment, (**e**, **f**) close-up before and after treatment; demarcation between healthy skin (with needle marks) and necrotic tumor tissue is clearly seen, which shows the sparing of healthy tissue

Necrotic Tissue

Necrosis is often observed after treatment of large metastases with electrochemotherapy and can be the cause of malicious odor, probably due to anaerobic bacterial colonization. Patients should be affiliated to local caretaker units that are used to manage malignant wounds and debridement as well as cleansing, according to the patients needs. If necessary, surgical debridement can be performed. In our experience, this has been applied successfully in cases where retreatment could be provided in an operating theater. Prior to retreatment, the necrotic tissue having arisen from the previous treatment is surgically debrided to allow for better wound management and more effective treatment of residual tumor tissue.

Skin Penetration

Previously irradiated or tumor-invaded skin that is fibrotic can be difficult to penetrate with commercially available needle electrodes, both in our own and others' experience [10]. It is necessary to penetrate the skin in order to obtain a sufficient electric field strength that will reach the deepest part of the tumor or at least as deep as possible. We have attempted to use one application followed by another in the exact same spot in order to overcome the skin barrier, but have only had moderate success. Combination with surgery can also be attempted. It should be kept in mind that electrochemotherapy to areas where the skin is not yet ulcerated will accelerate ulceration and necrosis of the skin [3], which can make it easier to retreat the area but will not necessarily give the patient symptomatic relief.

Vital Structures

Cutaneous and subcutaneous tumors can be located close to vital structures such as large vessels and nerves and even surround these structures. Experience with electrochemotherapy close to such structures is sparse. Ultrasound guidance can help to avoid perforation of vital structures, but treatment to metastases surrounding these structures cannot be recommended with needle electrodes. Use of plate electrodes can carefully be attempted.

Combination with Other Treatment Modalities

For selected patients with large tumors having a narrow pedunculated base, we have opted to surgically resect the tumor with a narrow margin to allow primary closure of the defect. The wound is then treated with a safety margin with electrochemotherapy and closed with sutures thereafter. This approach needs further investigation and follow-up but has the potential of successfully getting rid of tumor volume and concentrating the electrochemotherapy treatment to the tumor base.

As in the primary management of large volume disease, it is clear that in patients with large metastases, a combination approach of electrochemotherapy, surgery, chemotherapy, and other modalities such as isolated limb infusion and perfusion will increase the likelihood of tumor control.

The intriguing possibility of the use of electrochemotherapy to induce tumor necrosis with a lower recurrence rate brings about the potential possibility of reducing tumor volume, which can then be followed by surgery or chemotherapy in a neo-adjuvant type model.

Pain Management

Pain after treatment is normally not described as a problem and can be controlled with mild pain-killers. In our experience, some patients developed neuralgia-like pain sensations after treatment, which has been difficult to control. Expertise in pain management has been necessary in such cases. The pain could be due to irritated nerve ends, and further investigation is needed to clarify this matter.

Guidelines

Before Treatment

Treatment of patients with cutaneous or subcutaneous metastases from primary tumors is palliative and an understanding of the palliative goals in the care of such patients is essential in developing a treatment plan aimed toward decreasing the effect that these lesions have on the patient's quality of life. Some patients are desperate and will push for treatment, and it is the physician's job to assess if the patient will benefit from the treatment and exclude those patients who will not.

Some patients are in antineoplastic treatment when the need for electrochemotherapy arises. The antineoplastic treatment can either continue or be paused while receiving electrochemotherapy, depending on toxicity and interference with anesthesia, as well as expected degree of neutropenia in light of the infection risk.

Treatment

ESOPE Guidelines

The ESOPE guidelines, although developed for use in treatment of small nodules, can also be used for treating larger cutaneous or subcutaneous metastases. For details on the ESOPE guidelines, please refer to Chap. 8. Specifics pertaining to the treatment of larger tumors will be discussed in the following sections.

Chemotherapy

When treating larger metastases that may be a confluent mass or without sharp demarcation, it is preferable to use intravenous (i.v.) injection in order to obtain sufficiently high drug concentrations in the whole tumor. Bleomycin is therefore the drug of choice, since cisplatin can only be administered intratumorally, and the dosage used is in accordance with the ESOPE guidelines.

Bleomycin has low myelotoxicity but can induce lung fibrosis. Lung fibrosis occurs sporadically at doses between 100,000 and 450,000 International Units [one unit (1 U) contains 0.56–0.66 mg of bleomycin and is equivalent to 1,000 international units (1000 IU)] [15].

Single-breath carbon monoxide diffusing capacity test (DLCO) can be performed if the patient has a history of lung disease or if retreatment is expected. According to guidelines for testicular cancer and Hodgkin's disease, treatment with bleomycin should be discontinued if a linear fall in DLCO of more than 25% compared to the baseline value before bleomycin treatment or other signs that indicate pulmonary toxicity are observed [16, 17]. Bleomycin dose should be reduced in patients with reduced renal function and the cumulative dose should be adjusted to age [15].

Oxygen exposure is a potential risk factor for the development of bleomycin-induced lung damage [18]; it is therefore recommended that the patient should not be exposed to oxygen concentrations in the inspired air (FiO_2) higher than 25–30% [19]. Delivery of bleomycin should not be given during induction of anesthesia as the high oxygen concentrations used for the intubation procedure may increase the risk of inducing lung damage.

Electrodes and Pulse Delivery

Commercially available electrode devices come as either plate or needle electrodes. If not completely superficial, a tumor should be treated with needle electrodes in order to ensure penetration of the tumor tissue and as deep reaching a treatment as possible. Ultrasound guidance can be used if the treatment is to take place close to vital structures. More than one electrode type can be used for the same treatment in order to provide the best coverage with as little damage to healthy tissue as possible.

Multiple applications can safely be applied in one treatment session [3], and our own experience is that more than 100 applications of pulse delivery can easily be used. The main limitation on the number of pulses that can be applied is a 20-min window for treatment [20]. This is based on experience from a single study [3]. In this study, it was found that nodules treated sooner than 8 min or later than 28 min after bleomycin administration had a lower response rate. The study was very small and has not been repeated. However, since a certain time for tissue distribution of bleomycin is to be expected, the 8 min dogma has stuck. In addition, the elimination of bleomycin happens in two phases, of which one takes approximately 24–30 min [15]. Therefore, a 28-min time limit is assumed to be reasonable, but further exploration may prove that a longer window for treatment exists.

Anesthesia

Depending on the size, location, and shape of the tumor, anesthesia can be given as local or general anesthesia. Local anesthesia is preferable for the patient if the tumor is well demarcated and superficial. When multiple applications are needed in order to cover the tumor metastases, demarcation is vague, or the tumor is close to structures where treatment will be painful (e.g., bone), it is preferable to have the patient fully anesthetized (Fig. 9.3). This allows for many applications of electric pulses, and as pulses may be applied quickly, the window of 20 min may be sufficient to treat a large volume.

Dressing

After treatment, the wound should be covered if ulcerated. Nonadherent dressings should be applied for the primary contact layer, since this will allow for atraumatic dressing removal. Dressings that absorb exudate can be placed on top of that. Depending on the wound, different dressing choices can be made (see next section).

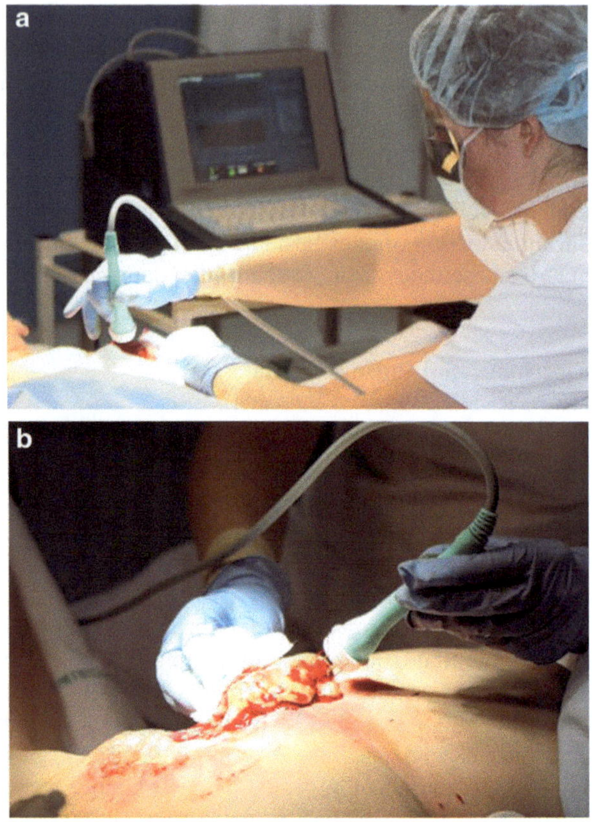

Fig. 9.3 Example of treatment with electrochemotherapy in general anesthesia to a patient with chest wall recurrence of breast cancer. Bleomycin is given intravenously before the electric pulses are applied. Electric pulses are administered using a square wave electroporator (**a**). Eight pulses at a frequency of 5 kHz are used for each application and the needle electrode is placed multiple times until the entire tumor is covered (**b**)

After Treatment

Management of the Treated Area

A patient being treated for large volume ulcerated cancer lesions requires specialized care. The patient should be affiliated to a caretaking unit that can manage wounds. Necrotic tissue should be removed using autolytic and/or gentle mechanical methods or sharp debridement by a trained clinician [21].

Dressings should be changed depending on the exudation and odor; normally every second day, but more often if wounds are malodorous and highly exudative. Nonadherent contact layers can be used to prevent adherence and bleeding when removing it. Topical metronidazole, charcoal dressings, and silver-based dressings can be used to prevent odor and colonization of anaerobic bacteria. Concealing and collecting dressings can be placed on top in order to avoid drainage on clothing or bedding.

If anaerobic colonization arises locally, there can be problems with loathsome odor. In that case, topical cleansing, debridement, and treatment with a local antibacterial agent (e.g., metronidazole gel) can be performed. Systemic antibacterial treatment should be reserved for systemic infections.

Pain should be controlled with either local or systemic painkillers. Topical application of lidocaine, benzocaine, or opioids can help improve pain control [21].

Evaluation

Electrochemotherapy is evaluated by measuring the longest and the second longest diameter of the lesion. The response is evaluated using the RECIST criteria [22] and documented with photography; however, large cutaneous metastases are frequently a confluent mass of tumor tissue with varying depth and chronic ulceration/fungation making the conventional evaluation methods difficult to apply. Therefore, new methods for evaluation of electrochemotherapy given to larger tumors are to be investigated. In our unit, we are currently investigating combined positron emission tomography (PET) and computed tomography (CT) scans as a tool for documentation of response in such tumors and as a tool to help determine the optimal time for retreatment (Fig. 9.2a, b).

Patient Satisfaction

In order for electrochemotherapy to be justifiable as a palliative treatment, the patient should experience rapid relief from symptoms and also be satisfied with the treatment.

In a study by Campana et al. [10], 36 of 52 patients completed questionnaires for evaluation of perception. Overall, 34 of the 36 patients were satisfied, 1 uncertain, and 1 dissatisfied, and in the ESOPE study [2], 93% of patients reported that they would opt for another treatment should this be indicated. When treating larger nodules, the same CR rate cannot be expected as in the ESOPE study and the study from Campana et al., but patients may still benefit due to a reduction in bleeding, oozing, and progression. Further studies are needed to elucidate this issue.

Retreatment

If only a PR is obtained or new lesions arise, retreatment can be safely administrated. Responses have been observed in metastases that did not respond when treated the first time [9], and deeper parts of the metastases can usually be reached in a second session.

There are reports of retreatment safely administrated up to 6 times [6] but the recommended cumulative dose of bleomycin should not be exceeded, and DLCO may be performed in order to ensure that bleomycin-induced toxicity is not developing.

The optimal time for retreatment is not known, but bleomycin should not be administrated i.v. more than once a week [20], and the patient should be systemically fit for another treatment session under general anesthesia before retreatment is provided. On the other hand, the time period between treatment sessions should not be too long if only a PR is obtained in the first session, because regrowth of the metastases may occur.

Summary of Treatment for Larger Cutaneous Metastases

Electrochemotherapy for cutaneous metastases larger than 3 cm is not as well investigated as electrochemotherapy for metastases smaller than 3 cm. However, some points in the treatment of large metastases evidently differ from the treatment of small metastases:

- Multiple applications are often necessary in order to treat as large a volume as possible. General anesthesia is preferred because it allows the physician to carry out the treatment undisturbed by the patient and therefore to work faster. Furthermore, local anesthesia can be difficult to obtain in a larger area.

- I.v. injection of bleomycin will be the choice of chemotherapy administration in most cases, as it will ensure better distribution of the drug in the metastases to be treated. Also, if a large tumor volume needs to be treated, the amount of bleomycin needed for local injection may sum up to what equates to an i.v. dose of bleomycin, anyway.
- Before treatment, it is important to consider what can be achieved. The goal is palliation, and the benefit for the patient should always be weighed against the costs to the patient, especially in case of thick fibrotic skin that is hard to penetrate, where there is a risk of inducing morbidity to the patient due to subsequent ulceration and necrosis.
- There are cases where electrochemotherapy is not the treatment of choice, for example, deep tumors close to or surrounding vital structures, or if there is no palliative need. Other treatment opportunities must be considered in these cases.
- A multidisciplinary caretaker team should be available for the patient, when larger cutaneous metastases are treated with electrochemotherapy, for the purpose of managing wound dressings as well as for cleansing, surgical debridement, and infection and pain management.
- Surgical debridement of necrotic tumor can be considered prior to further treatment in order to increase wound control and target retreatment to residual tumor tissue.
- Retreatment is often necessary and can be safely administered if the recommended cumulative dose of bleomycin is not exceeded and there are no signs of bleomycin-induced lung toxicity. The optimal time for retreatment is not defined but can be decided on an individual basis.

Conclusion

Electrochemotherapy for larger cutaneous metastases can offer symptomatic relief for patients in the palliative setting; however, the benefit should always be weighed against any disproportionate burdens to the patient.

The high CR rates seen in the treatment of smaller cutaneous and subcutaneous metastases cannot be expected when treating larger metastases, but the clinician should not hesitate to use electrochemotherapy for larger cutaneous metastases if it will improve the quality of life for patients with a malignant wound. Electrochemotherapy that achieves only a PR may still alleviate symptoms and improve the well-being of the patient. In particular, patients may benefit from decreased secretion or hemorrhage from the cancerous wound.

Further investigation is needed to address some of the problems associated with electrochemotherapy for larger metastases: (1) How to reach the inner portion of metastases with varying depth and close proximity of vital structures; (2) penetration of fibrotic, thick skin; and (3) the role of surgical tumor debulking prior to electrochemotherapy as well as the potential of post-electrochemotherapy application of further surgery or chemotherapy if a significant reduction in tumor volume can be achieved.

References

1. Rolz-Cruz G, Kim CC. Tumor invasion of the skin. Dermatol Clin 2008;26(1):89–102, viii.
2. Marty M, Sersa G, Garbay JR, Gehl J, Collins CG, Snoj M, et al. Electrochemotherapy, an easy, highly effective and safe treatment of cutaneous and subcutaneous metastases: results of ESOPE (European Standard Operating Procedures of Electrochemotherapy) study. EJC Suppl. 2006;4(11):3–13.
3. Domenge C, Orlowski S, Luboinski B, De BT, Schwaab G, Belehradek Jr J, et al. Antitumor electrochemotherapy: new advances in the clinical protocol. Cancer. 1996;77(5):956–63.
4. Rols MP, Bachaud JM, Giraud P, Chevreau C, Roche H, Teissie J. Electrochemotherapy of cutaneous metastases in malignant melanoma. Melanoma Res. 2000;10(5):468–74.

5. Whelan MC, Larkin JO, Collins CG, Cashman J, Breathnach O, Soden DM, et al. Effective treatment of an extensive recurrent breast cancer which was refractory to multimodal therapy by multiple applications of electrochemotherapy. EJC Suppl. 2006;4(11):32–4.
6. Garbay JR, Billard V, Bernat C, Mir LM, Morsli N, Robert C. Successful repetitive treatments by electrochemotherapy of multiple unresectable Kaposi sarcoma nodules. EJC Suppl. 2006;4(11):29–31.
7. Byrne CM, Thompson JF, Johnston H, Hersey P, Quinn MJ, Michael HT, et al. Treatment of metastatic melanoma using electroporation therapy with bleomycin (electrochemotherapy). Melanoma Res. 2005;15(1):45–51.
8. Curatolo P, Mancini M, Clerico R, Ruggiero A, Frascione P, Di Marco P, et al. Remission of extensive merkel cell carcinoma after electrochemotherapy. Arch Dermatol. 2009;145(4):494–5.
9. Larkin JO, Collins CG, Aarons S, Tangney M, Whelan M, O'Reily S, et al. Electrochemotherapy: aspects of preclinical development and early clinical experience. Ann Surg. 2007;245(3):469–79.
10. Campana LG, Mocellin S, Basso M, Puccetti O, De Salvo GL, Chiarion-Sileni V, et al. Bleomycin-based electrochemotherapy: clinical outcome from a single institution's experience with 52 patients. Ann Surg Oncol. 2009;16(1):191–9.
11. Quaglino P, Mortera C, Osella-Abate S, Barberis M, Illengo M, Rissone M, et al. Electrochemotherapy with intravenous bleomycin in the local treatment of skin melanoma metastases. Ann Surg Oncol. 2008;15(8):2215–22.
12. Gehl J, Geertsen PF. Efficient palliation of haemorrhaging malignant melanoma skin metastases by electrochemotherapy. Melanoma Res. 2000;10(6):585–9.
13. Gehl J, Geertsen PF. Palliation of haemorrhaging and ulcerated cutaneous tumours using electrochemotherapy. EJC Suppl. 2006;4(11):35–7.
14. Sersa G, Cemazar M, Miklavcic D, Chaplin DJ. Tumor blood flow modifying effect of electrochemotherapy with bleomycin. Anticancer Res. 1999;19(5B):4017–22.
15. Gothelf A, Mir LM, Gehl J. Electrochemotherapy: results of cancer treatment using enhanced delivery of bleomycin by electroporation. Cancer Treat Rev. 2003;29(5):371–87.
16. Perez-Guerra F, Harkleroad LE, Walsh RE, Costanzi JJ. Acute bleomycin lung. Am Rev Respir Dis. 1972;106(6):909–13.
17. Comis RL, Kuppinger MS, Ginsberg SJ, Crooke ST, Gilbert R, Auchincloss JH, et al. Role of single-breath carbon monoxide-diffusing capacity in monitoring the pulmonary effects of bleomycin in germ cell tumor patients. Cancer Res. 1979;39(12):5076–80.
18. Goldiner PL, Schweizer O. The hazards of anesthesia and surgery in bleomycin-treated patients. Semin Oncol. 1979;6(1):121–4.
19. Mathes DD. Bleomycin and hyperoxia exposure in the operating room. Anesth Analg. 1995;81(3):624–9.
20. Mir LM, Gehl J, Sersa G, Collins CG, Garbay JR, Billard V, et al. Standard operating procedures of the electrochemotherapy: Instructions for the use of bleomycin or cisplatin administered either systemically or locally and electric pulses delivered by the Cliniporator™ by means of invasive or non-invasive electrodes. EJC Suppl. 2006;4(11):14–25.
21. Seaman S. Management of malignant fungating wounds in advanced cancer. Semin Oncol Nurs. 2006;22(3):185–93.
22. Eisenhauer EA, Therasse P, Bogaerts J, Schwartz LH, Sargent D, Ford R, et al. New response evaluation criteria in solid tumours: revised RECIST guideline (version 1.1). Eur J Cancer. 2009;45(2):228–47.

Chapter 10
Cell Electroporation in Bone Tissue

Milena Fini, Matilde Tschon, Marco Alberghini, Giuseppe Bianchi, Mario Mercuri, Laura Campanacci, Francesco Cavani, Mattia Ronchetti, Francesca de Terlizzi, and Ruggero Cadossi

Abstract Electroporation in the cell membrane occurs following exposure to a high-intensity electric field. Electroporation can be used to introduce large molecules into the cell or to induce cell apoptosis by the application of the electric field alone, provided that the cell damage is such that it cannot be recovered. Electroporation use in clinical practice is standardized in association with drugs, electrochemotherapy, for the treatment of cutaneous and subcutaneous tumor nodules. Effective tumor ablation requires complete membrane electroporation of all malignant cells to allow drug diffusion into the cytoplasm. We investigated the impact of the presence of bone trabeculae on electric field effect and whether the mineralized component of the bone prevented the use of electroporation to eradicate tumor cells in bone tissue. We evaluated the possibility of efficiently performing electroporation of osteoblasts and osteocytes, as well as of cells interspersed among bone trabeculae. On healthy rabbits, the effect of electroporation on the distal femoral epiphysis, an area of high osteogenetic activity, was investigated by histological and functional analysis. In bone tissue, complete cell ablation by electroporation was achieved when the absorbed energy dose in the tissue exceeded 3,500 J/Kg. This threshold value was reached with all electric fields tested by increasing the number of pulses delivered. The results of the preclinical investigation set the rationale for the use of electrochemotherapy in patients with bone metastases. Preliminary experience with the use of electrochemotherapy for bone metastases in patients will be discussed.

Keywords Electroporation • Electrochemotherapy • Bone • Osteoblasts • Bone metastasis

Introduction

Primary bone tumors are rare (less than 1% of all malignant tumors with 2,400 new cases in Europe per year) and are mostly found in young men. However, bone metastases are a frequent complication of many primary cancers including breast, prostate, lung, kidney, and thyroid. In Europe, the number of new cases of bone metastases per year is about 1,100,000.

Bone cancers greatly impacts patients' quality of life due to associated symptoms such as pain, pathological fractures, spinal cord compression, hypercalcemia, and reduction of movement and performance status.

Standard treatment of bone metastases includes radiotherapy and rarely surgery. Surgical excision is generally reserved for smaller or more accessible lesions. Radiofrequency thermal ablation

R. Cadossi (✉)
Laboratory of Clinical Biophysics, IGEA, 41012 Carpi, Italy
e-mail: r.cadossi@igea.it

S. Kee et al. (eds.), *Clinical Aspects of Electroporation*,
DOI 10.1007/978-1-4419-8363-3_10, © Springer Science+Business Media, LLC 2011

(RFA) has also been used; however, there are concerns that heat dissipation is associated to connective and vascular structure degeneration [1, 2]. Furthermore, when RFA is applied to bone tissue, it leaves the trabecular structure brittle and not mechanically competent. Cryosurgery is particularly time consuming, requires multiple probes, and has a number of side effects. Furthermore, all therapies have to be weighed against the need to obtain radical margins that cannot always be achieved because of the presence of structures (vessels, nerves) that must be preserved. This is particularly relevant for vertebral body metastasis, especially when the posterior lamina is involved, due to its proximity to the spinal cord.

Electrochemotherapy has proven effective in the treatment of metastases from solid tumors located in the skin or subcutaneous tissue. The ESOPE trial (see Chap. 8) demonstrated that electrochemotherapy can obtain 74% complete response and 85% objective response of treated tumor nodules [3, 4]. Since the publication of the Operating Standard Procedures, the electrochemotherapy technology has been disseminated and is already successfully used in more than 60 hospitals in the EU for cutaneous and subcutaneous tumor nodule treatment. Furthermore, long-term histological results show that after nodule complete response to electrochemotherapy, no tumor cells are locally detected [5].

On the basis of the high efficacy of electrochemotherapy [6–11], clinicians and researchers are developing strategies to extend the use of electrochemotherapy to the treatment of visceral and deep-seated tumors. Electroporation combined with methotrexate has been employed with success in tumor-bearing mice with implanted osteosarcoma cells [12]. Electrochemotherapy for bone metastasis ablation is certainly appealing because of its efficiency and lack of structural damage to the tissue. For example, electrical pulses applied to meninges covering the spinal cord did not cause structure denaturation at the transmission electron microscopy analysis (Fig. 10.1).

Electrochemotherapy efficacy requires that all cells in the target volume are exposed to an electric field strength sufficient to cause pore formation [13]. The presence of bone trabeculae may have an impact on the electric field distribution and prevent the use of electrochemotherapy to eradicate

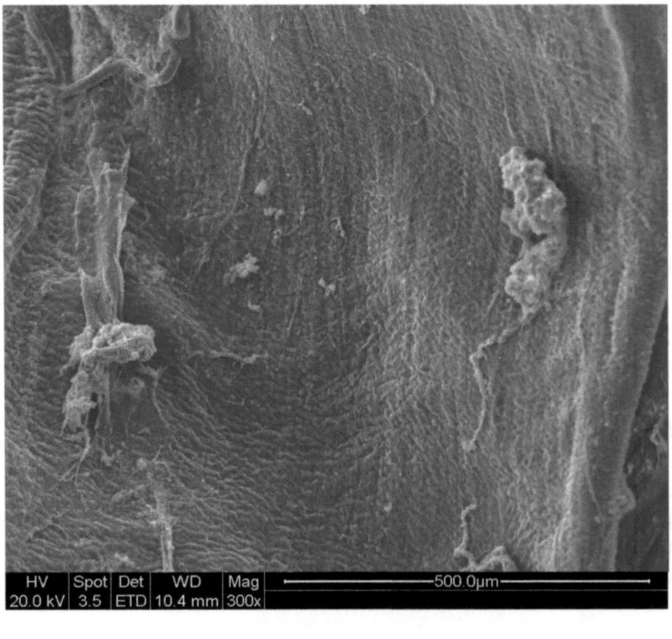

Fig. 10.1 Transmission electron microscopy image of electroporated spinal cord meninges, no collagen denaturation or structural damage are observed

tumor cells inside and among trabeculae. To the best of the authors' knowledge, the possibility of safely and effectively electroporating bone tissue has never been studied in depth. In rabbits, we have investigated the possibility of effectively electroporating osteoblasts and osteocytes as well as cells interspersed among bone trabeculae.

Employing an in vivo animal model of healthy rabbit, the effects of electroporation on femoral distal epiphysis, an area of high osteogenetic activity, were investigated by histological and functional analysis. Healthy animals were used to assess the effect of electroporation on bone tissue in a model representative of the heterogeneities of human bone tissue. In small animals with bone tumors, the tumor tissue will usually dominate to the extent that treating such an area will similar to treating a deep-seated soft tissue tumor. For the purpose of this initial study, electroporation was therefore performed on healthy bone tissue.

We attempted to:

- Develop a reproducible technique to introduce electrodes into the target bone tissue.
- Identify the electroporation protocols (voltage applied and numbers of pulses) sufficient to ablate all bone cells in the target area.
- Investigate biological activity in the electroporation area 30 days after complete cell ablation.
- Test the mechanical competence of mineralized bone trabeculae after electroporation.

If analyses were to show that the bone tissue was able to withstand and eventually recover following the electroporation procedures used in this study, with parameters aimed at inducing irreversible electroporation (see Chaps. 19–21), it would be reasonable to assume that parameters for reversible electroporation could safely be used in applications to bone tissue in patients. Thus, the information gathered during this preclinical study would set the basis to extend electrochemotherapy to the treatment of bone metastasis in clinical settings.

Electric Pulse Delivery to Bone Tissue

According to a protocol approved by the Institutional Review Board and strictly following Italian Laws on animal experiments, adult male rabbits were used. The distal femur condyles were exposed, and using a plexiglass guide, four holes were drilled across the bone to allow the insertion of four stainless steel electrodes (0.7 mm diameter) separated by 4 mm. After electric pulse delivery, the electrodes were cut flush to the cortical bone surface and left in place until sacrifice, to allow exact identification of the treated area (Fig. 10.2a, b).

Animals were sacrificed either 7 or 30 days after electroporation by pharmacological euthanasia. The femoral condyles were recovered and sectioned. Half of each sample was embedded in polymethylmethacrylate, microradiographed, and evaluated under fluorescent light, methylmethacrylate embedded sections were further processed and stained with toluidine blue and fast green for histological analysis; the other half was decalcified and stained with haematoxylin and eosin (H&E) for histological analysis (Fig. 10.2b–d).

A custom tissue electroporation device derived from the Cliniporator™ (see Chap. 5) was employed. Electric pulses were delivered between two electrodes at a time in the six possible combinations: four sides and two diagonals (Fig. 10.3a).

Square-wave 100-μs pulses at 4 Hz were applied (Fig. 10.3b). The voltage applied is expressed in V/mm, and the actual electric field applied to the electrodes was adjusted for the electrode separation. For example, the electric field applied between electrodes was 700 V/4 mm and 1,000 V/5.7 mm (square diagonal). This yielded a nominal electric field of 1,750 V/cm. In addition to 1,750, 1,300 and 1,000 V/cm were also used. In the different electroporation protocols tested, the number of pulses varied from a minimum of 50 up to 240 pulses per electrode couple.

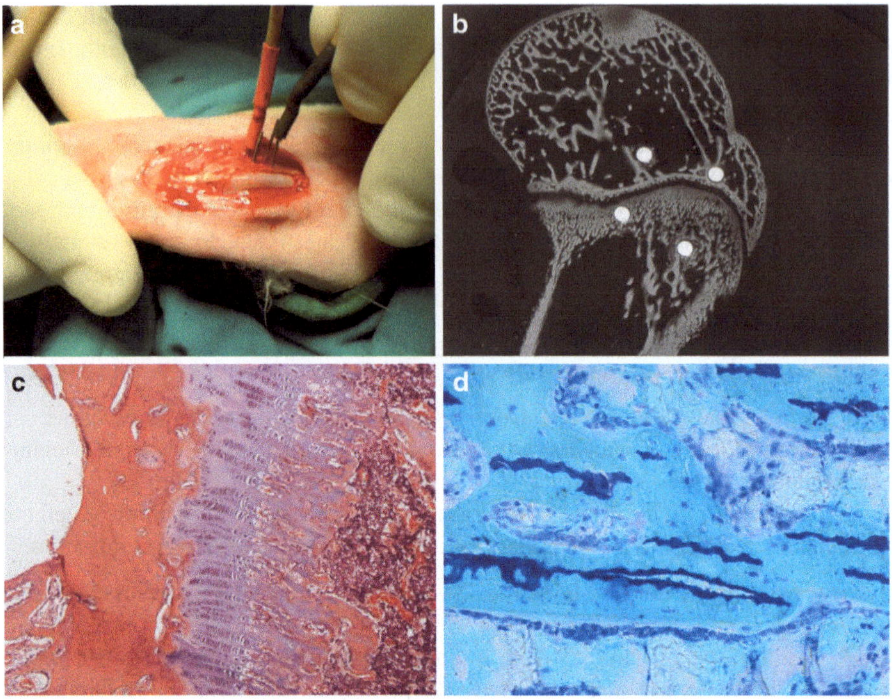

Fig. 10.2 (**a**) Electrode insertion and connection to the pulse generator; (**b**) microradiograph of the distal epiphysis of the femur with the four electrodes left inside; bone structure is maintained; (**c**) histology (H&E staining) of the bone tissue after electrode insertion; cartilage and bone tissue appear normal; (**d**) toluidine blue staining of the trabeculae showing the osteoblast aligned on the surface

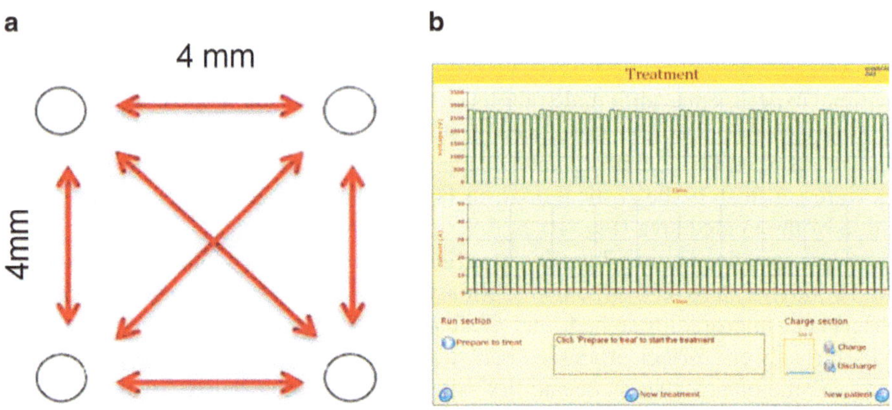

Fig. 10.3 (**a**) Combinations among the electrodes during pulse delivery; (**b**) shape of electric pulses; *top*: voltage applied, *bottom*: measure of the electrical current flowing between two electrodes

Effect of Electroporation on Osteoblast Activity

Osteoblasts are located on the trabeculae surface and are responsible for new bone deposition. Their activity can be monitored by means of tetracycline that is incorporated within the new bone (osteoid) matrix, fluoresces when exposed to UV light microscopy, and stains yellow in new bone. Oxytetracycline 30 mg/kg was injected i.m. on the second and third day after surgery in animals sacrificed on day 7, and the 27th and 28th day after surgery in animals sacrificed on day 30. To investigate bone fluorescence and, indirectly, the metabolic activity of osteoblasts, the lateral condyles were processed undecalcified and embedded in polymethylmethacrylate. Seven days after electroporation, tetracycline incorporation between the four electrodes was completely absent at electric field values applied (1,000, 1,300, and 1,750 V/cm) when at least 240, 180, and 80 pulses were delivered to all couples of the four electrodes, respectively (Figs. 10.4 and 10.5).

The same analysis was performed in animals sacrificed 30 days after electroporation and with tetracycline injected 2 and 3 days before sacrifice. A strong vital reaction was present in the area around/between the electrodes, with intense fluorescence and osteoblast activity on the trabeculae surface with new bone formation, suggestive that the bony cells ablated by electroporation recovered by 30 days (Fig. 10.6).

Histology of Electroporated Bone and Cartilage

Polymethylmethacrylate-embedded femur blocks were further cut to 5-μm thick sections before toluidine blue and fast green staining, and the presence of osteoblasts on trabeculae surface was investigated.

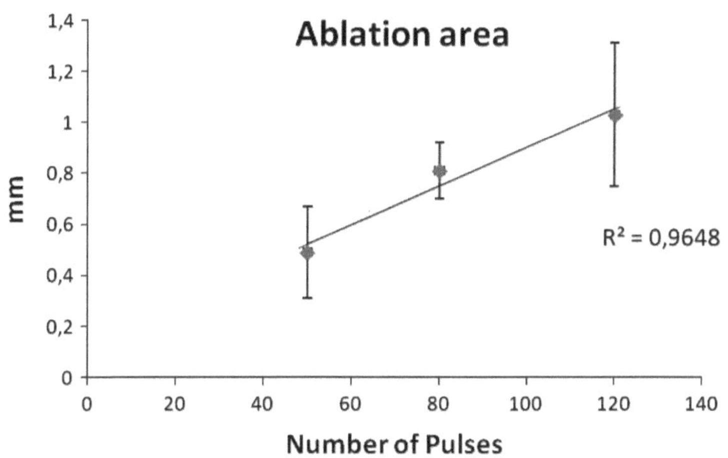

Fig. 10.4 Area ablated using 1,750 V/cm using increasing number of pulses

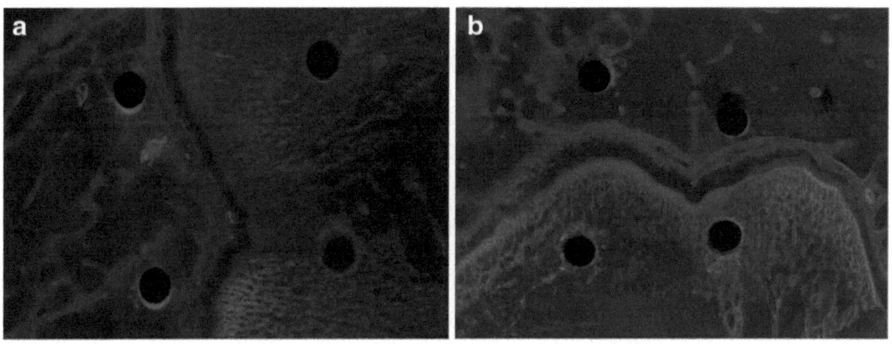

Fig. 10.5 Bone fluorescence following the delivery of 120 pulses at 1,300 V/cm (**a**) or 1,000 V/cm (**b**)

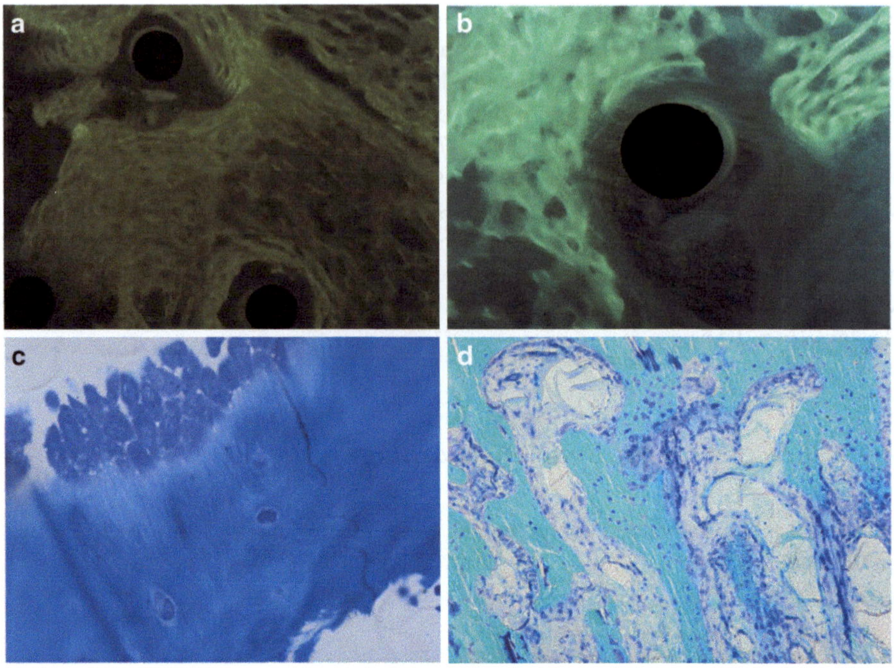

Fig. 10.6 (**a, b**) Strong fluorescence of bone tissue around/between the electrodes 30 days after electroporation with 120 pulses at 1,750 V/cm. (**c, d**) Toluidine blue staining shows the presence of osteoblasts and new bone apposition

Medial femoral condyles at sacrifice were decalcified, and 4-μm sections were stained routinely with H&E. The same electroporation protocols that prevented bone labeling by tetracycline effectively ablated cells from trabeculae surface and removed bone marrow cells. The few apoptotic osteoblasts identified on the trabeculae surface showed irregular shape and vacuoli in the cytoplasm and stained positive to Bcl-2 like osteocytes (Fig. 10.7). Transmission electron microscopy investigation showed the presence of chromatin disaggregates in osteocytes present in the lacunae (Fig. 10.8) consistent with osteocytes cell death induced by the application of electric pulses. Cartilage extracellular matrix did not stain, while chondrocytes nuclei appeared picnotic (Fig. 10.9). The application of appropriate combination of electric pulses (pulse amplitude and number) causes complete ablation of the cellular component in the bone tissue regardless of the presence of mineralized matrix and extracellular matrix (i.e., cartilage).

Effect of Electroporation on Bone Trabeculae Microhardness

Mechanical competence of electroporated bone tissue was investigated by microhardness (Vickers Hardness, HV) using a Leitz-Durimet equipped with a Vickers indenter on polymethylmethacrylate-embedded specimens' sections. Imprints were performed under a load of 25 g for each specimen, and the length of the diagonals of the imprint was measured by a screw micrometric eye-piece at a magnification of 40×. The microhardness number was calculated by the formula $HV = 1854.4 * L/d^2$ where L is the load in grams and d is the mean length of the diagonals of the imprint measured in microns, and it is expressed in kg/mm^2.

Microhardness data is a viable means of estimating the Young's modulus of specimens [14].

Trabeculae microhardness, the value of which reflects bone tissue Young's modulus, indicator of the mechanical competence of the bone, was unchanged both 7 and 30 days after treatment compared to control nonelectroporated bone (Fig. 10.10).

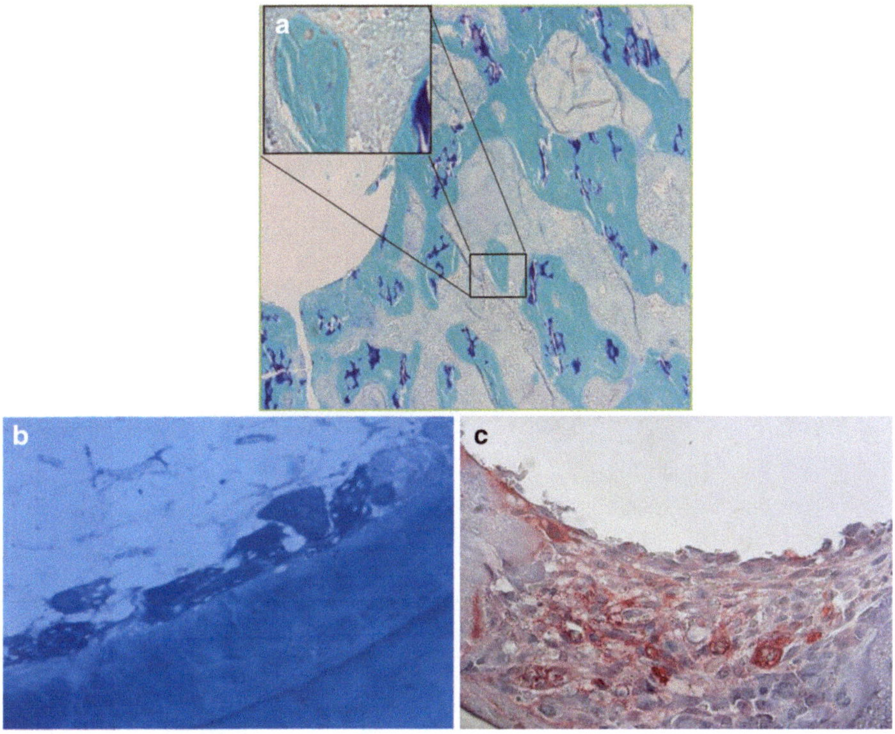

Fig. 10.7 Seven days after electroporation (1,750 V/cm and 120 pulses). (**a**) Toluidine blue staining of ablated bone tissue; the *insert* shows the absence of the osteoblasts on the trabeculae surface and picnotic osteocytes. (**b**) Few osteoblasts present on the trabeculae surface show large vacuoli in the cytoplasm. (**c**) Positive staining to Bcl-2 of cells present in the ablated area

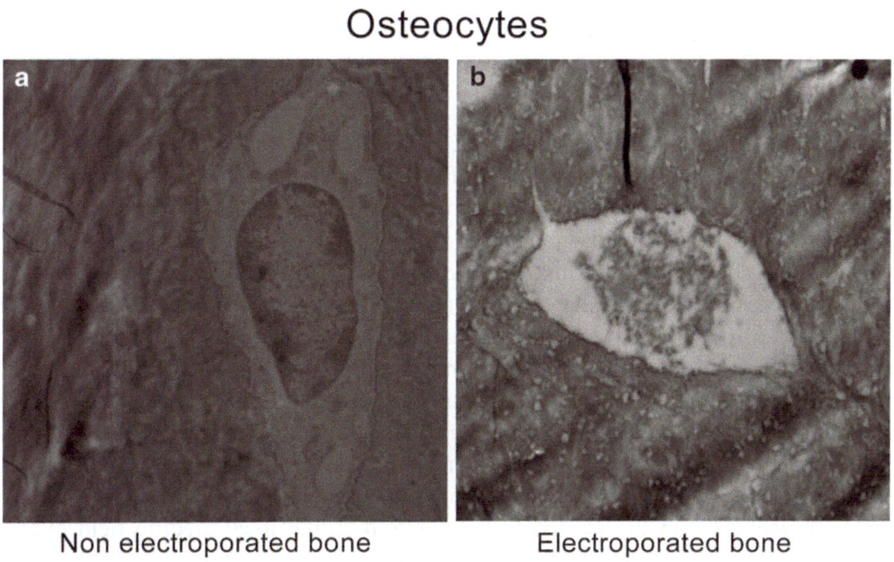

Fig. 10.8 Transmission electron microscopy images of osteocytes in control bone (**a**) and in the electroporation area (**b**) 7 days after 1,750 V/cm and 120 pulses. Magnification × 7,000

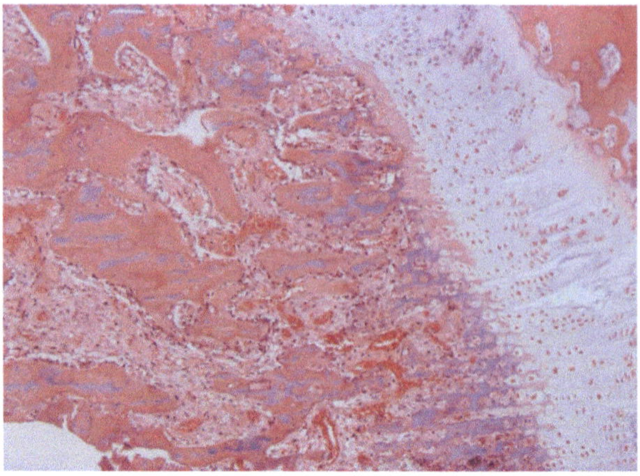

Fig. 10.9 Cartilage in the electroporated area; extracellular matrix does not stain, and chondrocytes appear picnotic with small nuclei and unstained cytoplasm

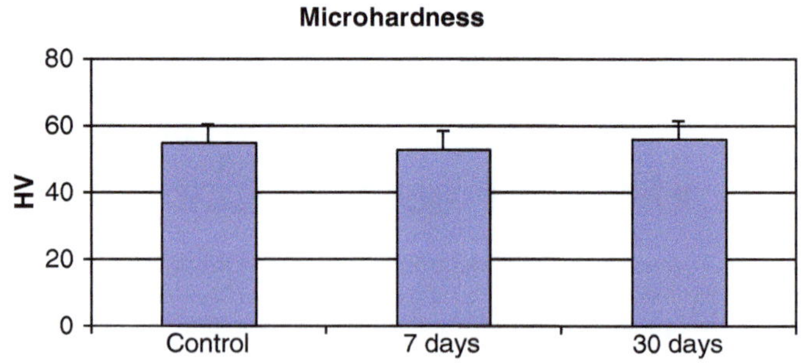

Fig. 10.10 Microhardness of bone trabeculae 7 and 30 days after electroporation, and in control nonelectroporated bone

Combined Effect of Electric Field Amplitude and Number of Pulses: Absorbed Dose in Bone Tissue

Several pulse protocols were effective in ablating all bone cells within the area covered by the electrodes. Our experiments clearly show that complete tissue ablation can be obtained with decreasing values of electric field provided that the number of pulses delivered is increased. These findings show the importance of the amount of energy delivered to the tissues; a similar observation has been made by Ibey et al. for ultra short pulses demonstrating that the key parameter is the absorbed dose (AD) [15].

To calculate the AD in our conditions, the electric field distribution in the bone tissue was simulated using the COMSOL Multiphysics software (COMSOL Inc., Burlington, MA, US), based on a finite element method. This method solves partial differential equations by dividing the model into small elements, where the quantity to be determined is approximated with a function or is assumed to be constant throughout the element. In this study, we modeled the local electric field by means of 2D numerical models. Four stainless steel electrodes were modeled in a target bone region: four stainless steel electrodes (0.7 mm diameter) were used and 4 mm-square-positioned. In order to quantify and compare different electrical conditions and applied voltages, we visualized the regions around/between electrodes in the treated tissue exposed to the local electric field exceeding the value E_0 by keeping this value constant for all conditions, so that the electric field distribution could be directly compared. Model geometries were meshed by triangular finite elements. The final mesh models were obtained by refining the mesh until the discrepancies between two consecutive meshes were negligible.

For calculations, conductivity values of 4.032×10^{6} [S/m] and 0.02 [S/m] were used for electrodes and bone, respectively [15]. The minimum electric field threshold E_0 was settled at 900 V/cm, as this is reported as the highest irreversible electroporation threshold for tissues [16].

The AD (J/kg) was calculated using the following formula:

$$\mathrm{AD} = \sigma \frac{E^2}{\rho} \tau,$$

where σ is the material conductivity, E is the local electric field, ρ is the material density, and τ is the total duration of the applied pulses.

Our calculations show that for all electric fields used, complete tissue ablation around/between the electrodes could be obtained only when the AD value exceeded 3,500 J/kg.

Clearly, the maps of the electric field and AD are not the same. Figure 10.11 shows the electric field gradient at 1,000 and 1,750 V. However, when different numbers of pulses were applied to the tissue (240 and 80 pulses, respectively), the same AD gradient was calculated in the tissue, and both pulse protocols effectively ablated all cells in rabbit femurs.

Clinical Relevance

The above results show that different pulse protocols can be used to permeabilize bone tissue. This information is of great importance when treating bone malignancies: tissue inhomogeneities, local necrosis, and areas with high local conductivity (low tissue impedance) may prevent the applications of sufficiently intense electric fields to achieve electroporation with a limited number of pulses (i.e., 8 square wave pulses of 100 μs duration with a nominal electric field of 1,000 V/cm: ESOPE protocol standard electroporation conditions). An attractive way to overcome this limitation is to apply an electric field of lower amplitude and increase the number of pulses with the intent to deliver an ESOPE-equivalent pulse protocol based on AD values.

This finding is of fundamental importance as bone metastases are neither visible nor readily accessible: the target volume to be treated needs to be identified and electrodes applied using medical imaging techniques (e.g., CT, MRI). An accurate preoperative study of the tumor geometry is required to define electrode position and achieve complete electroporation of tumor cells, including

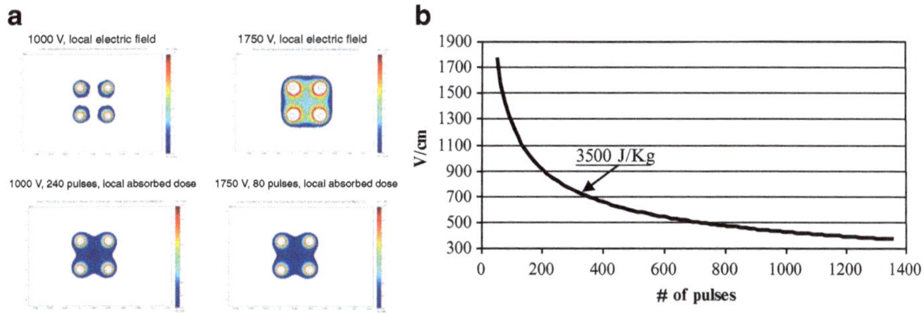

Fig. 10.11 (**a**) Electric field gradient around/between the electrodes when 1,000 or 1,750 V/cm are applied. The *blue* corresponds to 400 V/cm value. (**b**) AD around/between the electrodes when either 1,000 V/cm, 240 pulses or 1,750 V/cm, 80 pulses are applied. The *blue* color corresponds to 3,500 J/Kg value

enough surrounding healthy tissue as safety margins. The interventional access route, the maximum voltage and current that can be sustained during treatment, and number of electrodes to be used have to be taken into account. Nevertheless, early clinical experiences show that in deep-seated large tumors, electrical characteristics of the tissue (impedance) may differ significantly between different parts of the nodule and between tumor and healthy tissue. As a consequence, under some conditions, the ESOPE electroporation protocol, that is currently recognized as the gold standard in electrochemotherapy treatments, may not be delivered because of limitations in the maximum amount of current the device can supply, thus requiring a reduction in the applied voltage (Fig. 10.12).

Currently, a phase I–II clinical trial has been approved by Istituto Ortopedico Rizzoli (Bologna, Italy) ethical committee, and patients are actively being recruited [17]. Main inclusion criteria are no local treatment of target lesion in the 3 months before electrochemotherapy and maximum tumor volume of 100 cm^3. Pathological fracture is a contraindication. Two treatment groups are considered. Group 1 enrolls patients with resectable tumors (1 electrochemotherapy application), and group 2 includes unresectable tumors (2 electrochemotherapy applications with a 4-week interval). Electrochemotherapy feasibility, safety, and efficacy will be evaluated after resection at 4 weeks with histological review of the surgical specimen in group 1. Electrochemotherapy response in group 2 will be carried out with MRI/CT evaluation 4 and 8 weeks after the first and second application. Pain

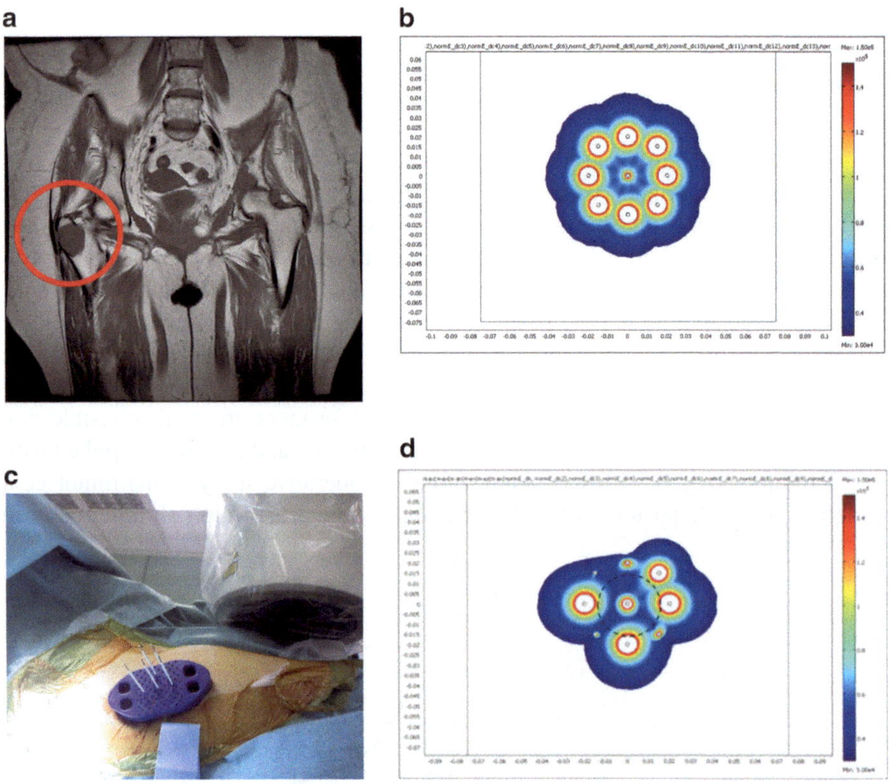

Fig. 10.12 (**a**) MRI image of a carcinoma metastasis in the femur (within the *red circle*). (**b**) Numerical calculations showing the electrode position able to cover the whole tumor and the safety margins. (**c**) In the operating theater, electrodes are inserted percutaneously according to the preoperative treatment plan. (**d**) Electric field distribution was recalculated based on the actual voltage applied. Between some electrodes, the electrical current would exceed 50 A, and the standard ESOPE pulse protocol could not be delivered. In this case the whole tumor volume was still covered by a minimum electric field of 300 V/cm (*blue*) that is considered the effective threshold to achieve electroporation. Nevertheless, if fewer electrodes were energized, the result would be an incomplete tumor electroporation and treatment unless an ESOPE-equivalent pulse protocol would be applied

relief will be evaluated with VAS score and EORTC QLQ-C30 questionnaire. Patients are discharged the day after treatment. As of May 2010, two patients have been enrolled in treatment group 2. Figure 10.13 shows an example of how the electrodes can be placed properly in the proximal femur to treat a metastasis. No complications were reported, and fast patient recovery was assessed.

Evaluation with MRI before and at 4 weeks after electrochemotherapy (Fig. 10.14) showed promising results. More patients will be enrolled in our study and longer follow-up is needed. Once efficacy of electrochemotherapy treatment for bone metastasis will be demonstrated, its use could be extended to treat spine, sacrum, or pelvic metastases under appropriate intraoperative guidance, reducing tumor volume, providing effective palliation of symptoms, and improving the quality of life of metastatic patients.

Conclusions

To an extent, the structure and inhomogeneity of bone tissue could interfere with and limit the use of electroporation technology for bone cell ablation. The effectiveness of the electric field in inducing cell membrane permeabilization in bone has never before been investigated in vivo. We have

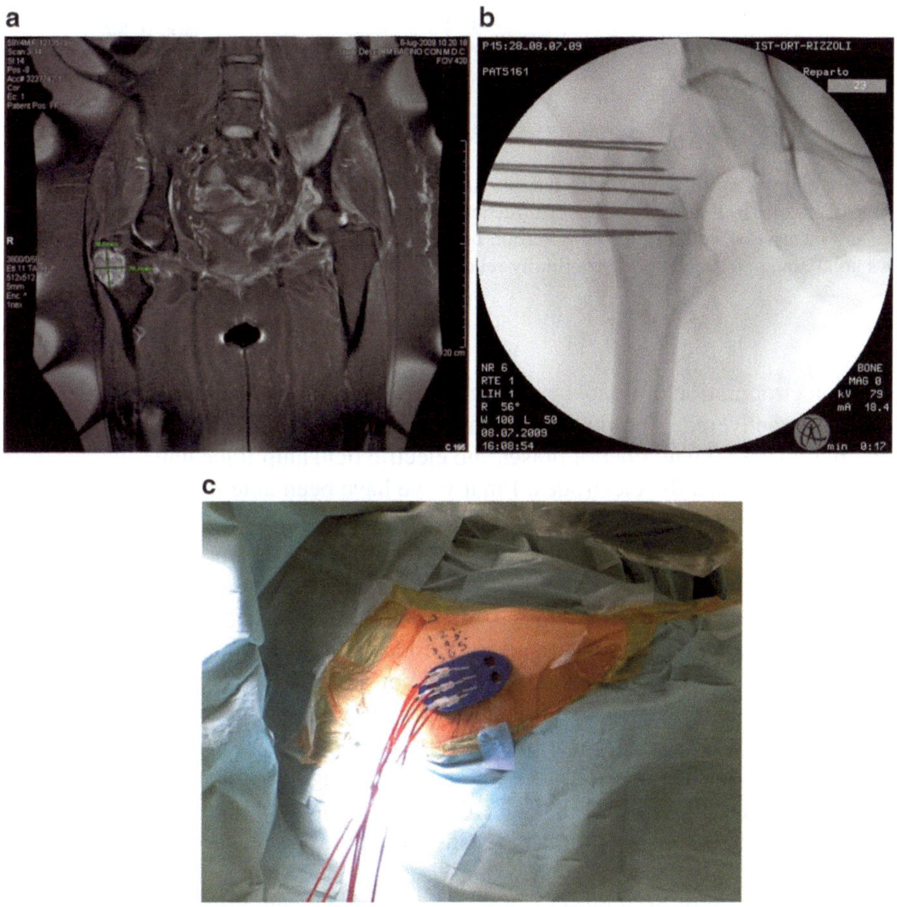

Fig. 10.13 Fifty-eight-year-old female with right intratrochanteric breast cancer metastasis. (**a**) MRI showing bone metastasis at the proximal femur. (**b**) X-ray image after insertion of 9 needle electrodes. (**c**) Electrodes connected to the pulse generator during treatment

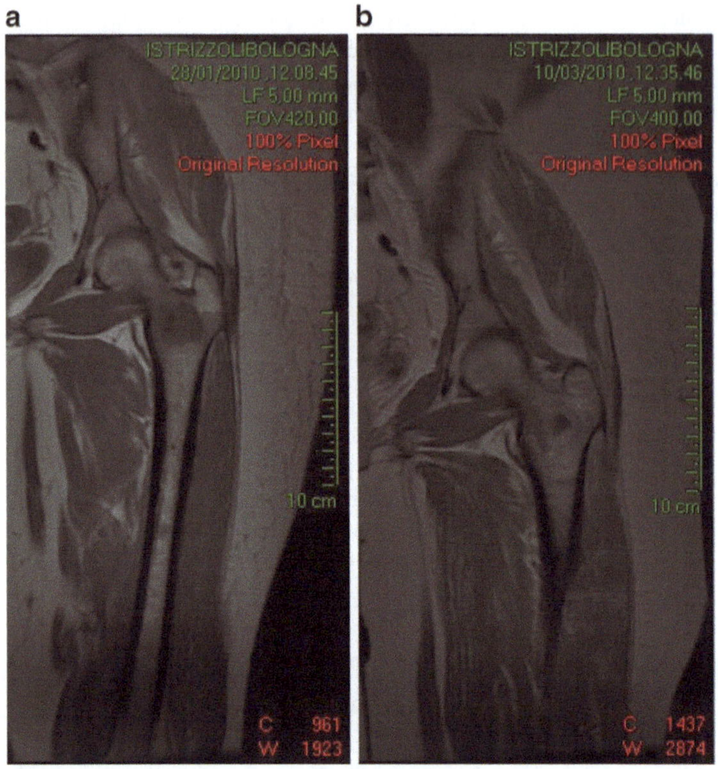

Fig. 10.14 Fifty-eight-year-old female with left intratrochanteric breast cancer metastasis. (**a**) Preoperative MRI imaging of target lesion. (**b**) Four weeks after electrochemotherapy treatment of breast cancer metastasis, MRI shows shrinking of the metastasis with a thin osteosclerotic border at the periphery. Normal bone (cortex and cancellous bone) shows no alteration of signal or discontinuity related to side effect of the procedure

tested several electroporation protocols by using different combinations of electric field strength and number of pulses delivered. The distance from the electrode surface at which cell ablation was observed increased with the number of pulses and electric field amplitude until all cells were ablated in the area around/between the electrodes. Finally, we have been able to identify the AD threshold of 3,500 J/Kg, above which cell damage becomes irreversible and leads to cell death in the area around/between the electrodes. The structural integrity of the bone and of the extracellular matrix and its mechanical competence were maintained with all electroporation protocols used.

The effect of electroporation is generally so rapid that on the second day after treatment, osteoblasts stop depositing bone as demonstrated by the lack of fluorescence upon addition of tetracycline. However, the effect of electroporation is not necessarily consequent to cell lysis as hypothesized by other authors. The histological fields observed at day 7 show the presence of picnotic osteocytes within bone trabeculae and the almost complete absence of osteoblasts: the few cells observed on the surface of the trabeculae have an irregular shape with large vacuoli in the cytoplasm. Positive staining to Bcl-2 indicates that cells are undergoing apoptosis.

Recovery from the electroporation-induced damage is already observed 30 days after treatment.

The reparative activity of osteoblasts is not present immediately around the electrodes, the area that experienced the highest AD values, where a significant temperature increase and associated thermal effect may occur.

Altogether the findings demonstrate that cell membrane electroporation can be induced in bone tissue and provide the preclinical information necessary to extend the use of electrochemotherapy to the treatment of metastases in the bone tissue.

The identification of a threshold AD value that has to be overcome to achieve complete effective electroporation-induced ablation in the bone environment, and the relationship between potential applied, number of pulses, and tissue AD lays the foundation for the development equivalent electroporation protocols for effective bone electroporation. However, the identification of a specific threshold AD value for reversible electroporation, to be used in electrochemotherapy clinical practice, will need to be further addressed to develop ESOPE-equivalent pulse protocols. These ESOPE-equivalent protocols will allow complete and effective electroporation of the target lesions even when tissue electrical characteristics may prevent the application of the standard ESOPE protocol and guarantee the delivery of an effective electrochemotherapy treatment.

References

1. Callstrom MR, Charboneau JW. Image-guided palliation of painful metastases using percutaneous ablation. Tech Vasc Interv Radiol. 2007;10:120–31.
2. Capanna R, De Biase P, Sensi L. Minimally invasive technique for treatment of metastatic cancers. Orthopade. 2009;38(4):343–7.
3. Marty M, Sersa G, Garbay JR. Electrochemotherapy – an easy, highly effective and safe treatment of cutaneous and subcutaneous metastases: results of ESOPE (European Standard Operating Procedures of Electrochemotherapy) study. EJC Suppl. 2006;4:3–13.
4. Giardino R, Fini M, Bonazzi V, et al. Electrochemotherapy a novel approach to the treatment of metastatic nodules on the skin and subcutaneous tissues. Biomed Pharmacother. 2006;60:458–62.
5. Quaglino P, Mortera C, Osella-Abate S, Barberis M, Illengo M, Rissone M, et al. Electrochemotherapy with intravenous bleomycin in the local treatment of skin melanoma metastases. Ann Surg Oncol. 2008;15(8):2215–22.
6. Neumann E, Schaefer-Ridder M, et al. Gene transfer into mouse lyoma cells by electroporation in high electrical fields. EMBO J. 1982;1:841–5.
7. Mir LM, Belehdradek M, Domenge C, et al. Electro-chemotherapy, a new antitumor treatment: first clinical trial. C R Acad Sci III. 1991;313:613–8.
8. Orlowski S, Behradek Jr J, Paoletti C. Transient electropermeabilization of cells in culture. Increase in the cytotoxicity of anticancer drugs. Biochem Pharmacol. 1988;37:4724–33.
9. Belehradek M, Domenge C, Luboinski B, et al. Electro-chemotherapy, a new antitumor treatment. First clincal phase I-II trial. Cancer. 1993;72(12):3694–700.
10. Gothelf A, Mir LM, Gehl J. Electrochemotherapy: results of cancer treatment using enhanced delivery of bleomycin by electroporation. Cancer Treat Rev. 2003;29(5):371–87.
11. Sersa G, Miklavcic D, Camazar M, Rudolf Z, Pucihar G, Snoj M. Electrochemotherapy in treatment of tumor. EJSO. 2008;34:232–40.
12. Isobe K, Shimizu T, Nikaido T, Takaoka K. Low voltage electrochemotherapy with low dose methotrexate enhances survival in mice with osteosarcoma. Clin Orthop Relat Res. 2007;426:226–31.
13. Corovic S, Pavlin M, Miklavcic D. Analytical and numerical quantification and comparison of the local electric field in the tissue for different electrode configurations. Biomed Eng Online. 2007;6:37–51.
14. Boivin G, Bala Y, Doublier A, Farlay D, Ste-Marie LG, Meunier PJ, et al. The role of mineralization and organic matrix in microhardness of bone tissue from controls and osteoporotic patients. Bone. 2008;43:532–8.
15. Ibey BL, Xiao S, Schoenbach KH, Murphy MR, Pakhomov AG. Plasma membrane permeabilization by-60-and 600 ns electric pulses is determined by the absorbed dose. Bioelectromagnetics. 2009;30(2):92–9.
16. Gabriel S, Lau RW, Gabriel C. The dielectric properties of biological tissues: II. Measurements in the frequency range 10 Hz to 20 GHz. Phys Med Biol. 1996;41:2251–69.
17. Bianchi G, Campanacci L, Fini M, Alberghini M, Mercuri M. Electrochemotherapy for the treatment of osteolytic bone metastasis: a phase I/II clinical trial. EMSOS 2010 Annual Meeting, Birmingham, UK; 2010.

Chapter 11
Drug and Gene Electrotransfer to the Brain

Birgit Agerholm-Larsen, Mette Linnert, Helle K. Iversen, and Julie Gehl

Abstract Applying drugs and genes to brain tissue using electroporation is a new and upcoming field of research. Because of the blood brain barrier (BBB), the access of agents from the blood into brain tissue is restricted. This could theoretically be overcome by the use of electroporation. In the early 1990s, the first pre-clinical experiments using electrochemotherapy in brain tissue were conducted in rats with inoculated brain tumours; however, the technique has not yet been further explored and applied in humans. This chapter will focus on the pre-clinical experience with drug and gene electrotransfer in the brain, the clinical experience with use of bleomycin in the brain, and the following clinical perspectives. Further discussion of central issues, such as safety and the BBB, will also be discussed.

Keywords Brain • Tumour • Bleomycin • Blood brain barrier • Electrode • Pre-clinical • Electrochemotherapy • Gene electrotransfer

Introduction

This chapter will address the pre-clinical experience with drug and gene electrotransfer in the brain and the following clinical perspectives.

Primary and Secondary Brain Cancer

In the US, around 170,000 cancer patients each year will suffer from brain metastases [1]. We have estimated that in the European Union 72,000 patients per year will develop primary brain cancer and 240,000 patients per year will develop brain metastases. Patients with lung cancer, breast cancer and malignant melanoma are at most risk for developing metastases to the brain. Clinical-, imaging- and autopsy series have shown that about half of brain metastases will be solitary and

J. Gehl (✉)
University of Copenhagen, Copenhagen, Denmark
and
Center for Experimental Drug and Gene Electrotransfer (C*EDGE), Department of Oncology 54B1,
Copenhagen University Hospital Herlev, Herlev Ringvej 75, 2730 Herlev, Denmark
e-mail: juge@heh.regionh.dk

S.T. Kee et al. (eds.), *Clinical Aspects of Electroporation*,
DOI 10.1007/978-1-4419-8363-3_11,

half will be multiple [1]. The most common symptoms of brain metastases are headaches, altered mental status and focal weakness, but seizures and gait ataxia are also observed [1]. The prognosis is dependent on factors such as performance status, control of primary cancer, age, number of metastases and presence of midline shift and post-WBRT response. WBRT, short for whole-brain radiotherapy, is the treatment of choice for patients with multiple brain metastases. Unfortunately, WBRT is a palliative treatment, and the median survival time is 4–6 months. About half of the patients experience an improvement in their neurological symptoms after WBRT [1]. Selected patients can be treated with surgery and stereotaxic radiotherapy. Still, the majority of patients do not achieve local control and frequently succumb to the progressive brain disease [1]. Therefore, there is a desperate need for new treatments that can provide better results.

Brain Diseases

Diseases of the brain cause considerable morbidity, at great cost for the individual patient and for society as a whole [2]. Gene therapy is one of the avenues being investigated for brain diseases, and one of the most investigated disease targets has been Parkinson's disease [3]. The first clinical results of gene therapy with viral vectors show promising results [4]. However, it would be an advantage to perform non-viral gene therapy from a patient safety, treatment cost and an environmental point of view. Since treatment of, e.g. Parkinson's disease involves transfer to a defined target region (the substantia nigra), it would be a valid goal for the use of gene electrotransfer.

There is no clinical experience with the electrotransfer of drugs or genes to the brain yet, thus, the following paragraphs will summarize the pre-clinical experience in this area.

Electrochemotherapy to Treat Brain Tumours: In Vivo

Electrochemotherapy is dealt with in detail in other chapters (Chaps. 6, 8 and 9). In essence, the cytotoxicity of the anti-cancer drug, bleomycin, may be augmented more than 300 times by enabling the permeability of the membrane by application of electric pulses [5–7].

Pre-Clinical Studies on Electrochemotherapy in the Brain

In 1993, the first reported pre-clinical experiments were made by using the principles of electropermeabilization to achieve improved uptake of bleomycin into brain tumours in vivo. The experiments were performed in Fischer 344 rats inoculated with tumour cells and treated with electrochemotherapy. The end point was survival time to observation of symptoms of severe tumour growth (e.g. the rats moving in circles, hemiparesis or drowsiness), and consequently termination after appearance of symptoms. This association study indicated that rats treated with electrochemotherapy (bleomycin) had a better mean survival time (days ± SD) of 10.3 ± 4.7 ($n = 17, p = 0.015$) than untreated 6.3 ± 3.2 ($n = 13, p = 0.005$) [8].

Electrochemotherapy has also been given to Fischer 344 rats inoculated with brain tumour cells, with the end point to look for pathological necrotic tissue in the target area suggesting successful elimination of target cells in the treated area [9]. We have experience with the treatment of brain tissue and inoculated brain tumours in Fisher 344 rats with electroporation, bleomycin and electrochemotherapy. In initial studies, nine out of ten rats treated with an eight-electrode device had severely affected and necrotic brain tissue in the target areas. Post-treatment rats showed no obvious adverse behavioural effects. Some of the rats were monitored in vivo by magnetic resonance imaging (MRI) to confirm presence of tumour and treatment [9].

Bleomycin and the Blood Brain Barrier

The blood brain barrier (BBB) is made of non-fenestrated endothelial cells, which makes it highly impermeable, allowing only the passage of small, hydrophobic and uncharged molecules such as water. The BBB is disrupted to different degrees by pathological processes, such as in instances of stroke, a malignant brain tumour, infection, or trauma. After cranial irradiation (WBRT), the BBB is damaged for weeks to months [10].

Bleomycin has been used in the treatment of human brain tumours for several years, but with limited effectiveness. If bleomycin is to be given intravenously, it is essential that the drug passes the BBB and leaves the vascular system, in order to obtain an effect in the target area of the brain. Bleomycin, at its best, is inadequately effective, and at worst is not capable of passing the BBB under normal circumstances, because it is a large, hydrophilic and charged molecule. Electroporation may cause an increased BBB permeabilization. An improved mean survival time was reported for intravenously administered bleomycin and electroporation in rats [8], suggesting that the BBB can be altered to allow penetration of bleomycin through the simultaneous process of electroporation. The observations from intra-cranially administered bleomycin and electroporation in rats [9] suggest that for bleomycin to be effective, it is necessary to use additional methods to alter the BBB. Intra-cranially administered bleomycin had no effect on target brain tissue unless electroporation was also performed.

Particular Considerations for Electrodes Used in the Brain

Previous chapters have dealt in detail with questions on electric field distribution and electrode design (Chaps. 4 and 5). What needs to be mentioned here is that the anatomical constraints associated with electrotransfer in the brain present some additional challenges to electrode versatility.

It is desirable that the electrode may be inserted with minimal damage to healthy tissues. This includes making insertion through a burr hole if possible, and using a relatively small calibre for insertion through normal tissue between the brain surface and the target region (Fig. 11.1).

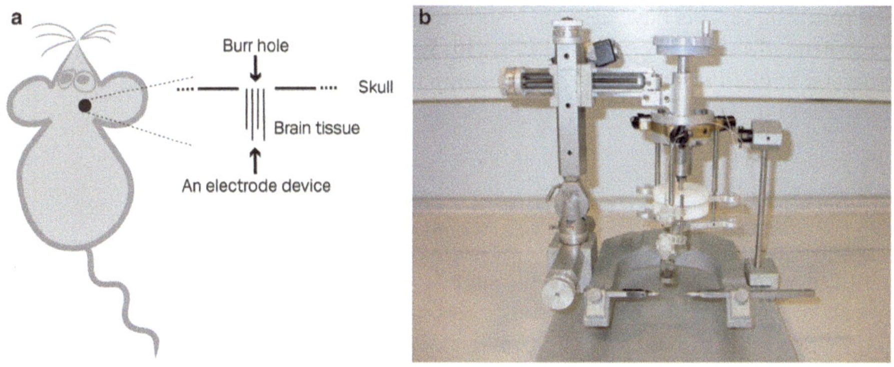

Fig. 11.1 Experimental setup for electroporation in a rat brain. (**a**) Sedated rat with a burr hole in the skull for intra-cranial injection of tumour cells, drugs and genes, and for insertion of an electrode device for electroporation in soft tissue. (**b**) Stereotaxic equipment for precise and accurate intra-cranial placement of needles and electrodes in an electroporation setup. The stereotaxic equipment is supplemented by a carousel with three working positions for needles or electrodes useful for electroporation with drug or genes

For example, when treating skin metastatic lesions, treatment failures can easily be handled by re-treatment. Since electrotransfer to the brain is an invasive procedure, one-time-only treatment is the goal, and therefore optimal field distribution for the intended procedure is crucial. Additionally, field distribution should be adequate with a high level of predictability. Accurate positioning of the electrode device is possible by mounting on stereotaxic frames, as those used in neurosurgery, and the equipment will have to be put in neurosurgical units.

Gene Electrotransfer in the Brain

In Vivo Pre-Clinical Studies

Pre-clinical studies have shown that the electroporation technology can be used for gene transfer in vivo [3, 9–15] [17]. The results are obtained at many different conditions depending on the choice of electrode device (invasive or non-invasive, electrode configuration etc.), injection of the gene, pulse generator features, voltage amplitude, and the frequency, number and duration of applied pulses. Results also vary with the choice of species (mice, rats, chickens or hamsters) and the state of the animal (newborn or adults). It is also dependent on the procedures used to evaluate transfection efficiency (fluorescence imaging, protein expression, immunohistochemical staining). As expected within a new scientific field, data is still limited.

In gene electrotransfer studies so far, there have mainly been reports of the green fluorescent protein (GFP) reporter gene transfected into brain tissue by electrotransfer [3, 9–12, 14, 15] [17]. The results were qualitative and, in a few cases, also quantitative based on the expression of GFP measured by fluorescent imaging. The positive results demonstrating expression of GFP signals that the involved cells have been transiently permeabilized, and that the plasmid with the GFP gene has gained access to the cell cytosol and further to the cell nucleus to be expressed. Alterations in the cell membrane must only have been temporary in order to achieve expression of the protein GFP (see Chap. 2).

The gene electrotransfer results were achieved by injection of 0.5–40 μg DNA and using 1–5 pulses at 100–1,000 V/cm for 2–50 ms at 1–10 Hz, and by using invasive as well as non-invasive electrodes. All these heterogeneous parameters suggest that gene electrotransfer can be achieved under several different conditions. From a clinical point of view, the invasive technology may be the most relevant, as treatment of a specific region of the brain will not be achievable with external electrodes. Promising reports have also been shown using genes other than GFP, where gene expression from the gene of interest is obtained [18, 19]. It is also possible to see a "dose-response" relationship between applied voltage and the efficiency of GFP transfected into brain cells [9].

Which Brain Cells Were Susceptible to Gene Electrotransfer?

The different cell types in the brain may have slightly different thresholds for transient permeabilization due to cell size, shape, and basic resting membrane potential. So far the aim of most studies is fulfilled simply by successful gene electrotransfer, but further studies may show evidence of cell type sensitivity and specificity when variable electroporation parameters are used. Meningeal cells and oligodendrocytes [11], neurons and microglia [11], neuronal cells (17), cells in the suprachiasmatic nucleus [12], ependymal cells (in ventricles), putative neural stem or progenitor cells and neuroblasts [9] have all been listed as brain cell types suitable for gene electrotransfer in animal models.

Transgene Expression over Time

The brain tissue is known for its many cells that, once differentiated, principally survive the entire lifetime of the organism. It is also known for its low mitotic activity. Compared to other body cell types like skin and muscle, the brain has the potential for long-term expression of transfected genes beyond weeks, months or even a few years. However, the anti-pathogenic systems may have to be circumvented to avoid elimination of the gene and immediate degradation of the gene product. Among the reports using invasive electrodes for gene electrotransfer, gene expression was shown to last up until 45 days from electrotransfer [12].

Since most papers report visual observations of GFP after termination of the animal, one would hope for new future long-term studies using the available in vivo fluorescent technologies.

Safety Issues

For gene electrotransfer in the brain tissue to become a successful technology, there are several safety issues that have to be met. The use of invasive electrodes raises the risks of bleeding and infection. When the electrodes are inserted, there is risk of damage to healthy tissue. There are also the toxic effects of DNA to consider. As an example, when targeting dopamine-producing cells in the substantia nigra of a Parkinson's disease patient with gene electrotransfer, the consequences of non-target cell damage could cause clinical deterioration.

In pre-clinical studies, photomicrographs and pathological staining for gliafilaments, neurofilaments and necrotic cells have revealed that the physical damage as a result of the needles and electrodes is in fact relatively small and basically restricted to areas where these items have passed through brain tissue on their way to the target area. Not surprisingly, smaller electrodes make less damage [11]. Necrotic cells are found along the electrode traces [11], as well as astrocytes and lymphocytes [13]. Gliafilaments are more affected by electrochemotherapy than neurofilaments, as the effect on neurofilaments is restricted to the target area, whereas it goes beyond the target area for the gliafilaments [9]. Behavioural observations in a single pre-clinical study showed no signs of adverse behavioural effect after application of electroporation and inoculation of the gene [3].

Only a few of these safety issues concerning electroporation of brain tissue are relevant to virus-mediated gene therapy, which has other major safety concerns, such as strong immune response to vira, toxicity and limitations in restricting vira to the target area.

Clinical Perspectives on Drug and Gene Electrotransfer in Brain Tissue

Where Are We Now

The future holds a lot of challenges for electrotransfer of drugs and genes to the brain. Among these are the electrodes. Electrodes need to be physically flexible in length, shape and selection (see Chap. 5). For gene electrotransfer, the demands of the electrodes primarily focus on their ability to be selective, in order to obtain gene transfer in highly restricted areas of the brain.

In the clinic, neurosurgeons have the necessary technology available to target any area for gene electrotransfer by coordinating using stereotaxy. Only the prospect of severe and non-recoverable brain damage made in the attempt to reach the target by the electrodes may withhold the surgeons from using the available technology. Figure 11.2 shows a schematic view of the Ellisphere brain electrode in action in the clinical setting.

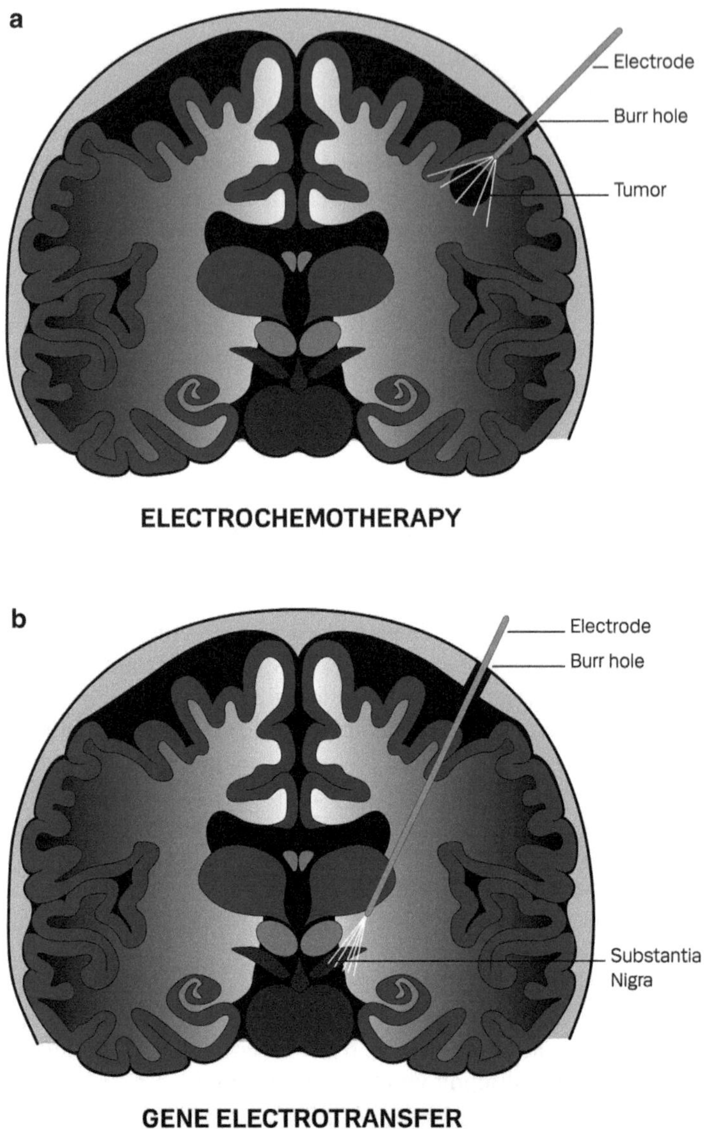

Fig. 11.2 Schematic drawing of methods for applying electrochemotherapy (**a**) and gene electrotransfer (**b**) to brain tissue in the clinical setting. A more detailed description of the concept behind this electrode device can be found in Chap. 5, Sect. 5.2, the Ellisphere system

With regard to electrochemotherapy, there are relevant data from clinical experience with bleomycin directly injected into a brain tumour or cyst. Bleomycin is a drug often used for electrochemotherapy, and has been used in the treatment of brain tumours for selected cases for more than 30 years as single drug injections. This experience can be used to evaluate the toxicity of bleomycin in brain tissue for future use of electrochemotherapy in the brain. Currently, there are two major indications for the use of bleomycin in the brain: solid tumours, such as glioblastoma, and cystic tumours in the form of craniopharyngiomas [14]. Unfortunately, the clinical benefit has been limited, but that is probably due to the nature of bleomycin and the BBB. Bleomycin is a hydrophilic and charged molecule, which poorly passes the intact plasma membrane [15]. The BBB is nonpermeable to many types of chemotherapy, and that is certainly true for a large molecule such as bleomycin with characteristics as mentioned above. This is reflected by the clinical results, because local bleomycin treatment works better on a thin-walled cyst and practically not on solid tumours [23–26]. The clinical effect on brain tissue is also dose dependent, which is also true for the adverse effects. In a review of the adverse effects of bleomycin used in the treatment of solid and cystic brain tumours, there were only a few cases of serious adverse effects [14].

A future clinical trial is planned, with the purpose of investigating the efficacy and safety of electrochemotherapy using bleomycin in the treatment of secondary brain tumours. The rationale behind this protocol is that clinical trials have shown improvement in neurocognitive function and survival with tumour volume reduction [27–29]. The total tumour volume is therefore an important clinical parameter and could be diminished by electrochemotherapy.

No clinical studies have yet been performed for brain tissue gene therapy, but Parkinson's disease is an obvious candidate for gene therapy. It represents a disease where the dopamine production is disturbed, and where dopamine level restoration is an acknowledged and eligible treatment of Parkinson's disease symptoms [3]. The target of gene therapy would be the substantia nigra, to attain regeneration and control of the dopamine production in vivo (Fig. 11.2b). The ability to be target specifically with gene electrotransfer may therefore make it the method of choice for gene therapy in highly restricted and small target areas.

Treatment of brain disorders is a major challenge, and it will be highly interesting to see the future research in the area of gene and drug electrotransfer to the brain.

References

1. Videtic GM, Gaspar LE, Aref AM, et al. American College of Radiology appropriateness criteria on multiple brain metastases. Int J Radiat Oncol Biol Phys. 2009;75(4):961–5.
2. Andlin-Sobocki P, Jonsson B, Wittchen HU, Olesen J. Cost of disorders of the brain in Europe. Eur J Neurol. 2005;12 Suppl 1:1–27.
3. Burton EA, Glorioso JC, Fink DJ. Gene therapy progress and prospects: Parkinson's disease. Gene Ther. 2003;10(20):1721–7.
4. Christine CW, Starr PA, Larson PS, et al. Safety and tolerability of putaminal AADC gene therapy for Parkinson disease. Neurology. 2009;73(20):1662–9.
5. Orlowski S, Belehradek Jr J, Paoletti C, Mir LM. Transient electropermeabilization of cells in culture. Increase of the cytotoxicity of anticancer drugs. Biochem Pharmacol. 1988;37(24):4727–33.
6. Gehl J, Skovsgaard T, Mir LM. Enhancement of cytotoxicity by electropermeabilization: an improved method for screening drugs. Anticancer Drugs. 1998;9(4):319–25.
7. Jaroszeski MJ, Dang V, Pottinger C, Hickey J, Gilbert R, Heller R. Toxicity of anticancer agents mediated by electroporation *in vitro*. Anticancer Drugs. 2000;11(3):201–8.
8. Salford LG, Persson BR, Brun A, Ceberg CP, Kongstad PC, Mir LM. A new brain tumour therapy combining bleomycin with *in vivo* electropermeabilization. Biochem Biophys Res Commun. 1993;194(2):938–43.
9. Larsen BA, Iversen H, Ibsen P, et al. Electrochemotherapy for brain tumors investigated *in vivo*. Neuro Oncol. 2009;11(5):597.
10. De Vita V, Hellmann S, Rosenberg S. Cancer, principles and practice of oncology. 5th ed. Philadelphia, PA: Lippincott-Raven; 1993.
11. Kondoh T, Motooka Y, Bhattacharjee AK, Kokunai T, Saito N, Tamaki N. *In vivo* gene transfer into the periventricular region by electroporation. Neurol Med Chir. 2000;40(12):618–22.
12. Wang H, Ko CH, Koletar MM, Ralph MR, Yeomans J. Casein kinase I epsilon gene transfer into the suprachiasmatic nucleus via electroporation lengthens circadian periods of tau mutant hamsters. Eur J Neurosci. 2007;25(11):3359–66.
13. Nishi T, Yoshizato K, Yamashiro S, et al. High-efficiency *in vivo* gene transfer using intraarterial plasmid DNA injection following *in vivo* electroporation. Cancer Res. 1996;56(5):1050–5.
14. Linnert M, Gehl J. Bleomycin treatment of brain tumors: an evaluation. Anticancer Drugs. 2009;20(3):157–64.
15. Poddevin B, Orlowski S, Belehradek J, Mir LM. Very high cytotoxicity of bleomycin introduced into the cytosol of cells in culture. Biochem Pharmacol. 1991;42:S67–75.

Chapter 12
Minimally Invasive Intraluminal Tumor Ablation

Patrick F. Forde, Michael G. Bourke, Slawomir Salwa, Gerald C. O'Sullivan, and Declan M. Soden

Abstract Surgery is the standard modality for the removal of tumors, either alone or in combination with other therapies such as radiotherapy and chemotherapy. These treatment adjuncts can be associated with significant toxicity, may not be appropriate at the time of diagnosis, and do not necessarily reduce the risk of metastasis. Consequently, a considerable volume of research has focused on the identification, validation, and refinement of alternative approaches and therapies. Here we outline a novel treatment for intraluminal tumors via an endoscopic device that delivers an electroporating pulse, resulting in enhanced tumor-targeted therapeutic absorption. This device has been demonstrated to be highly effective in the curative treatment of canine intraluminal tumors and has also been demonstrated to successfully deliver DNA in a targeted manner to intraluminal porcine tissues.

Keywords Electroporation • EndoVe • Electrochemotherapy • Gene therapy • Gastrointestinal cancers

Background

Removal of the primary tumor mass remains a critically important element in the treatment of solid malignant tumors, as it has the potential to significantly relieve symptoms, forestall complications, and facilitate responsiveness to multimodal systemic therapies [1–4]. However, many cancers are resistant to current multimodal treatment regimens, creating a need for therapeutic innovations and discovery. The causes of this intractability may include advanced stage disease at presentation, which limits the application or effectiveness of treatments, resistance of tumor cells to chemotherapy or radiation therapy, anatomical locations of the cancer which preclude either complete excision or ablation by radiotherapy, and the presence of inter-current illnesses, which may limit therapeutic options or adversely affect the risks and benefits of treatment [1, 5–7]. Poor quality of life and the intrusion on their valuable remaining time resulting from invasive or toxic therapies are a major problem for many patients with incurable tumors [8–10]. In this context, an ideal cancer treatment should effectively control local disease, be applicable to a diversity of tumor types

---

D.M. Soden (✉)
Cork Cancer Research Centre, Leslie C. Quick Jnr. Laboratory, BioSciences Institute, University College Cork, Cork, Ireland
e-mail: d.soden@ucc.ie

S.T. Kee et al. (eds.), *Clinical Aspects of Electroporation*,
DOI 10.1007/978-1-4419-8363-3_12, © Springer Science+Business Media, LLC 2011

and anatomical locations, be effective against locally recurrent disease, facilitate multimodal and systemic therapies, be minimally intrusive, and improve patient well-being and life expectancy by tumor control or cure.

Electroporation

Electroporation makes use of an externally applied electric field to increase the permeability of plasma membranes, thus achieving highly efficient gene and/or drug transfer [11–15]. Through a variety of processes, electroporation temporarily disrupts membrane stability, causing pores to form within the membrane. With careful control of the electric field strength and the duration of the cell's exposure to it, these pores reseal after a short period of time [11]. Many chemotherapeutic drugs, including bleomycin and cisplatin, are poorly permeant at the cell membrane under physiologic conditions. Electropermeabilization therefore offers a novel means of increasing delivery of these drugs into cancer cells, with a consequent improvement in antitumor effect [13, 15–17]. This approach is known as electrochemotherapy. Now that the efficacy, safety, and clinical utility of electrochemotherapy have been established for skin-based tumors, there is continued impetus to modify and further develop the clinical potential of this technology.

Endoscopic Electroporation with the EndoVe Device

Minimally Invasive Procedures

There are many advantages to the use of minimally invasive surgical options, including reduced pain, a frequently reduced hospital stay, a more rapid return to normal activity, and, in the case of gastrointestinal surgery, reduced ileus [18–21]. Used appropriately, minimally invasive techniques therefore have the potential to lead to an overall improved standard of patient care.

In the context of malignant disease, several minimally invasive techniques have been developed, employing a range of energy-based methods for in situ tumor destruction. These include targeted radiofrequency ablation, laser ablation, cryoablation, photodynamic therapy, high-intensity focused ultrasound (HIFU), and techniques that allow for enhanced targeting of radiotherapy [22–31]. Oncologic surgical principles require that neoplastic tissue is excised with a margin sufficient to ensure tumor clearance. If a minimally invasive technique employing an energy-based treatment can destroy equivalent neoplastic tissue volumes with an equivalent margin of normal tissue, then the outcome in terms of disease-free survival should be at least equal to that following conventional open surgery. However, the benefits associated with the use of minimally invasive techniques set them apart, as there is the potential to achieve similar outcomes of patient survival but with reduced treatment-associated morbidity.

The Endoscopic Electrode: EndoVe

The ability to localize and treat internal cancerous tissue with electrochemotherapy, without disrupting nontarget tissues or their physiological function, presents a number of challenges.

Overcoming these requires both a means of delivering chemotherapeutic agents specifically to the diseased tissue and the development of minimally invasive options to facilitate targeted pulse delivery.

The available technology for delivery of electrochemotherapy has to date been reliant on macroelectrodes, such as calipers and needles, thus limiting its application to surface tumors. Efficient and safe electroporation of internal cancers, especially luminal tumors, have therefore not been possible thus far. However, electrode modification raises the potential for endoscopic, laparoscopic, or image-guided delivery of electric current to more deep-seated internal tumors [17]. For example, were it possible to deliver permeabilizing electric pulses to intra-abdominal, intra-thoracic, or genitourinary tumors, many lesions that have previously been deemed inoperable would be amenable to treatment with electrochemotherapy. It is also likely that electrode modification would allow electrochemotherapy to treat many, currently inoperable or incurable, primary cancers with curative intent. In particular, cancers of the foregut and bladder, which are often either incurable at presentation or unsuitable for conventional therapies due to a lack of patient fitness, are often readily accessible to endoscopes, making them ideal targets for electrochemotherapy delivered via an endoscopic device. Electrochemotherapy could also be added to many current systemic multidrug chemotherapy regimens to improve their efficacy. Similarly, electrochemotherapy could also be applied to sensitize recalcitrant cancers to radiation therapy, thus allowing a more targeted tumoricidal therapy with less collateral tissue injury. The EndoVe device has been developed to deliver electroporation endoluminally.

The EndoVe was designed using principles common to all electroporation devices; however, it fits on the end of a conventional endoscope, thereby allowing both direct tumor visualization and targeting. It has a flexible end, which attaches to the endoscope but also sits apart from it, in order to maximize luminal visualization (Fig. 12.1). The creation of a vacuum effect draws tissue into a chamber within the EndoVe, thus bringing the tumor into contact with plate electrodes contained within this chamber, allowing for electric field application. This chamber, which has a transparent

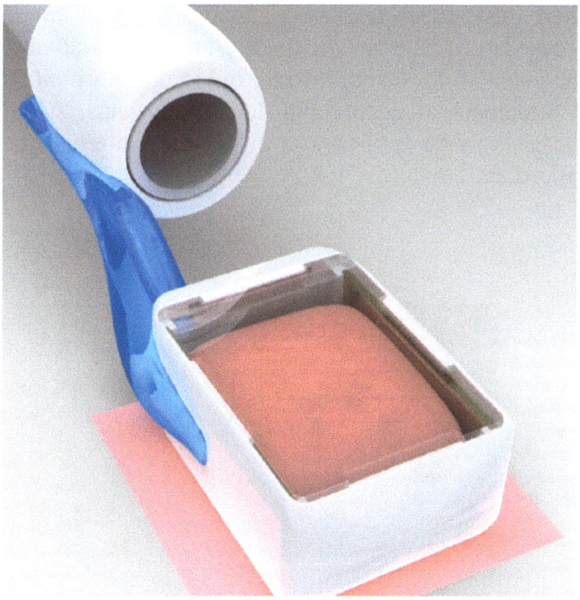

Fig. 12.1 EndoVe device which attaches to the end of an endoscope

roof that allows for tissue capture to be confirmed visually, also facilitates targeted drug delivery. The design and size of the chamber can be altered based on tumor size and location to allow for optimum tumor accessibility and tumor-electrode contact.

The EndoVe has already been applied to the treatment of tumors in small and large animals, and has been approved for a phase 1 clinical trial. It also has the potential to deliver gene therapy to nonskin-based tumors and to deliver both anticancer drugs and genes in either the adjuvant or neo-adjuvant setting.

Preclinical Case Study

A 14-year-old Scottie terrier was brought to a local veterinary surgeon with per rectum bleeding and loss of condition, including significant recent weight loss. Colonoscopy revealed a nonobstructing, 5 cm long, circumferential rectal tumor, situated approximately 3 cm from the anal margin (Fig. 12.2a). Histopathological analysis determined that this lesion was a moderately differentiated rectal adenocarcinoma. The tumor was deemed unsuitable for surgical resection and the dog was referred for electrochemotherapy. Bleomycin was delivered intravenously. Using successive EndoVe applications, the entire lesion was treated with electrochemotherapy. Follow-up colonoscopy 5 weeks following treatment demonstrated significant regression of the tumor, in association with a marked improvement in the dog's clinical condition (Fig. 12.2b).

Conclusion

Electrochemotherapy is an effective drug delivery system, which acts by greatly enhancing the local cytotoxicity of the chemotherapeutic drug. The advantages of this therapy are its simplicity, the short duration of treatment sessions, with an associated reduction in anesthetic requirements, reduced chemotherapeutic dosages, the comparatively low costs, its minimal side effects, as well as the potential for a significantly reduced in-hospital stay, both before and after treatment. With the development of endoscopic delivery systems, such as the EndoVe, electrochemotherapy could increasingly be applied to a diversity of internal cancers as a minimally invasive tumor ablation procedure.

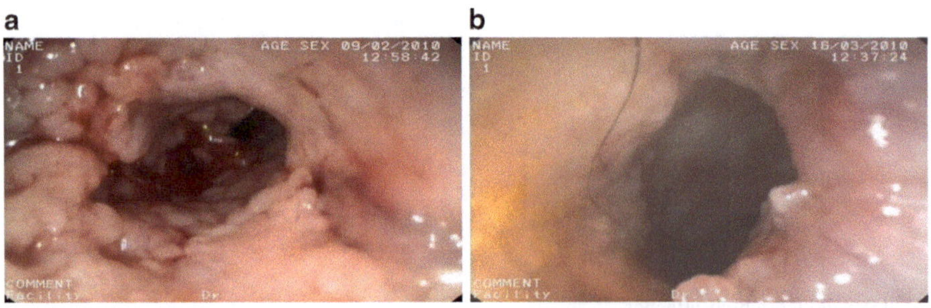

Fig. 12.2 Preclinical electrochemotherapy of a rectal adenocarcinoma. (**a**) Before treatment. (**b**) Five weeks after treatment

References

1. Termuhlen PM, Kemeny MM. Surgery in the older patient. Oncology (Williston Park) 2002;16(2):183–9; discussion 194–6, 199.
2. Easson AM, Asch M, Swallow CJ. Palliative general surgical procedures. Surg Oncol Clin N Am. 2001;10(1):161–84.
3. Shi Y, Zhou Y. The role of surgery in the treatment of gastric cancer. J Surg Oncol. 2010;101(8):687–92.
4. Wasserberg N, Kaufman HS. Palliation of colorectal cancer. Surg Oncol. 2007;16(4):299–310.
5. Weichselbaum RR, Dahlberg W, Little JB. Inherently radioresistant cells exist in some human tumors. Proc Natl Acad Sci USA. 1985;82(14):4732–5.
6. Voltz E, Gronemeyer H. A new era of cancer therapy: cancer cell targeted therapies are coming of age. Int J Biochem Cell Biol. 2008;40(1):1–8.
7. Kreeft A et al. The surgical dilemma of 'functional inoperability' in oral and oropharyngeal cancer: current consensus on operability with regard to functional results. Clin Otolaryngol. 2009;34(2):140–6.
8. McLarnon C et al. Quality-of-life considerations in treatment of unresectable, recurrent head and neck cancer. Expert Rev Anticancer Ther. 2010;10(3):345–52.
9. Mastracci TM et al. The impact of surgery for colorectal cancer on quality of life and functional status in the elderly. Dis Colon Rectum. 2006;49(12):1878–84.
10. Gunnars B, Nygren P, Glimelius B. Assessment of quality of life during chemotherapy. Acta Oncol. 2001;40(2–3):175–84.
11. Tsong TY. Electroporation of cell membranes. Biophys J. 1991;60(2):297–306.
12. Somiari S et al. Theory and *in vivo* application of electroporative gene delivery. Mol Ther. 2000;2(3):178–87.
13. Sadadcharam M, Soden DM, O'Sullivan GC. Electrochemotherapy: an emerging cancer treatment. Int J Hyperthermia. 2008;24(3):263–73.
14. Jaroszeski MJ et al. *In vivo* gene delivery by electroporation. Adv Drug Deliv Rev. 1999;35(1):131–7.
15. Heller R, Gilbert R, Jaroszeski MJ. Clinical applications of electrochemotherapy. Adv Drug Deliv Rev. 1999;35(1):119–29.
16. Larkin JO et al. Electrochemotherapy: aspects of preclinical development and early clinical experience. Ann Surg. 2007;245(3):469–79.
17. Soden DM et al. Successful application of targeted electrochemotherapy using novel flexible electrodes and low dose bleomycin to solid tumours. Cancer Lett. 2006;232(2):300–10.
18. Choh MS, Madura JA, II. The role of minimally invasive treatments in surgical oncology. Surg Clin North Am. 2009;89(1):53–77, viii.
19. Greene FL et al. Minimal access cancer management. CA Cancer J Clin. 2007;57(3):130–46.
20. Greene FL. Minimal access surgery alters approach to cancer. J Surg Oncol. 2007;95(4):276–7.
21. Robinson TN, Stiegmann GV. Minimally invasive surgery. Endoscopy. 2004;36(1):48–51.
22. Kennedy JE. High-intensity focused ultrasound in the treatment of solid tumours. Nat Rev Cancer. 2005;5(4):321–7.
23. Curley SA et al. Radiofrequency ablation of hepatocellular cancer in 110 patients with cirrhosis. Ann Surg. 2000;232(3):381–91.
24. Zlotta AR et al. Percutaneous transperineal radiofrequency ablation of prostate tumour: safety, feasibility and pathological effects on human prostate cancer. Br J Urol. 1998;81(2):265–75.
25. Posteraro AF, Dupuy DE, Mayo-Smith WW. Radiofrequency ablation of bony metastatic disease. Clin Radiol. 2004;59(9):803–11.
26. Robertson CA, Evans DH, Abrahamse H. Photodynamic therapy (PDT): a short review on cellular mechanisms and cancer research applications for PDT. J Photochem Photobiol B. 2009;96(1):1–8.
27. Zhou XD et al. The role of cryosurgery in the treatment of hepatic cancer: a report of 113 cases. J Cancer Res Clin Oncol. 1993;120(1–2):100–2.
28. Lezoche E, et al. Ultrasound-guided laparoscopic cryoablation of hepatic tumors: preliminary report. World J Surg. 1998;22(8):829–35; discussion 835–6.
29. Chung DE, Te AE. High-power 532 nm laser prostatectomy: an update. Curr Opin Urol. 2010;20(1):13–9.
30. Grant DG et al. Transoral laser microsurgery for early laryngeal cancer. Expert Rev Anticancer Ther. 2010;10(3):331–8.
31. Moran MS, Haffty BG. Radiation techniques and toxicities for locally advanced breast cancer. Semin Radiat Oncol. 2009;19(4):244–55.

Part III
Gene Electrotransfer

Chapter 13
Electrotransfer of Plasmid DNA

Jean-Michel Escoffre, Marie-Pierre Rols, and David A. Dean

Abstract Various vectors have been developed in the field of gene transfer. However, important unresolved problems persist such as secondary toxicity or low gene transfer efficiency of viral as well as nonviral vectors. Therefore, an efficient and safe method of DNA delivery needs to be found. DNA electrotransfer is a physical method that consists of the local application of electric pulses after the introduction of DNA into the extracellular medium. Electrotransfer has proven to be one of the most efficient and simple nonviral methods of delivery. Moreover, it may provide an important alternative technique in the field of cell and gene therapies. The present chapter focuses on questions related to the mechanism of DNA electrotransfer, i.e., the basic processes responsible for membrane electropermeabilization, interaction of plasmid DNA with the plasma membrane, and its transport through the cytoplasm and into the nucleus.

Keywords Electroporation • Plasmid DNA • Plasma membrane • Intracellular trafficking • Nuclear envelope • DNA targeting sequence

Introduction

Gene therapy involves the delivery of therapeutic genes into the target cells in order to prevent, treat, or cure genetic and acquired human diseases. The administration of naked plasmid DNA into target cells and tissues can be considered as the simplest and safest method for gene delivery [1]. Historically, naked plasmid DNA has not been the choice vector for gene therapy because of the variable and relatively low transfection efficiencies compared to those achieved with viral vectors [2]. Unfortunately, viral proteins can induce specific immune responses that can limit the ability to readminister the viral vectors [3]. Moreover, viral vectors, like retrovirus or lentivirus, can evoke insertional mutations during their integration into the host genome [4, 5]. As a result, these adverse events may pose a danger for the patient. In contrast, naked plasmid DNA is composed entirely of covalently closed circles of double-stranded DNA with no associated protein [6]. Moreover, naked plasmid DNA is simple to manipulate and can easily be produced in large pharmaceutical grade quantities [7]. These properties highlight why plasmid DNA is an attractive molecule for human clinical applications. However, the current challenge consists of developing an efficient and safe method for gene delivery.

M.-P. Rols (✉)
Centre Nationale de la Recherche Scientifique (CNRS), IPBS (Institut de Pharmacologie et de Biologie Structurale), Université de Toulouse, UPS, IPBS, 205 route de Narbonne, 31077, Toulouse, France
e-mail: Rols@ipbs.fr

S.T. Kee et al. (eds.), *Clinical Aspects of Electroporation*,
DOI 10.1007/978-1-4419-8363-3_13, © Springer Science+Business Media, LLC 2011

The controlled use of electric pulses as a safe tool to deliver therapeutic molecules to tissues and organs has been developed over the last decade [8, 9]. This method refers to the transient increase in the permeability of the cell membrane when exposed to electric field pulses. This process is commonly known as electropermeabilization or electroporation [10, 11]. Nowadays, electropermeabilization represents one of the most widespread techniques to transfer genetic material. In vivo gene electrotransfer is of special interest since it is the most efficient nonviral strategy for gene delivery and also because of its low cost, ease of realization, and safety [11]. Moreover, gene delivery is limited to the volume of tissue localized between the electrodes, where the electric field pulses are applied. In contrast to viral vectors, this method allows the delivery of large plasmid DNA (range from 3 to 5 kbp), which greatly expands research and clinical applications. As a result, gene electrotransfer has now been applied to a wide variety of tissues including muscle [12, 13], skin [14, 15], liver [16], lung [17, 18], kidney [19], eyes [20, 21], brain [22], joints [23], and tumors [24, 25]. This strategy is not only promising for the treatment of genetic and acquired diseases, but also for the systemic secretion of therapeutic proteins [26]. Genetic vaccination and cancer gene therapy are also additional fields of application [27, 28]. Therefore, electrogenetherapy is relevant in a variety of research and clinical settings including cancer therapy, modulation of pathogenic immune responses, and treatment of infectious diseases [29]. A phase I dose escalation trial of electroporation of a plasmid expressing interleukin-12 (IL-12) has been carried out in patients with metastatic melanoma. Biopsies showed plasmid dose proportional increases in IL-12 protein levels as well as marked tumor necrosis and lymphocytic infiltrate, indicating this modality to be safe, effective, and titratable [30].

However, the mechanisms underlying DNA electrotransfer are not completely known. The comprehension of these mechanisms is necessary for the rational use (i.e., efficiency and safety) of the method, in vitro and in vivo [31]. Successful electrotransfer of plasmid DNA into target cells depends on the ways the cell membrane has been permeabilized, as well as how the DNA molecules interact with and are transported from the plasma membrane towards the nuclear envelope. The focus of this review is to describe the different aspects of these processes.

Membrane Electropermeabilization

Basic Aspects: Modulation of Membrane Potential Difference

The key effect of an electric field on cells is a position-dependent change in the resting transmembrane potential difference, $\Delta\Psi_0$, of their plasma membrane. If the cell membrane is modeled as a thin spherical dielectric shell, the electrically induced potential difference, $\Delta\Psi_E$, which is the difference between the potential inside the cell, Ψ_{in}, and the potential outside the cell, Ψ_{out}, at a point M on the cell surface, is given by:

$$\Delta\Psi_E(t) = \Psi_{in} - \Psi_{out} = -g(\lambda)r\, E\cos(\theta_M)\left[1 - e^{(-\frac{t}{\tau})}\right], \tag{13.1}$$

where t is the time after the onset of the electric pulse, g depends on the conductivities λ of the membrane, of the cytoplasm, and of the extracellular medium, r is the radius of the cell, E the field strength, θ_M is the angle between the normal to the membrane at the position M and the direction of the field, and τ is the membrane charging time (Fig. 13.1a) [32]. The field-induced potential difference adds to the resting potential $\Delta\Psi_o$ [33].

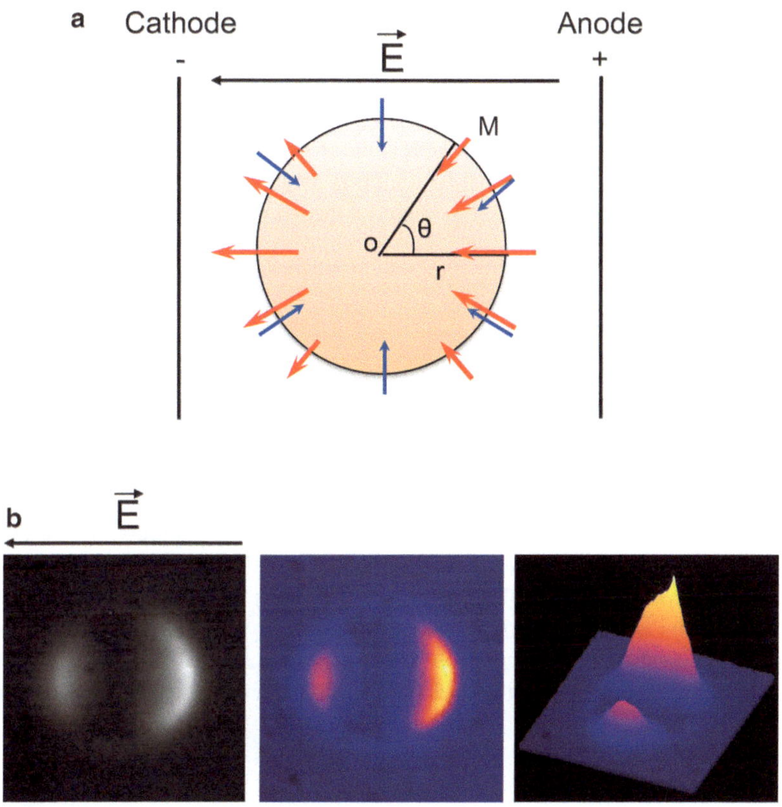

Fig. 13.1 Physical principle of electropermeabilization. (**a**) The plasma membrane is the site of native transmembrane potential difference, $\Delta\psi_0$ (*blue arrow*). If we consider the cell like a sphere and the plasma membrane like a dielectric spherical shell, when we apply an electric pulse, an induced transmembrane voltage, $\Delta\psi_E$, is created (*red arrow*). Being dependent on the angular parameter θ, the $\Delta\psi_E$ effect is position-dependent on the cell surface; therefore, the side of the cell facing the anode is hyperpolarized, while the side of the cell facing the cathode is depolarized. (**b**) The localization and asymmetry of electropermeabilization can be detected by propidium iodide uptake in a CHO cell submitted to a train of 10 pulses, 5 ms, 1 Hz at 0.7 kV/cm. Propidium iodide uptake is visualized by fluorescence microscopy. Pseudocolor image and 3D graph are obtained by Image J software

$$\Delta\Psi = \Delta\Psi_0 + \Delta\Psi_E \tag{13.2}$$

Being dependent on the angular parameter θ, the field effect is position-dependent on the cell surface. Therefore, the side of the cell facing the anode is going to be hyperpolarized, while the side of the cell facing the cathode is depolarized (Fig. 13.1b). This theoretical prediction has been experimentally validated by using a voltage-sensitive fluorescent dye [34]. Therefore, the transmembrane potential difference of a cell exposed to an electric field defines the sites (location, extend) where molecule uptake can take place.

Scaling of Electropermeabilization

Therefore, membrane permeabilization occurs only on the part of the cell membrane where the potential difference has been brought to its critical value [35]. This value has been evaluated to be on the order of 200–300 mV regardless of the cell type [36]. Field intensities, E, larger than a critical value, E_p, must be applied where E_p is dependent on the size of the target cells. This value ranges from 200 V/cm in the case of large cells such as mice myotubes to 1–2 kV/cm in the case of bacteria. Therefore, electric field values have to be adapted to each cell line. Membrane permeabilization is controlled by the field strength (Fig. 13.2), which is the trigger of permeabilization: when E is larger than E_p, it controls the area of the cell surface which is affected [37]. Membrane permeabilization only occurs for electric field values, E, higher than the threshold value, E_p, regardless of the number and duration of electric pulses. Increasing E above E_p leads to an increase in the area where permeabilization takes place and, in that particular area, the extent of permeabilization is determined by the number and duration of electric pulses (Fig. 13.2). As a whole, these data led to the concept of membrane domains, where macrodomains are regions where permeabilization can take place and in which an area is determined by the pulse intensity according to:

$$\frac{A}{2}\left(1-\frac{E_p}{E}\right), \tag{13.3}$$

where A is the cell surface. Within macrodomains, microdomains (defects, pores, permeant structures, etc.) exist as areas where permeabilization actually takes place and in which density depends on the number of pulses and on the pulse duration [37]. However, the molecular characteristics of these domains in terms of composition, structures, and dynamics remain an open question. Theoretical models have been proposed to explain the mechanism of this reversible membrane electropermeabilization. Nevertheless, the molecular definition of the transient permeable structures is not yet known.

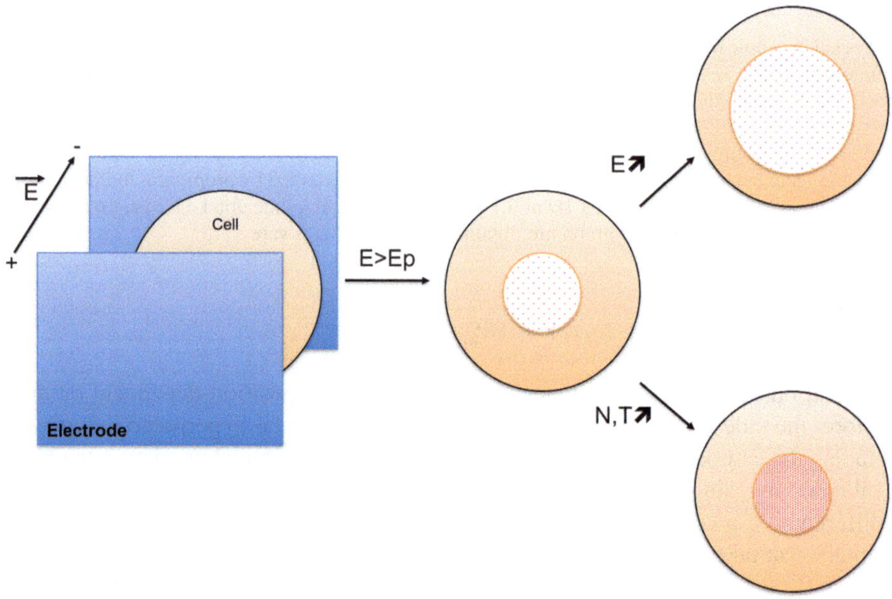

Fig. 13.2 Effect of the electric field parameters on membrane permeabilization. The electric field E leads to the induction of a transmembrane potential difference, $\Delta\psi_E$, which sur-imposes to the resting $\Delta\psi_0$. Cells are hyperpolarized at the anode-facing side, while depolarized at the cathode side. The *pink area* represents the area where the resulting potential is higher than the threshold value, so where permeabilization is present when $E > E_p$. Increasing E above E_p leads to an increase in this area. At a constant E value, increasing the pulse number N or the pulse duration T does not lead to any increase of that area, but leads to a increase in permeabilization efficiency as shown here by a *red color*. *Blue squares* represent the electrodes

Electropermeabilization, A Fast and Localized Process

The use of video microscopy allows visualization of the permeabilization phenomenon at the single cell level. Propidium iodide uptake in the cytoplasm is a fast process that can be detected seconds after the application of electric pulses (Fig. 13.1b). Exchange across the permeabilized membrane is not homogeneous on the whole cell membrane. It occurs at the sides of the cells facing the electrodes in an asymmetrical way where it is more pronounced at the anode-facing side of the cells than at the cathode, i.e., in the hyperpolarized area than in the depolarized area [38], which is in agreement with the above theoretical considerations.

Electropermeabilization can be described as a three-step process in respect with electric field: (1) Before electropulsation, the plasma membrane acts as a physical barrier that prevents the free exchange of hydrophilic molecules between the cell cytoplasm and external medium; (2) during electropulsation, the transmembrane potential increases which induces the formation of transient permeable structures facing the electrodes and allows the exchange of molecules; (3) after electropulsation, membrane resealing occurs.

Gene Electrotransfer

Basic Aspects: Scaling of Gene Expression

Membrane permeabilization is the first step of gene electrotransfer. However, this step, although necessary, is not sufficient to obtain gene expression. Millisecond pulses are generally required to obtain efficient gene expression by preserving cell viability and limiting the electric field intensities required when short pulses are used [39, 40]. Nevertheless, gene electrotransfer can be obtained with short strong pulses [41]. The transfection efficiency obeys the following equation:

$$\text{Expr} = KNT^{2,3}\left(1-\frac{E_{\text{p}}}{E}\right)f(\text{DNA}) \tag{13.4}$$

where K is a constant, N the number of pulses, and T is the pulse duration. The dependence on the plasmid concentration $f(\text{DNA})$ is rather complex, and it is observed that high levels of plasmids are toxic [42]. The effect of pulse duration also appears to be essential as it is a key parameter for efficient gene expression in target cells and tissues [41].

Additionally, the polarity of the electric field has a direct effect on transfection. This dependence of the transfection efficiency on the direction of the field might be due to the involvement of the electrophoretic force in the translocation of the negatively charged plasmid DNA [43]. While cell permeabilization is only slightly affected by reversing the polarity of the electric pulses or by changing the orientation of pulses, increased transfection levels are observed where these last effects are due to an increase in the cell membrane area where plasmid DNA interacts [44].

Gene Electrotransfer: A Multistep and Localized Process

Fluorescent plasmids allow monitoring of the interaction of DNA molecules with permeabilized cells [45]. DNA molecules, which are negatively charged, migrate electrophoretically when subjected to the electric field. Under electric fields, which are too small to permeabilize the membrane, the DNA simply flows around the membrane in the direction of the anode. However, beyond a critical field value, above which cell permeabilization occurs, the DNA interacts with the plasma membrane. This interaction only occurs at the pole of the cell opposite the cathode and demonstrates the importance of electrophoretic forces in the initial phase of the DNA/membrane interaction. When the DNA/membrane interaction occurs, one observes the formation of microdomains whose dimensions lie between 0.1 and 0.5 μm. Also seen are clusters or aggregates of DNA, which grow during the application of the field. However, once the field is cut, the growth of these clusters stops. DNA electrotransfer can be described as a multistep process with respect to electropulsation. First, the negatively charged DNA migrates electrophoretically towards the plasma membrane on the cathode side, where it accumulates. For electric field values above a certain threshold, the plasma membrane is permeabilized, thereby allowing the accumulated plasmid DNA to be inserted into it. This interaction, which is observed for several minutes, lasts much longer than the duration of the electric field pulse. Translocation of the plasmid from the plasma membrane to the cytoplasm and its subsequent passage towards the nuclear envelope takes place with kinetics ranging from minutes to hours. When the plasmid has reached the nucleus, gene expression can take place and can be detected for up to several weeks afterwards. Due to the good correlation between visualization of DNA/membrane interaction and gene expression, these results are consistent with a multistep process of DNA electrotransfer: (1) Before electropulsation: plasma membrane acts as a physical barrier that prevents the entrance of plasmid DNA into the target cells (Fig. 13.3a); (2) during electropulsation, the plasma membrane is permeabilized on the cell sides facing the electrodes. Negatively charged plasmid DNA migrates electrophoretically towards the permeabilized membrane on the cathode side, where it is inserted in membrane competent sites (Fig. 13.3a). Nevertheless, DNA/membrane interaction can be obtained on the whole cell membrane perimeter by changing the polarity of electric pulses [44]. (3) After electropulsation, plasmid translocation through the cytoplasm to the nucleus takes place, eventually leading to gene expression. This final step, including plasmid DNA trafficking in the cytosol and its passage through the nuclear pore, can limit gene expression. The challenge is to overcome these limiting steps. An alternative approach comes from nanosecond pulsed electric fields (nPEFs). New findings indeed indicate that very short (10–300 ns) but high (up to 300 kV/cm) pulses extend classical electropermeabilization to include events that primarily affect intracellular structures and functions. As the pulse duration is decreased below the plasma membrane charging time constant (see equation 13.1 [12]), plasma

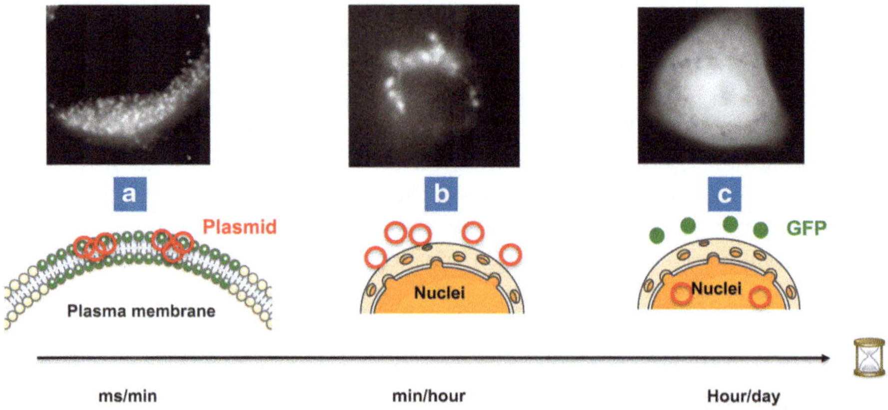

Fig. 13.3 The different steps involved in DNA electrotransfer. (**a**) During the application of the electric field, DNA molecules (labeled with a fluorescent marker, TOTO-1) migrate towards the electropermeabilized cell plasma membrane where they interact with and can become inserted in the membrane. This interaction proceeds from a few ms to a few minutes. (**b**) After the electric field application, transport of DNA in the cytoplasm takes place with kinetics ranging from minutes to hours, finally leading to (**c**) gene expression lasting several days to weeks

membrane effects decrease and intracellular effects predominate [46, 47]. When used in conjugation with classical electropermeabilization, nanopulses can increase gene expression. The idea is to perform classical membrane permeabilization and allow plasmid DNA electrotransfer and then, 30 min later, permeabilize the nuclear envelope by using short nPEFs. Thus, it is possible to not only electropermeabilize cells, but also electromanipulate them.

Cytoplasmic Trafficking

Once the membrane has been destabilized allowing for DNA entry, plasmids are confronted by a number of barriers that must be overcome in order for gene expression to occur, none of which depend on the electrical field. Studies with fluorescently labeled plasmids show that the DNA crosses the plasma membrane, but remains near the inner surface of the membrane for a period of time. Since cortical actin forms a meshwork beneath the plasma membrane in order to provide structure to the cell and connections between surface proteins and intracellular networks, it is likely that the entering DNA becomes "trapped" within this area for a brief amount of time. Similar findings have been reported for the entry of a number of viral particles, including HIV and Semliki Forest virus [48, 49]. How the DNA escapes this region is unclear, but the meshwork is not uniform and areas with a larger mesh size may allow for localized diffusion of the DNA out of this region and toward the interior.

How DNA, or any molecule for that matter, moves through the cytoplasm to the nucleus has long been assumed to be by means of diffusion. However, a number of studies have elegantly shown that the cytoplasm is relatively stiff and does not allow for a great deal of free diffusion of large molecules. Using a combination of cell-free extracts, microinjected cells, and fluorescence recovery after photobleaching experiments, Verkman and colleagues demonstrated that DNA fragments longer that 2,000 bp do not diffuse to any significant degree within a biologically relevant time frame [50]. Indeed, while 1,000 bp DNA fragments diffuse relatively freely in cytoplasm, 2,000 bp fragments show greatly reduced movement, and 6,000 bp fragments are immobile. The reason for this limited diffusion is that the cytoplasm is not simply an aqueous environment, but rather a complex system with visco-elastic properties which is composed of multiple cytoskeletal elements, including microfilaments, microtubules, and intermediate filaments. These elements are organized into a complex, crowded latticework that is constantly remodeling itself in response to a variety of internal and external stimuli. This lattice is a barrier to the movement of DNA toward the nucleus, which is evident from the fact that disruption of the actin cytoskeleton using latrunculin B or cytochalasin D resulted in greatly enhanced diffusion of large DNA fragments within the cytoplasm of microinjected cells [51].

If, then, DNA cannot diffuse to any extent through the cytoplasm, how does it reach the nucleus? It has been demonstrated that, like many viruses and cellular proteins, plasmids move through the cytoplasm along the microtubule network using dynein as a microtubule motor protein [52, 53]. Unlike many proteins that are trafficked along microtubules, DNA does not bind directly to either dynein or the microtubules themselves. Rather, it is thought to interact with the motor proteins through adapter proteins that bind to the DNA once it enters the cytoplasm [52, 53]. While it is "naked" DNA that is electroporated into the cell, any plasmid or DNA fragment very quickly becomes associated with a number of cations, peptides, and proteins that interact electrostatically and/or sequence-specifically with the DNA. The resulting protein–DNA complex is the form of DNA that traffics through the cell. Although the exact nature of the protein complement that binds to the DNA to mediate interactions with the microtubule motors to facilitate movement is unknown, several recent studies have used a proteomics approach to begin to address this question [54, 55]. Taking an in vitro approach to identify proteins in cytoplasmic extract, which bind to plasmids that traffic and enter the nuclei of either all cells or specific cell types, a number of proteins have been identified. These include a number of proteins that bind directly, but nonspecifically, to DNA as well as a number of general and cell-specific transcription factors that recognize unique sequences within the plasmids. While both studies focused on the ability of these plasmids to enter the nuclei of nondividing cells, all DNA that enters the nucleus must also be able to move through the cytoplasm, so it is likely that many of the proteins identified may also play a role in cytoplasmic trafficking as well as nuclear import. Since many proteins that bind DNA are nuclear proteins, when they bind to the DNA, the DNA becomes partially coated with nuclear localization signals (NLSs), the small amino acid postal code that directs proteins to the nucleus. Both studies found the small GTPase RAN and several importin β family members that bind to the DNA, supporting previous studies showing that these proteins are necessary for nuclear import of plasmids [56]. Further, coprecipitation assays of cells that had been electroporated with these plasmids demonstrated that both proteins formed complexes in transfected cells following electroporation. RNA interference-mediated reduction of these proteins confirmed that importin β was indeed needed for cytoplasmic movement and nuclear import in living cells. Taken together with several studies demonstrating that importin β can bind to NLSs on proteins destined for the nucleus and at the same time bind to dynein for movement along microtubules [52, 57–59], these findings support the model for trafficking of plasmids (Fig. 13.4).

Additionally, the speed with which plasmids move to the nucleus has not been directly measured, but in static cells, once DNA is free in the cytoplasm, nuclear DNA can be detected within 1 h in many cell types [60, 61]. Further, in cells electroporated with plasmid, gene expression can be detected within several hours [61], suggesting that movement can be relatively rapid, although much slower than the millisecond timescale needed for transport across the plasma membrane. The rates of plasmid movement through the cytoplasm also can be increased by manipulation of the microtubule network. In initial studies designed to look at how stretching the basement membrane of lung epithelial cells in a cyclic manner to represent tidal breathing in the lung affected the intracellular trafficking of plasmids, it was found that cyclic stretch increased microtubule acetylation and that cells with elevated levels

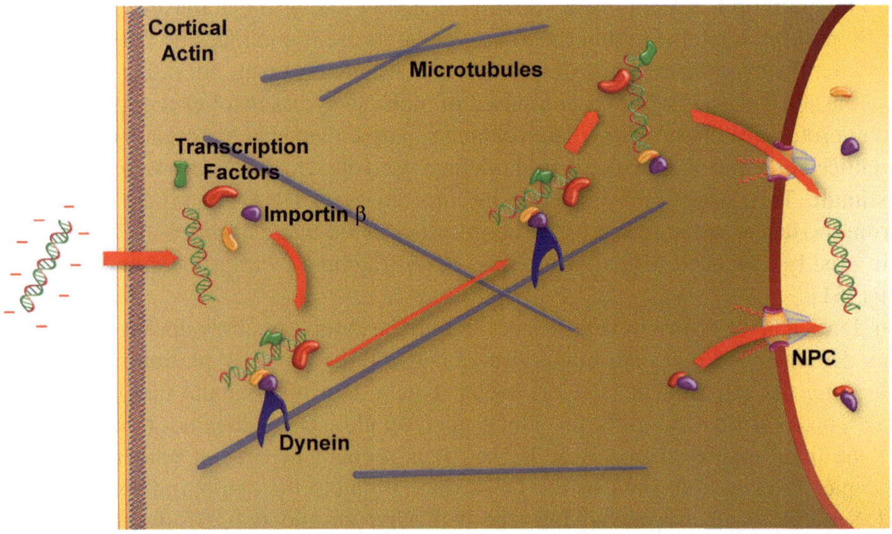

Fig. 13.4 Intracellular trafficking of plasmids. Following electropermeabilization of the plasma membrane and translocation through the cortical actin layer, plasmids associate with a number of DNA-binding proteins present in the cytoplasm to form DNA–protein complexes. At least some of the NLSs present on these DNA-binding proteins are accessible to the importin machinery and are bound by importin β or transportin, which then interacts with the microtubule motor protein dynein to move the DNA through the cytoplasm toward the nucleus. The motor–cargo complex then falls apart, allowing the DNA to enter the nucleus in a DNA-sequence- and importin-dependent process

of acetylated microtubules showed greater and more rapid gene expression following transfection [62, 63]. This effect was mediated through the major tubulin deacetylase, HDAC6, whose activity was inhibited by cyclic stretch. When the level of acetylated microtubules increased by the application of cyclic stretch, drug inhibition of HDAC6, or siRNA-mediated silencing of HDAC6, plasmids trafficked along microtubules to the nucleus much faster than in untreated cells, resulting in up to an almost 30-fold increase in transfection efficiency by 24 h postelectroporation [61].

Nuclear Import

Plasmid movement through the cytoplasm toward the nuclear envelope does not guarantee that the plasmid will be translocated across the nuclear envelope into the nucleus for gene expression. Indeed, it has been shown that in the absence of cell division, nuclear import of plasmid DNA is a sequence-specific process that requires binding of specific transcription factors and other proteins to the DNA in order for nuclear translocation to occur. In most laboratory transfections, actively dividing cells are used. Since one of the hallmarks of mitosis is nuclear envelope breakdown, any DNA that has entered the cytoplasm prior to mitosis would gain access to the nuclear compartment once cells enter the M phase. Indeed, it has been repeatedly shown that nonviral transfections, and transductions by numerous viruses, are cell cycle dependent [64–68]. Although it has been shown that mitosis-associated nuclear envelope breakdown greatly enhances nuclear localization of plasmids and transfection efficiency, it is not required.

Numerous groups have demonstrated that plasmids can enter the nuclei through nuclear pore complexes (NPCs) in the absence of cell division, although the efficiency of such transfection is usually much lower than in dividing cells [69–71]. Moreover, certain DNA sequences can increase this nuclear targeting of plasmids prior to mitosis. This nuclear import of plasmid DNA through the NPCs is a sequence-specific process, mediated by specific eukaryotic sequence elements [69]. When delivered side-by-side, plasmids containing as little as 72 bp of the SV40 enhancer target the nucleus of most cells within several hours, whereas an isogenic plasmid lacking this 72 bp sequence remains cytoplasmic until cell division (or indefinitely if the cell is nondividing) [69, 72]. This sequence, termed the SV40 DNA nuclear targeting sequence (DTS), has been shown to mediate plasmid nuclear import in all primary cells and cell lines tested, as well as in tissues of living animals [69, 71–77]. Apart from this SV40 sequence, several other DTSs have been identified and shown to mediate plasmid nuclear import in either all or specific cell types [71, 78–80]. For example, Reich and colleagues have shown that plasmids containing multiple NF-κB binding sites had increased levels of gene transfer compared to identical plasmids lacking NF-kB binding sites, due to more efficient transfer across the nuclear envelope [52, 81]. Further, several DTSs have been shown to act only in specific cell types due to the fact that they bind to transcription factors expressed only in those cells. Two such sequences are the smooth-muscle-cell-specific SMGA DTS, whose activity is dependent on the smooth-muscle-specific transcription factors SRF and Nkx3.1 [71, 76, 78, 79], and the alveolar epithelial type II cell-specific SPC DTS, whose activity requires several transcription factors expressed together in alveolar epithelial type II cells [80]. In all cases, inclusion of the DTS on a plasmid greatly increases nuclear import and gene expression in cells.

The defining feature of the DTS is that it contains binding sites for a number of transcription factors. Because transcription factors act in the nucleus, they contain NLSs that target them to the nucleus through interactions with receptor proteins. Although transcription factors function in the nucleus, they spend a fair amount of time in the cytoplasm, either after their translation or as part of their normal regulation (many factors, such as NF-kB, are sequestered in the cytoplasm as a way of controlling their access to genes in the nucleus). When plasmids carrying a DTS are delivered into the cytoplasm by any method, some of these transcription factors can bind to the DTS, thereby coating a region of the plasmid with NLSs, at least some of which are oriented away from the DNA itself. These DNA-bound NLSs can be recognized by importin β or transportin and transported into the nucleus through the NPC [54, 56, 69, 70, 82, 83].

Although the function of the DTS is mediated by binding of NLS-containing transcription factors, it would seem that any eukaryotic regulatory sequence could function similarly for DNA nuclear import. Surprisingly, this is not the case and although half a dozen or so DNA nuclear targeting sequences have been identified, most promoters and enhancers, including the CMV immediate-early promoter/enhancer, the Herpes TK promoter, and the RSV LTR, have no import activity [72]. The likely explanation for this is that the transcription factors bound to these other promoters may not present their NLSs in an orientation that is accessible to the importins, as demonstrated by studies with GAL4 DNA-importin binding [84]. Further, while the dependence on the DTS for plasmid nuclear import appears almost absolute in cultured cells, a number of studies have shown that in many tissues, especially skeletal muscle, robust gene transfer and expression can be obtained using plasmids lacking any nuclear import sequence. It is likely that when the cytoplasm becomes filled with large concentrations of plasmids, at least some of the plasmids can randomly make their way to the nuclear envelope and be imported into the nucleus independent of any DTS. Indeed, when linear DNA is brought close enough to the nuclear envelope using laser tweezers, it is pulled in [85]. Further, it has been shown that when DTS-lacking plasmids are delivered to the cytoplasm of a mouse myotube in vivo, no gene expression is observed until 1,000,000 plasmids are injected, suggesting that mass action could account for the nuclear localization [86].

Conclusion

All in all, in addition to its potential use in gene therapy, gene electrotransfer is, because of its simplicity, a powerful laboratory tool to study gene expression and function in a given cell or a tissue. The processes by which molecules translocate across the electropermeabilized membrane are dependent on the size of the molecules. Small molecules can freely cross the permeabilized cell membrane, but plasmid DNA transfer involves complex steps including interaction with the permeabilized membrane. New directions of research are needed to characterize membrane competent sites involved in gene electrotransfer in terms of composition, structure, and dynamics. If the effects of the electric field parameters are about to be elucidated (electric pulse strength higher than a threshold value, millisecond pulse duration for efficient gene expression), the associated membrane destabilization, which is a stress for the cells and may affect the cell viability, has still to be clearly described. Moreover, it becomes evident that extracellular barriers (e.g., extracellular matrix and exogenous nucleases) and intracellular barriers (e.g., cytoplasm crowding, endogenous nucleases, nuclear envelope) compromise the transfection efficiency. Furthermore, studies will also be necessary to understand the cascade of events triggered by electropermeabilization at the tissue level where new constraints coming from tissue organization are present, such as the inhomogeneity of the electric field strength and the intracellular distribution of plasmid DNA [38, 87].

Acknowledgments Many thanks for the financial support from the CNRS, the Association Française sur les Myopathies, the Région Midi-Pyrénées, and NIH.

References

1. Wolff JA, Budker V. The mechanism of naked DNA uptake and expression. Adv Genet. 2005;54:3–20.
2. Wolff JA et al. Direct gene transfer into mouse muscle *in vivo*. Science. 1990;247:1465–8.
3. Couzin J, Kaiser J. Gene therapy. As Gelsinger case ends, gene therapy suffers another blow. Science. 2005;307(5712):1028.

4. Hacein-Bey-Abina S et al. LMO2-associated clonal T cell proliferation in two patients after gene therapy for SCID-X1. Science. 2003;302(5644):415–19.
5. Hacein-Bey-Abina S et al. Sustained correction of X-linked severe combined immunodeficiency by *ex vivo* gene therapy. N Engl J Med. 2002;346(16):1185–93.
6. Wells DJ. Gene therapy progress and prospects: electroporation and other physical methods. Gene Ther. 2004;11(18):1363–9.
7. Bower DM, Prather KL. Engineering of bacterial strains and vectors for the production of plasmid DNA. Appl Microbiol Biotechnol. 2009;82(5):805–13.
8. Neumann E, Sowers AE, Jordan CA. Electroporation and electrofusion in cell biology. New York: Plenum; 1989.
9. Weaver JC. Electroporation theory. Concepts and mechanisms. Methods Mol Biol. 1995;55:3–28.
10. Teissie J, Golzio M, Rols MP. Mechanisms of cell membrane electropermeabilization: a minireview of our present (lack of?) knowledge. Biochim Biophys Acta. 2005;1724(3):270–80.
11. Escoffre JM et al. Membrane perturbation by an external electric field: a mechanism to permit molecular uptake. Eur Biophys J. 2007;36(8):973–83.
12. Aihara H, Miyazaki J. Gene transfer into muscle by electroporation *in vivo*. Nat Biotechnol. 1998;16(9):867–70.
13. Mir LM et al. High-efficiency gene transfer into skeletal muscle mediated by electric pulses. Proc Natl Acad Sci USA. 1999;96:4262–7.
14. Titomirov AV, Sukharev S, Kistanova E. *In vivo* electroporation and stable transformation of skin cells of newborn mice by plasmid DNA. Biochim Biophys Acta. 1991;1088(1):131–4.
15. Vandermeulen G et al. Optimisation of intradermal DNA electrotransfer for immunisation. J Control Release. 2007;124(1–2):81–7.
16. Heller R et al. *In vivo* gene elctroinjection and expression in rat liver. FEBS Lett. 1996;389:225–8.
17. Dean DA et al. Electroporation as a method for high-level non-viral gene transfer to the lung. Gene Ther. 2003;10(18):1608–15.
18. Zhou R et al. Electroporation-mediated transfer of plasmids to the lung results in reduced TLR9 signaling and inflammation. Gene Ther. 2007;14(9):775–80.
19. Isaka Y et al. Electroporation-mediated HGF gene transfection protected the kidney against graft injury. Gene Ther. 2005;12(10):815–20.
20. Blair-Parks K, Weston BC, Dean DA. Gene delivery to the cornea by plasmid injection and electroporation. J Gene Med. 2002;4:92–100.
21. Bloquel C et al. Plasmid electrotransfer of eye ciliary muscle: principles and therapeutic efficacy using hTNF-alpha soluble receptor in uveitis. FASEB J. 2006;20(2):389–91.
22. Judkewitz B et al. Targeted single-cell electroporation of mammalian neurons *in vivo*. Nat Protoc. 2009;4(6):862–9.
23. Khoury M et al. A comparative study on intra-articular versus systemic gene electrotransfer in experimental arthritis. J Gene Med. 2006;8(8):1027–36.
24. Rols MP et al. *In vivo* electrically mediated protein and gene transfer in murine melanoma. Nat Biotechnol. 1998;16(2):168–71.
25. Cemazar M et al. Control by pulse parameters of DNA electrotransfer into solid tumors in mice. Gene Ther. 2009;16(5):635–44.
26. Bloquel C et al. Plasmid DNA electrotransfer for intracellular and secreted proteins expression: new methodological developments and applications. J Gene Med. 2004;6 Suppl 1:S11–23.
27. Hirao LA et al. Combined effects of IL-12 and electroporation enhances the potency of DNA vaccination in macaques. Vaccine. 2008;26(25):3112–20.
28. Rice J, Ottensmeier CH, Stevenson FK. DNA vaccines: precision tools for activating effective immunity against cancer. Nat Rev Cancer. 2008;8(2):108–20.
29. Gehl J. Electroporation for drug and gene delivery in the clinic: doctors go electric. Methods Mol Biol. 2008;423:351–9.
30. Daud AI et al. Phase I trial of interleukin-12 plasmid electroporation in patients with metastatic melanoma. J Clin Oncol. 2008;26(36):5896–903.
31. Escoffre JM et al. What is (still not) known of the mechanism by which electroporation mediates gene transfer and expression in cells and tissues. Mol Biotechnol. 2009;41(3):286–95.
32. Bernhardt J, Pauly H. On the generation of potential differences across the membranes of ellipsoidal cells in an alternating electrical field. Biophysik. 1973;10(3):89–98.
33. Kotnik T et al. Evaluation of cell membrane electropermeabilization by means of a nonpermeant cytotoxic agent. Biotechniques. 2000;28(5):921–6.
34. Hibino M, Itoh H, Kinosita Jr K. Time courses of cell electroporation as revealed by submicrosecond imaging of transmembrane potential. Biophys J. 1993;64(6):1789–800.
35. Kotnik T, Miklavcic D. Analytical description of transmembrane voltage induced by electric fields on spheroidal cells. Biophys J. 2000;79(2):670–9.

36. Teissie J, Rols MP. An experimental evaluation of the critical potential difference inducing cell membrane electropermeabilization. Biophys J. 1993;65(1):409–13.
37. Rols MP, Teissie J. Electropermeabilization of mammalian cells. Quantitative analysis of the phenomenon. Biophys J. 1990;58(5):1089–98.
38. Bureau MF et al. Intramuscular plasmid DNA electrotransfer: biodistribution and degradation. Biochim Biophys Acta. 2004;1676(2):138–48.
39. Rols MP, Teissie J. Electropermeabilization of mammalian cells to macromolecules: control by pulse duration. Biophys J. 1998;75(3):1415–23.
40. Kubiniec RT, Liang H, Hui SW. Effects of pulse length and pulse strength on transfection by electroporation. Biotechniques. 1990;8(1):16–20.
41. Neumann E et al. Gene transfer into mouse lyoma cells by electroporation in high electric fields. EMBO J. 1982;1(7):841–5.
42. Rols MP, Coulet D, Teissie J. Highly efficient transfection of mammalian cells by electric field pulses. Application to large volumes of cell culture by using a flow system. Eur J Biochem. 1992;206(1):115–21.
43. Klenchin VA et al. Electrically induced DNA uptake by cells is a fast process involving DNA electrophoresis. Biophys J. 1991;60(4):804–11.
44. Faurie C et al. Effect of electric field vectoriality on electrically mediated gene delivery in mammalian cells. Biochim Biophys Acta. 2004;1665(1–2):92–100.
45. Golzio M, Teissie J, Rols MP. Direct visualization at the single-cell level of electrically mediated gene delivery. Proc Natl Acad Sci USA. 2002;99(3):1292–7.
46. Schoenbach KH, Beebe SJ, Buescher ES. Intracellular effect of ultrashort electrical pulses. Bioelectromagnetics. 2001;22(6):440–8.
47. Beebe SJ et al. Diverse effects of nanosecond pulsed electric fields on cells and tissues. DNA Cell Biol. 2003;22(12):785–96.
48. Gruenheid S, Finlay BB. Microbial pathogenesis and cytoskeletal function. Nature. 2003;422(6933):775–81.
49. Marsh M, Bron R. SFV infection in CHO cells: cell-type specific restrictions to productive virus entry at the cell surface. J Cell Sci. 1997;110(Pt 1):95–103.
50. Lukacs GL et al. Size-dependent DNA mobility in cytoplasm and nucleus. J Biol Chem. 2000;275(3):1625–9.
51. Dauty E, Verkman AS. Actin cytoskeleton as the principal determinant of size-dependent DNA mobility in cytoplasm: a new barrier for non-viral gene delivery. J Biol Chem. 2005;280(9):7823–8.
52. Mesika A et al. Enhanced intracellular mobility and nuclear accumulation of DNA plasmids associated with a karyophilic protein. Hum Gene Ther. 2005;16(2):200–8.
53. Vaughan EE, Dean DA. Intracellular trafficking of plasmids during transfection is mediated by microtubules. Mol Ther. 2006;13(2):422–8.
54. Miller AM et al. Identification of protein cofactors necessary for sequence-specific plasmid DNA nuclear import. Mol Ther. 2009;17:1897–903.
55. Munkonge FM et al. Identification and functional characterisation of cytoplasmic determinants of plasmid DNA nuclear import. J Biol Chem. 2009;284:26978–87.
56. Wilson GL et al. Nuclear import of plasmid DNA in digitonin-permeabilized cells requires both cytoplasmic factors and specific DNA sequences. J Biol Chem. 1999;274:22025–32.
57. Roth DM et al. A microtubule-facilitated nuclear import pathway for cancer regulatory proteins. Traffic. 2007;8(6):673–86.
58. Salman H et al. Nuclear localization signal peptides induce molecular delivery along microtubules. Biophys J. 2005;89(3):2134–45.
59. Perlson E et al. Vimentin-dependent spatial translocation of an activated MAP kinase in injured nerve. Neuron. 2005;45(5):715–26.
60. Dean DA. Improving gene delivery and expression of GFP by cyclic stretch. In: Spector DL, Goldman RD, editors. Live cell imaging: a laboratory manual. Cold Spring Harbor, NY: Cold Spring Harbor Laboratory Press; 2004. p. 51–66.
61. Vaughan EE et al. Microtubule acetylation through HDAC6 inhibition results in increased transfection efficiency. Mol Ther. 2008;16(11):1841–7.
62. Geiger RC et al. Cyclic stretch-induced reorganization of the cytoskeleton and its role in enhanced gene transfer. Gene Ther. 2006;13(8):725–31.
63. Taylor W et al. Effects of cyclic stretch on gene transfer in alveolar epithelial cells. Mol Ther. 2003;7(4):542–9.
64. Fasbender A et al. A low rate of cell proliferation and reduced DNA uptake limit cationic lipid-mediated gene transfer to primary cultures of ciliated human airway epithelia. Gene Ther. 1997;4:1173–80.
65. Brunner S et al. Cell cycle dependence of gene transfer by lipoplex, polyplex and recombinant adenovirus. Gene Ther. 2000;7:401–7.
66. Brunner S et al. Overcoming the nuclear barrier: cell cycle independent nonviral gene transfer with linear polyethylenimine or electroporation. Mol Ther. 2002;5(1):80–6.

67. Escriou V et al. Critical assessment of the nuclear import of plasmid during cationic lipid-mediated gene transfer. J Gene Med. 2001;3(2):179–87.
68. Tseng WC, Haselton FR, Giorgio TD. Mitosis enhances transgene expression of plasmid delivered by cationic liposomes. Biochim Biophys Acta. 1999;1445(1):53–64.
69. Dean DA. Import of plasmid DNA into the nucleus is sequence specific. Exp Cell Res. 1997;230:293–302.
70. Dowty ME et al. Plasmid DNA entry into postmitotic nuclei of primary rat myotubes. Proc Natl Acad Sci USA. 1995;92:4572–6.
71. Vacik J et al. Cell-specific nuclear import of plasmid DNA. Gene Ther. 1999;6:1006–14.
72. Dean DA et al. Sequence requirements for plasmid nuclear entry. Exp Cell Res. 1999;253:713–22.
73. Blomberg P et al. Electroporation in combination with a plasmid vector containing SV40 enhancer elements results in increased and persistent gene expression in mouse muscle. Biochem Biophys Res Commun. 2002;298(4):505–10.
74. Li S et al. Muscle-specific enhancement of gene expression by incorporation of the SV40 enhancer in the expression plasmid. Gene Ther. 2001;8:494–7.
75. Young JL, Benoit JN, Dean DA. Effect of a DNA nuclear targeting sequence on gene transfer and expression of plasmids in the intact vasculature. Gene Ther. 2003;10(17):1465–70.
76. Young JL, Zimmer WE, Dean DA. Smooth muscle-specific gene delivery in the vasculature based on restriction of DNA nuclear import. Exp Biol Med. 2008;233(7):840–8.
77. Zhou R, Dean DA. Gene transfer of interleukin 10 to the murine cornea using electroporation. Exp Biol Med (Maywood). 2007;232(3):362–9.
78. Miller AM, Dean DA. Cell-specific nuclear import of plasmid DNA in smooth muscle requires tissue-specific transcription factors and DNA sequences. Gene Ther. 2008;15(15):1107–15.
79. Miller AM, Dean DA. Tissue-specific and transcription factor-mediated nuclear entry of DNA. Adv Drug Deliv Rev. 2009;61(7–8):603–13.
80. DeGiulio JV, Kaufman CD, Dean DA. Alveolar epithelial cell-specific plasmid nuclear import. Gene Ther. 2010;17(4):541–9.
81. Mesika A et al. A regulated NFkappaB-assisted import of plasmid DNA into mammalian cell nuclei. Mol Ther. 2001;3(5 Pt 1):653–7.
82. Sebestyén MG et al. DNA vector chemistry: the covalent attachment of signal peptides to plasmid DNA. Nat Biotechnol. 1998;16:80–5.
83. Lachish-Zalait A et al. Transportin mediates nuclear entry of DNA in vertebrate systems. Traffic. 2009;10(10):1414–28.
84. Chan CK et al. Mutual exclusivity of DNA binding and nuclear localization signal recognition by the yeast transcription factor GAL4: implications for nonviral DNA delivery. Gene Ther. 1998;5(9):1204–12.
85. Salman H et al. Kinetics and mechanism of DNA uptake into the cell nucleus. Proc Natl Acad Sci USA. 2001;98:7247–52.
86. Utvik JK, Nja A, Gundersen K. DNA injection into single cells of intact mice. Hum Gene Ther. 1999;10(2):291–300.
87. Wasungu L et al. A 3D *in vitro* spheroid model as a way to study the mechanisms of electroporation. Int J Pharm. 2009;379(2):278–84.

Chapter 14
Gene Electrotransfer to Tumor

Loree C. Heller and Richard Heller

Abstract In vivo electroporation is a versatile delivery method for gene transfer which can be applied to any accessible tissue. Delivery of plasmid DNA encoding therapeutic genes or cDNAs with in vivo electroporation has been tested extensively in preclinical cancer models. For cancer therapy, direct delivery to the tumor may be used to generate a direct antitumor effect or delivery to other sites may be performed to produce cancer vaccines. Many of the preclinical therapies tested have demonstrated therapeutic efficacy against several tumor types. Some of these therapies have advanced to cancer clinical trials. This chapter discusses both preclinically tested therapies with clinical potential and current cancer human trials.

Keywords Electroporation • Cancer gene therapy • Clinical trials

Introduction

Successful gene therapy is dependent on effective delivery of the desired gene or cDNA to the appropriate tissue, attaining the desired level of expression and, most importantly, the desired clinical response. The design of a therapy must take into account the advantages and disadvantages of the specific gene transfer technique being used. Different techniques may be optimal in different therapeutic situations. Viral delivery is the chief delivery method for long-term gene expression such as in gene replacement. However, short-term expression may be optimal when dealing with potentially toxic proteins such as cytokines. While both delivery methods have uses in gene therapy, depending on the location, level, and expression time course necessary for the therapeutic transgene, plasmid DNA-based gene transfer is an attractive approach because it removes the need for a biological vector. It has inherent advantages such as improved safety, reduced immunogenicity, reduced potential for integration into the genome, and reduced potential for environmental spread. However, plasmid DNA-based gene delivery is handicapped by the lack of efficient delivery across cell membranes and low levels of expression in many tissues, even when used with nonviral packaging [1–3]. Several physical methods of enhancing delivered DNA expression have been tested including lipid or polymer conjugation, particle-mediated delivery, hydrodynamic

R. Heller (✉)
Frank Reidy Research Center for Bioelectrics, Old Dominion University,
4211 Monarch Way, Suite 300, Norfolk, VA 23508, USA
e-mail: rheller@odu.edu

S.T. Kee et al. (eds.), *Clinical Aspects of Electroporation*,
DOI 10.1007/978-1-4419-8363-3_14, © Springer Science+Business Media, LLC 2011

delivery, ultrasound, and electroporation [4–6]. In vivo electroporation was initially evaluated as a means to effectively deliver chemotherapeutic agents to tumors in animals and in humans. Clinical trials have been performed to test this therapy on multiple tumor types including melanoma, squamous cell carcinoma, and basal cell carcinoma [7, 8]. The discovery that electroporation could be used effectively in vivo to deliver chemotherapeutics combined with the demonstration that electroporation could deliver plasmid DNA to cells in vitro provided the basis for utilizing electroporation to deliver plasmid DNA in vivo. The first observations of this concept were in skin, liver, and orthotopic brain tumors [9–11]. Since then, this technique has been applied to many other tissues and animal models including skin, kidney, liver, testes, brain, cartilage, arteries, prostate, cornea, skeletal muscle, and many tumor types in rodents, guinea pigs, dogs, rabbits, and nonhuman primates [12, 13]. This chapter will focus on delivery of plasmid DNA to tumors. Studies that have demonstrated potential therapeutic or prophylactic responses will be discussed.

Therapeutic Approaches to Cancer

Recent advances in cancer biology have resulted in an increase in potential therapeutic targets. With these advances, gene therapy remains a promising approach to fix aberrantly overexpressed, mutated, or inactivated genes. However, because there are still issues with effective delivery of genes to specific target tissues for obtaining consistent expression, gene therapy has not reached this potential. Nevertheless, therapeutic approaches have been tested with many potential candidate genes including tumor suppressor genes, inhibitors of critical oncogenic pathways, tumor antigens, and secreted proteins that can inhibit the growth of cancer cells. In addition, immunotherapy has been utilized by many investigators as a potential therapeutic approach for cancer. Stimulation of both adaptive and innate immunity is accomplished through an intricate cascade of docking molecules and cytokines and may need to be selectively and precisely targeted to be effective. Since tumor necrosis and apoptosis releases tumor antigens, it has been hypothesized that concurrent expression of the appropriate cytokine or chemokines in tumor tissue can trigger a more vibrant immune response.

Preclinical Studies

The focus of this chapter will be on studies utilizing electroporation-mediated delivery of plasmid DNA that have demonstrated therapeutic potential. The first demonstration of tumor regression utilizing electroporation was after delivery of a plasmid DNA encoding dominant negative Stat 3 as a means of interference with several tumor-signaling pathways [14] in a mouse melanoma model [15]. The HIV protein VPR [16] was also used in the same model to induce tumor regression. Delivery of antisense oligonucleotides to polo-like kinase 1 was shown to induce tumor regression in several tumor types implanted subcutaneously in nude mice [17]. In a rat mammary adenocarcinoma model, intratumoral delivery of an MHC gene-liposome complex with electroporation enhanced tumor antigenicity and resulted in complete tumor regression [18].

Similarly, immunotherapy approaches have been extensively studied in a variety of tumor models [12, 19]. Intratumoral delivery of IL-12 in a mouse melanoma model resulted in long-term complete regression and resistance to the formation of new tumors [20, 21]. In those studies, this approach was used to block lung colonization as well as induce regression of an untreated cutaneous tumor. IFNα has induced long-term tumor regression as a single therapy for melanoma [22] or squamous cell carcinoma [23], although side effects such as cachexia may be produced. Delivery of IL-21 in mouse rectal carcinomas [24] or IL-15 in melanomas [25] has induced long-term tumor regression. Combinations of immune modulators have also been evaluated. Complete regression in a subcutaneous mouse fibrosarcoma model was obtained following the intratumoral delivery of plasmids encoding GM-CSF and B7.1 [26]. Intratumoral delivery of IL-12 and B7.1 eradicated 80% of tumors in mice bearing TRAMP or squamous cell carcinoma tumors [27].

Moreover, delivery of plasmids encoding immune modulators has been tested in combination with electroporation-mediated delivery of chemotherapeutics (electrochemotherapy). Plasmids encoding IL-2 or GM-CSF were originally combined with electrochemotherapy to induce long-term complete regression in a mouse melanoma model [28]. Electrochemotherapy with bleomycin has also been combined with plasmids encoding IL-12. Tumor eradication was demonstrated in mouse melanomas [29] and squamous cell carcinomas and mammary tumors [30] when the IL-12 plasmid was delivered with electroporation. In another study, electrochemotherapy was combined with the electroporation-mediated delivery of a plasmid encoding p53 delivery to induce tumor regression in a mouse sarcoma model [31]. When combining electrochemotherapy and plasmid DNA delivery, it is important to evaluate the timing of when each component of the combination is delivered, particularly if both agents are being delivered to the same site. The chemotherapeutic agent will kill the majority of the cells at the site which could lead to a decrease or elimination of expression of the delivered gene. Additionally, electrochemotherapy has also been combined with another immune modulator, CpG oligodeoxynucleotides, inducing regression in both treated and distant untreated mouse fibrosarcomas and ovalbumin antigen-modified melanomas [32]. Complete tumor regression in a pancreatic model was observed utilizing the combination of delivery of a plasmid encoding herpes simplex virus thymidine kinase and gancyclovir injection [33]. This combination was also used together with a plasmid encoding IL-12 to induce regression in a colon carcinoma model [34].

Electroporation has been used to deliver many different genes with therapeutic potential and has been tested in several animal cancer models. A number of studies have reported the efficacy of these approaches and illustrated the potential for human trials. These studies have included both single and combination therapies. Immunotherapy has been the predominant approach utilized for cancer therapy and has primarily used tumor or muscle as the target tissue. These preclinical investigations are fair models for the protocols already being tested in the clinic. While there are many more studies being conducted to test this delivery method for potential anticancer protocols, in this chapter, only the potential therapies that have demonstrated a clear therapeutic response were included.

All in all, the results obtained in these preclinical studies clearly demonstrated the efficacy of utilizing electroporation for gene delivery and its potential for clinical utility. Although clinical utility may have been demonstrated in animal studies, the potential for toxicity must be evaluated prior to the translation of this approach to the clinic where the specific gene is to be delivered and the target tissue must be considered. Furthermore, multiple time points should be evaluated after delivery of relevant doses or treatments and should include hematological and histological data [35]. Additional studies may be required to determine the distribution and persistence of the plasmid within the animal following therapy. If the preclinical studies demonstrate effectiveness and safety, the protocol can be submitted to the appropriate regulatory agencies for approval to initiate the clinical trial.

Clinical Trials Using In Vivo Electroporation

The first clinical trial using gene therapy delivered by in vivo electroporation (www.clinicaltrials.gov identifier *NCT00323206*) was performed in patients with metastatic melanoma [36]. This was a Phase I trial for safety and tolerability following the electroporation-mediated delivery of a plasmid encoding human interleukin 12 (hIL-12). Treatment was administered directly into two to four surface tumors. After administration of lidocaine, six 100 μs pulses at a nominal field strength of 1,300 V/cm were applied with a 6-needle array using a Medpulser DNA EPT System Generator (Inovio Biomedical Inc., San Diego, CA). These deliveries were performed three times over eight days. Treatment was well tolerated and only Grade 1 and Grade 2 toxicity was reported and no laboratory abnormality was noted following electroporation. Each patient reported transient pain and/or discomfort at the site of electroporation, but all stated it was tolerable. Tumor necrosis was observed in most electroporated lesions by day 11 and IL-12 expression was detected at all electroporation sites including at the lowest dose tested (0.1 mg/mL). In addition to the localized response, two patients of the 19 patients with untreated lesions had a complete response in distant nontreated metastases. A third patient who received chemotherapy with DTIC following the IL-12 gene therapy also had a complete response in distant nontreated metastases. These responses have persisted to date (>2 years in all cases). Seven patients had stable disease where tumor progression was halted, but no shrinkage of existing tumors was seen. No new lesions at any site appeared in the complete responders or those with stable disease.

In another trial, intramuscular delivery with electroporation of a DNA vaccine was evaluated. The long-term goal of this delivery was to prevent tumor recurrence rather than a direct intratumor cancer therapy [37]. The plasmid used in this study encoded a tetanus toxin domain fused to prostate-specific membrane antigen (PSMA). The plasmid was delivered to patients with recurrent prostate cancer. The apparatus used included a two-needle array which facilitated both injection and administration of pulses.

Following injection, a train of five 20 ms pulses at 8.3 Hz was delivered with a maximum current of 250 mA using an Elgen Twinjector device (Inovio Biomedical Inc., San Diego, CA). Five deliveries were administered to patients over a 48-week period. Brief pain was observed at the delivery site. Antibody responses to the tetanus toxin persisted up to 18 months. However, data on anti-PSMA antibodies and possible clinical efficacy have not yet been published.

As of early 2010, four additional active and/or recruiting cancer gene therapy clinical trials are registered in the www.clinicaltrials.gov database when "electroporation" or "electropermeabilization" is used as a search term. The cancer trials include direct tumor delivery of a plasmid encoding IL-2 (identifier *NCT00223899*) as well as delivery of DNA vaccines encoding rhesus prostate-specific antigen (*NCT00859729*), a xenogeneic tyrosinase (*NCT00471133*), or human telomerase reverse transcriptase (*NCT00753415*) for several solid tumors. These trials have been extensively reviewed elsewhere [19].

Conclusion

Electroporation-mediated delivery of plasmid DNA has seen a great deal of growth during the past 5 years [12, 13, 38]. Published studies have documented it as an important tool for performing effective gene transfer studies. The growth is directly related to the versatility inherent in this delivery system as it can be used to deliver plasmid DNA to a variety of tissue types and expression can be controlled through variation of electroporation parameters. Successful translation of clinical protocols utilizing electroporation is dependent on understanding the type of expression that is needed for the specific therapeutic application being investigated. Careful selection of tissue target and delivery parameters including electrical conditions allows an investigator to obtain the type of transgene expression necessary for a particular therapeutic application. The increased use of electroporation as a tool for gene therapy for cancer will be dependent on the results from clinical studies. Several clinical trials utilizing electroporation to deliver plasmid DNA have been initiated over the past several years, and when the results from these studies are released, additional trials will commence. The published results from these two trials are very encouraging and indicate that the results observed in the preclinical studies may translate well to clinical applications.

References

1. Li SD, Huang L. Gene therapy progress and prospects: non-viral gene therapy by systemic delivery. Gene Ther. 2006;13(18):1313–9.
2. Gao X, Kim KS, Liu D. Nonviral gene delivery: what we know and what is next. AAPS J. 2007;9(1):E92–104.
3. Braun S. Muscular gene transfer using nonviral vectors. Curr Gene Ther. 2008;8(5):391–405.
4. Niidome T, Huang L. Gene therapy progress and prospects: nonviral vectors. Gene Ther. 2002;9(24):1647–52.
5. Wells DJ. Gene therapy progress and prospects: electroporation and other physical methods. Gene Ther. 2004;11(18):1363–9.
6. Lavigne MD, Gorecki DC. Emerging vectors and targeting methods for nonviral gene therapy. Expert Opin Emerg Drugs. 2006;11(3):541–57.
7. Mir LM, Glass LF, Sersa G, Teissie J, Domenge C, Miklavcic D, et al. Effective treatment of cutaneous and subcutaneous malignant tumours by electrochemotherapy. Br J Cancer. 1998;77(12):2336–42.
8. Gothelf A, Mir LM, Gehl J. Electrochemotherapy: results of cancer treatment using enhanced delivery of bleomycin by electroporation. Cancer Treat Rev. 2003;29(5):371–87.
9. Titomirov AV, Sukharev S, Kistanova E. *In vivo* electroporation and stable transformation of skin cells of newborn mice by plasmid DNA. Biochim Biophys Acta. 1991;1088(1):131–4.
10. Heller R, Jaroszeski M, Atkin A, Moradpour D, Gilbert R, Wands J, et al. *In vivo* gene electroinjection and expression in rat liver. FEBS Lett. 1996;389(3):225–8.
11. Nishi T, Yoshizato K, Yamashiro S, Takeshima H, Sato K, Hamada K, et al. High-efficiency *in vivo* gene transfer using intraarterial plasmid DNA injection following *in vivo* electroporation. Cancer Res. 1996;56(5):1050–5.
12. Heller LC, Heller R. In vivo electroporation for gene therapy. Hum Gene Ther. 2006;17(9):890–7.
13. Favard C, Dean DS, Rols MP. Electrotransfer as a non viral method of gene delivery. Curr Gene Ther. 2007;7(1):67–77.
14. Kortylewski M, Yu H. Role of Stat3 in suppressing anti-tumor immunity. Curr Opin Immunol. 2008;20(2):228–33.
15. Niu G, Heller R, Catlett-Falcone R, Coppola D, Jaroszeski M, Dalton W, et al. Gene therapy with dominant-negative Stat3 suppresses growth of the murine melanoma B16 tumor *in vivo*. Cancer Res. 1999;59(20):5059–63.
16. Mccray AN, Cao CH, Muthumani K, Weiner DB, Ugen K, Heller R. Regression of established melanoma tumors through intratumoral delivery of HIV-1 Vpr using in vivo electroporation. Mol Ther. 2004;9:S363.
17. Elez R, Piiper A, Kronenberger B, Kock M, Brendel M, Hermann E, et al. Tumor regression by combination antisense therapy against Plk1 and Bcl-2. Oncogene. 2003;22(1):69–80.
18. Shimizu H, Nukui Y, Mitsuhashi N, Kimura F, Yoshidome H, Ohtsuka M, et al. Induction of antitumor response by *in vivo* allogeneic major histocompatibility complex gene transfer using electroporation. J Surg Res. 2009;154(1):60–7.
19. Bodles-Brakhop AM, Heller R, Draghia-Akli R. Electroporation for the delivery of DNA-based vaccines and immunotherapeutics: current clinical developments. Mol Ther. 2009;17(4):585–92.
20. Lucas ML, Heller L, Coppola D, Heller R. IL-12 plasmid delivery by *in vivo* electroporation for the successful treatment of established subcutaneous B16.F10 melanoma. Mol Ther. 2002;5(6):668–75.
21. Lucas ML, Heller R. IL-12 gene therapy using an electrically mediated nonviral approach reduces metastatic growth of melanoma. DNA Cell Biol. 2003;22(12):755–63.
22. Heller LC, Ingram SF, Lucas ML, Gilbert RA, Heller R. Effect of electrically mediated intratumor and intramuscular delivery of a plasmid encoding IFN alpha on visible B16 mouse melanomas. Technol Cancer Res Treat. 2002;1(3):205–9.
23. Li S, Xia X, Zhang X, Suen J. Regression of tumors by IFN-alpha electroporation gene therapy and analysis of the responsible genes by cDNA array. Gene Ther. 2002;9(6):390–7.
24. Hanari N, Matsubara H, Hoshino I, Akutsu Y, Nishimori T, Murakami K, et al. Combinatory gene therapy with electrotransfer of midkine promoter-HSV-TK and interleukin-21. Anticancer Res. 2007;27(4B):2305–10.
25. Ugen KE, Kutzler MA, Marrero B, Westover J, Coppola D, Weiner DB, et al. Regression of subcutaneous B16 melanoma tumors after intratumoral delivery of an IL-15-expressing plasmid followed by *in vivo* electroporation. Cancer Gene Ther. 2006;13(10):969–74.
26. Collins CG, Tangney M, Larkin JO, Casey G, Whelan MC, Cashman J, et al. Local gene therapy of solid tumors with GM-CSF and B7-1 eradicates both treated and distal tumors. Cancer Gene Ther. 2006;13(12):1061–71.
27. Liu J, Xia X, Torrero M, Barrett R, Shillitoe EJ, Li S. The mechanism of exogenous B7.1-enhanced IL-12-mediated complete regression of tumors by a single electroporation delivery. Int J Cancer. 2006;119(9):2113–8.
28. Heller L, Pottinger C, Jaroszeski MJ, Gilbert R, Heller R. In vivo electroporation of plasmids encoding GM-CSF or interleukin-2 into existing B16 melanomas combined with electrochemotherapy induces longterm antitumour immunity. Melanoma Res. 2000;10(6):577–83.

29. Kishida T, Asada H, Itokawa Y, Yasutomi K, Shin-Ya M, Gojo S, et al. Electrochemo-gene therapy of cancer: intratumoral delivery of interleukin-12 gene and bleomycin synergistically induced therapeutic immunity and suppressed subcutaneous and metastatic melanomas in mice. Mol Ther. 2003;8(5):738–45.
30. Torrero MN, Henk WG, Li S. Regression of high-grade malignancy in mice by bleomycin and interleukin-12 electrochemogenetherapy. Clin Cancer Res. 2006;12(1):257–63.
31. Grosel A, Sersa G, Kranjc S, Cemazar M. Electrogene therapy with p53 of murine sarcomas alone or combined with electrochemotherapy using cisplatin. DNA Cell Biol. 2006;25(12):674–83.
32. Roux S, Bernat C, Al Sakere B, Ghiringhelli F, Opolon P, Carpentier AF, et al. Tumor destruction using electrochemotherapy followed by CpG oligodeoxynucleotide injection induces distant tumor responses. Cancer Immunol Immunother. 2008;57(9):1291–300.
33. Cascante A, Huch M, Rodriguez LG, Gonzalez JR, Costantini L, Fillat C. Tat8-TK/GCV suicide gene therapy induces pancreatic tumor regression *in vivo*. Hum Gene Ther. 2005;16(12):1377–88.
34. Goto T, Nishi T, Kobayashi O, Tamura T, Dev SB, Takeshima H, et al. Combination electro-gene therapy using herpes virus thymidine kinase and interleukin-12 expression plasmids is highly efficient against murine carcinomas *in vivo*. Mol Ther. 2004;10(5):929–37.
35. Heller L, Merkler K, Westover J, Cruz Y, Coppola D, Benson K, et al. Evaluation of toxicity following electrically mediated interleukin-12 gene delivery in a B16 mouse melanoma model. Clin Cancer Res. 2006;12(10):3177–83.
36. Daud AI, DeConti RC, Andrews S, Urbas P, Riker AI, Sondak VK, et al. Phase I trial of interleukin-12 plasmid electroporation in patients with metastatic melanoma. J Clin Oncol. 2008;26(36):5896–903.
37. Low L, Mander A, McCann KJ, Dearnaley D, Tjelle TE, Mathiesen I, et al. DNA vaccination with electroporation induces increased antibody responses in patients with prostate cancer. Hum Gene Ther. 2009;20(11):1269–78.
38. Heller LC, Ugen K, Heller R. Electroporation for targeted gene transfer. Expert Opin Drug Deliv. 2005;2(2):255–68.

Chapter 15
Gene Electrotransfer to Lung

David A. Dean

Abstract Electroporation has proven to be a highly effective technique for the in vivo delivery of genes to a number of solid tissues. In most of the reported methods, DNA is injected into the target tissue and electrodes are placed directly on or in the tissue for application of the electric field. While this works well for solid tissues, the lung requires a different approach. We and others have developed safe, simple, and highly effective methods for DNA delivery to the lungs using electroporation. These methods have been used in both small and large animal models to transfer both reporter genes and therapeutic ones and have resulted in effective treatments for several pulmonary diseases in these models. The current chapter will discuss these methods and their applications.

Keywords Electroporation • Nonviral gene therapy • Plasmid • Lungs

Introduction

The lung is an attractive target for gene therapy. Multiple genetic, acquired, and infectious diseases are manifested in the lung and it is quite amenable to different delivery strategies [1]. Because of this, multiple techniques for gene delivery to the lung have been developed, including the use of adenoviruses, adeno-associated viruses, lipoplex, and polyethyleneimine [1, 2]. Further, vector administration has been achieved either by tracheal delivery to target the pulmonary epithelium or by vascular delivery to target the pulmonary endothelium. However, all of these approaches have limitations, including inefficiency of gene transfer, immunological responses, inflammation, nonspecificity of cell targeting, and low levels of gene expression. Based on the successful application of electroporation to multiple tissues in vivo, we and others have developed electroporation methods to transfer genes to the lung, both ex vivo and in vivo.

D.A. Dean (✉)
Department of Pediatrics, University of Rochester, 601 Elmwood Avenue, Box 850, Rochester, NY, USA
e-mail: david_dean@urmc.rochester.edu

S.T. Kee et al. (eds.), *Clinical Aspects of Electroporation*,
DOI 10.1007/978-1-4419-8363-3_15, © Springer Science+Business Media, LLC 2011

Ex Vivo Gene Transfer

Several groups have demonstrated effective gene delivery to excised rodent lungs using electric fields [3, 4]. These types of experiments using excised organs usually serve as exploratory studies to determine whether the technique can be applied to a given organ. However, they also may have clinical utility for organ transplantation. In one report, DNA was added to the lungs after removal from the animals, and in the other, DNA was administered intranasally prior to lung removal and subsequent electroporation. In the first case, immediately following removal of mouse or rat lungs *en bloc*, a solution of luciferase-expressing plasmid DNA or 10 mM Tris, pH 8, 1 mM EDTA, and 140 mM NaCl was administered into the bronchi of the lungs. For mice, 200 μL were delivered, and for rats, 500 μL were used. Flat, 0.7 cm diameter electrodes were placed on either side of each lobe and an electric field of 200 V/cm was applied in a series of 8 pulses of 10 ms duration, each using a BTX Instruments ECM830 electroporator. The lungs were maintained in growth medium for 24 h in a humidified CO_2 incubator and luciferase expression was then measured. Experiments using intranasal delivery were carried out in a similar manner, but 100 μL of plasmid in water were delivered to the lungs through the nose immediately prior to lung removal and electroporation. As in the first case, flat plate electrodes were placed on either side of the lungs for field delivery. Several field strengths were evaluated: 20, 200, and 800 V/cm; all using 8 pulses at 2, 20, or 200 ms each. In both studies, application of a 200 V/cm electric field gave approximately 100-fold more gene expression at 24 h compared to DNA alone. Further, the levels of expression were substantial: over 5 ng of gene product per gram wet weight of lung were expressed in the mouse following delivery of 20 μg of plasmid. Levels of expression in the rat lung were less efficient, requiring 0.5 mg of DNA to produce 1 ng of gene product per gram wet weight. One possible explanation for this difference is that the volume of plasmid delivered to the mouse lung was much higher relative to the lung itself than in the rat, and thus greater plasmid distribution could be achieved and result in transfer to a greater number of cells.

Transthoracic Electroporation

Based on the success of the ex vivo gene transfer, we tested whether genes could be transferred to the lung in living animals. While placement of electrodes directly on the surface of the lungs generated a high level of gene transfer and expression, we reasoned that this was too invasive an approach to be used routinely in animals. Thus, plasmids were suspended in saline or 10 mM Tris, pH 8 containing 1 mM EDTA, and 140 mM NaCl and delivered via the airways to the lungs of mice and rats. As such, several delivery methods have been used successfully by our lab and others. Also, injection of DNA into the trachea through cartilage rings following cutdown on the neck is a very effective way to achieve good distribution of the DNA. However, this requires an incision which can lead to infection and poor wound closure. Intubation of mice or rats using a small gauge catheter can be relatively easy to accomplish with practice and this method has been used successfully to deliver DNA into the airways. A benefit of this approach is that no incision is made, thus allowing faster recovery of the animals. Finally, aspiration has been used recently and results in a very good distribution of DNA within the lungs. The major benefit of this approach is that it is very fast and simple: animals are lightly anesthetized with isoflurane or halothane, held in a position resembling a standing human, and the tongue of the animal is pulled out of the mouth with pair of forceps. The DNA solution (50–100 μL for mice) is then delivered into the mouth using a pipettor such that the tip pushes down on the tongue, immobilizing it such that the animals aspirate the solution into the lungs. If a finger is placed over the nares, faster and more robust aspiration is achieved. After the solution has been aspirated, the animals are returned to a supine position and allowed to recover. This method has been used extensively for allergen administration such as ovalbumin-sensitization in mouse models of asthma. The major benefit is that it is also very fast, results in good distribution of DNA into all lobes of the lung, and allows the use of inhaled anesthetics creating faster recovery and no depression of the respiratory drive.

Once DNA has been delivered to the lungs, the animals are allowed to regain a normal breathing pattern (usually 15–30 s) and a series of electric pulses is applied to the chest. Flat electrodes are placed on either side of the chest, usually under the armpits of the animals (Fig. 15.1b). We have found that disposable, conformable, and pediatric pacemaker electrodes (Medtronics) work the best. A series of square wave electric pulses is then applied across the chest, which causes the animal to jump slightly. Following electroporation, the animals are placed on their side and allowed to recover. The animals recover and survive with no apparent trauma until the experiments are terminated at the desired times, typically between 1 and 21 days posttreatment.

We have had no mortality due to electroporation alone ($n = 30$ animals). However, we have seen up to 15% mortality due to drugs, surgery, endotracheal tube placement, or fluid delivery ($n \geq 400$ mice and/or rats). The greatest mortality appears to be when the interval between fluid delivery and electroporation is decreased to less than 15 s and seems to be related more to fluid delivery than application of the electric field. To decrease this, we have lengthened the interval

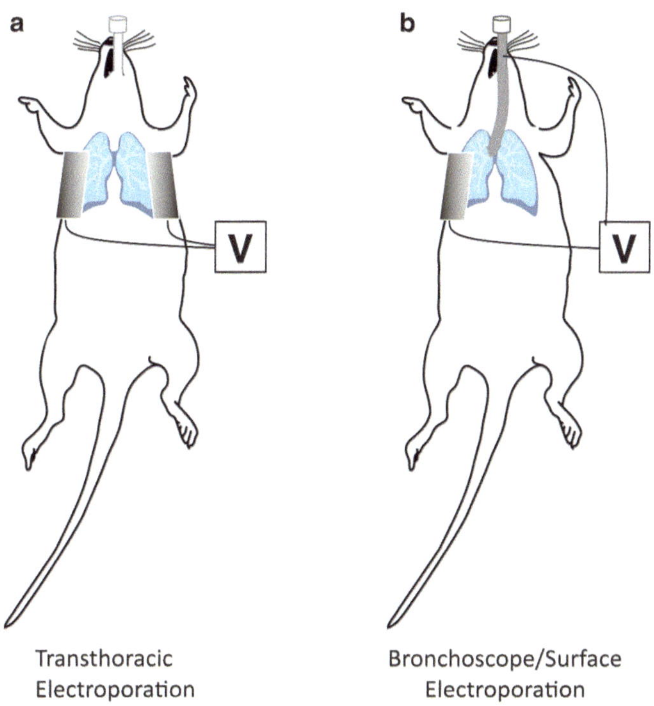

Fig. 15.1 Cartoon of electrode placement for pulmonary electroporation. For transthoracic electroporation (**a**), the DNA solution is delivered to the airways via an endotracheal tube or by aspiration. Electrodes are placed on either side of the chest, under the armpits, and immediately following DNA administration, the electric pulses are given. For bronchoscope-mediated delivery and electroporation (**b**), a bronchoscope is inserted into the airways, positioned in the desired lobe and location, and the DNA solution is delivered through the central channel. The port for the channel on the body of the bronchoscope is attached to the electroporator and a second surface electrode is placed on one side of the chest (same side as delivered DNA) for pulse delivery

between DNA delivery and application of the pulses to 30 s to allow the animals to distribute the DNA evenly within the lungs and regain a normal breathing pattern. We have also found that brief ventilation of the mice (less than 2 min) using room air immediately following electroporation reduced this mortality to about 5%. This is one benefit from using an endotracheal tube for delivery of DNA: it can be used for ventilation. Other labs have noted similar increases in mortality. Pringle and colleagues found up to 75% mortality using this approach [4]. Although anecdotal, in reports from other labs that have used these methods, we find that there is a steep learning curve with this technique in mice for the first 10–20 animals used and it is not uncommon for up to 75% of the animals to die. This is likely due to user training and getting used to the delivery techniques. However, after these initial attempts, mortality decreases substantially to the levels we have reported [3, 5].

Gene expression following transthoracic electroporation is dose-dependent. In the mouse, administration of 10 μg of a CMV promoter-driven, luciferase-expressing plasmid gives about 2 pg of gene product per lung, whereas administration of 40 or 100 μg yields 20 pg and 2 ng per lung, respectively, 2 days after electroporation [3]. Gene transfer and expression is also dependent on the field strength. These levels are very high compared to those achieved by other nonviral methods, including Polyethylenimine or DNA-liposome complexes [4, 6, 7]. In all of our experiments, we have used trains of 8 pulses between 10 and 20 ms duration each, based on early studies in skeletal muscle showing that this approach works well [8–10]. We have found very little, if any, gene expression in the lung when no electric field is applied following DNA delivery and seen optimal expression at 200 V/cm [3, 5]; very little expression was seen at 50 or 100 V/cm, and although expression was detected at 400 V/cm, the level was lower than that at 200 V/cm. Further, at 400 V/cm, tissue damage is observed in lungs and other tissues [3, 11, 12]. Other studies have seen detectable expression in the absence of electroporation, but have shown that the electric field can increase gene expression about 50-fold over DNA alone [4]. Similar damage is seen at higher field strengths [4]. There is also a direct relationship between pulse length and expression, with maximal expression being seen at 10–20 ms compared to 0.01 and 0.5 ms [5].

The duration of gene expression seen following electroporation-mediated delivery depends entirely on the cells being transfected and the promoter being used to drive transgene expression. Although the CMV promoter drives high-level, long-term expression in skeletal muscle [13], in the lung, it is silenced within 5 days [3, 5]. By contrast, the Ubiquitin C (UbC) promoter can be used in the lung following delivery by liposomes or electroporation and gives high-level gene expression for up to 6 months [4, 14, 15]. We have also found that cell-specific promoters can also be used to direct gene expression to specific cell types with success [16].

Perhaps the greatest advantage to pulmonary electroporation is that gene delivery and expression is seen throughout multiple cell layers in the lung (Fig. 15.2). While most gene expression is seen in the airway and alveolar epithelial cells, a significant amount of expression is seen in endothelial cells, vascular smooth muscle, and airway smooth muscle cells, all of which lie beneath the epithelium [3–5]. This makes electroporation the only method that can be used to deliver genes beyond the epithelium without damage to the epithelium itself. Further, the most exciting application of this is the ability to transfer genes to airway smooth muscle cells, a primary target for any gene therapy approach treating bronchoconstriction associated with asthma. However, this ability to transfect all cell types and layers in the lung should not imply that all cells in the lung receive transgenes. Rather, gene delivery and expression is controlled by two major factors: distribution of the delivered DNA and distribution of the applied field. We have found that if DNA is delivered only to one lobe of the lung and the field is applied across the entire lung, gene expression is detected only in the lung receiving the DNA. This results in nonuniform distribution of gene expression – some areas have a high percentage of transfected cells, while other areas show sparse expression. Further research is required to optimize these parameters to obtain uniform high-level delivery and expression.

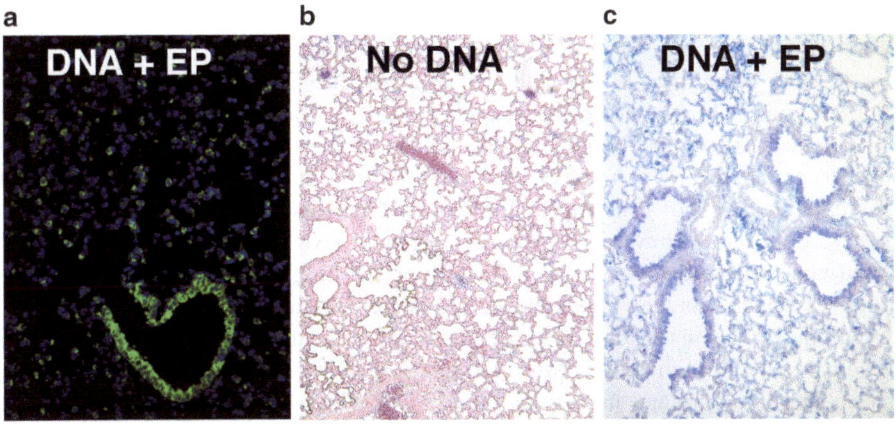

Fig. 15.2 Gene expression in the lung following electroporation. Plasmids expressing GFP (**a**) or LacZ (**b, c**) were delivered to the lungs through an endotracheal tube. Animals received a series of eight 10 ms long pulses of 200 V/cm each (**a, c**) or no electric pulses (**b**). Gene expression was visualized 2 days later directly using either fluorescence microscopy (*green*; **a**) or immunohistochemistry for LacZ (*blue*; **b, c**). Sections were counterstained with DAPI to visualize nuclei (*blue*; **a**) or with eosin (*pink*; **b, c**)

Invasive Thoracotomy-Mediated Electroporation

Several groups have also developed methods to transfer genes to the lungs using electroporation and more invasive approaches to apply the electric field. For instance, Schmid and colleagues routinely perform a thoracotomy to expose the lungs for electroporation. In some experiments, DNA in water or saline is delivered intranasally to the lungs of anesthetized mice and the mice are intubated and ventilated prior to thoracotomy and electroporation [4]. In other experiments, DNA is delivered to the left lung using a catheter following thoracotomy [15, 17]. In both cases, the electric field is then applied to the left lung using plate electrodes on either side of the exposed lung, a chest drain is placed into the hemithorax, and the chest is closed with sutures. The chest drain is removed when the animals resume spontaneous breathing, and the animals are extubated. One advantage to this approach is that no mortality was reported in three different studies, suggesting that it may be safer than the transthoracic method. However, the relative invasiveness of the approach may limit clinical acceptance.

As with transthoracic electroporation, gene delivery and expression is both DNA dose-dependent and field strength-dependent. When DNA is delivered to the entire lung and only the left lung is electroporated, there is between 100- and 1,000-fold more expression seen in the electroporated lobes [4, 15]. Although a field strength of 800 V/cm using 2 ms pulses gave the highest levels of gene expression, there was significantly more lung injury at this strength than at a field of 200 V/cm using 20 ms pulses. It should be pointed out, however, that in one study, even at 200 V/cm, there appeared to be a fair amount of lung injury, determined histologically [4]. By contrast, two other studies showed very little tissue damage or evidence of inflammation at these lower field strengths [15, 17]. It is possible that the tissue damage observed could have been close to the surface of the lungs and be the result of the electrodes being placed directly on the lungs themselves. Indeed, we and others have found that electroporation to skin can result in transient reddening and tissue damage reminiscent of a minor sun burn (at low field strengths) to more severe burns (at very high field strengths).

Gene expression following electroporation is detected in many cell types in the lung, including alveolar type I and type II epithelial cells, airway epithelial cells, endothelial cells, and vascular smooth muscle cells [15]. Further, as with every other delivery technique, the duration of gene expression was also dependent on the promoter used. Two studies used the UbC promoter to drive gene expression and detected significant levels of gene expression for up to 40 days [4, 15]. By contrast, expression using the CMV promoter peaked by one to two days and decreased immediately thereafter, giving almost undetectable levels by day 5. These are exactly the results we have seen in our studies. Unfortunately, gene expression in studies using thoracotomy-mediated electroporation was reported only as relative light units per mg protein, and consequently, cannot be directly compared to levels of gene expression reported in other studies, due to the intrinsic nature of the "relative light unit." However, in comparing our in vivo transthoracic delivery and ex vivo experiments (where electrodes were placed directly on the lungs), we found that expression in the in vivo lungs was much less than that achieved in our ex vivo lungs [3]. It is likely that when electrodes are placed directly on the lung, the lung "sees" all of the applied field. In contrast, in the case of in vivo delivery, the field must travel through multiple layers of different tissues, including skin, fat, muscle, bone, cartilage, and interstitial fluid, all of which have different resistive properties, prior to reaching the lungs. As such, it is not clear what field strength the lungs themselves actually see, but it is very possible that it is less than 200 V/cm. Thus, it is possible that higher levels of gene expression can be achieved using this more invasive approach, but further studies directly addressing this are needed.

Bronchoscope-Mediated Electroporation

Although several groups have had success using electroporation to transfer genes to the lungs of animals following thoracotomy and open-chest surgery [4, 15, 17], this relatively severe method would be unattractive to many physicians and patients. Over the past 5 years, we have developed less and less invasive methods for pulmonary electroporation. In our initial experiments, we delivered DNA following exposure of the trachea by incision, but required suturing of the animals [3]. We next simply intubated the animals and delivered DNA via an endotracheal tube which required no incision, and mice and rats recovered quicker and easier [5]. More recently, we have found that plasmid can be delivered efficiently to the lungs of mice and rats by placing the solution on the back of the tongue while the tongue is lightly pulled and held to the side. Along these same lines, although we know that application of the electric field to either side of the chest does not result in arrhythmia or fibrillation of the heart, does not cause any burning, and causes no inflammation, trauma, or injury to the animals, many people may perceive this as a harsh and dangerous method. If this promising approach is to be used in humans, we must have a method for electric field application that is less "scary" to people so that it will be accepted and used.

Pringle and colleagues were the first to develop a bronchoscope-based electrode that was able to deliver DNA (through its access channel) and an electrical field [4]. They did this by attaching two insulated wires to the outside of the bronchoscope and connecting them to the pulse generator. Sheep were anesthetized and ventilated in a negative pressure ventilation box and luciferase-expressing plasmid (30 mg) was delivered via the channel on the bronchoscope. The two wires, separated by a 0.5 cm gap, were placed on either side of an airway segment bifurcation, and the field was applied. Only fivefold more gene expression compared to DNA only was detected when a series of 800 V/cm pulses of 2 ms duration was applied to the segments, but almost 100-fold more expression was seen when a field of 200 V/cm (20 ms) was applied. This was approximately 50-fold greater than the level of expression seen following delivery of the same amount of identical plasmid using 25 kDa polyethyleneimine.

We have taken a different approach and used a bronchoscope-based electrode as a "point charge" inside the lung and then placed a plate electrode on the surface of the chest on the same side of the lung (Fig. 15.1b). In this way, the heart is isolated from the applied field. We should stress that even though the use of two surface plates as electrodes on either side of the chest may be seen as potentially dangerous, all of our data to date demonstrate that this is a safe procedure at the field strengths and pulse lengths used.

To carry out these experiments, we used pigs as a large animal model. The internal channel of most bronchoscopes, including ours, is stainless steel and the body is coated with an insulated polymer. The pigs (35–45 kg) were anesthetized, intubated, and ventilated. The bronchoscope was inserted through the endotracheal tube and directed to the right lower lobe (pigs have three lobes on the left side and four on the right, the largest of which is the right lower lobe). The total lung capacity of pigs of this size is approximately 1,200 mL, and we delivered 50 mg of plasmid in 50 mLof saline (a volume that would routinely be used for obtaining bronchoalveolar lavage fluid (BALF) in a human). Within 10 s of DNA delivery, the channel is connected to the pulse generator and a defibrillation electrode (10 × 15 cm) is placed on the chest under the armpits outside the right lung. Although application of the electric field caused the animals to jerk, no changes in cardiac rhythm or output were detected at fields lower than 250 V/cm using pulses of 10 ms duration. We did have several animals enter ventricular fibrillation when the field was raised to 400 V/cm using 10 ms pulses, but could go to higher field strengths with much shorter pulse lengths (0.1 ms) with no trauma. Gene expression was very high two days postelectroporation with most of the expression seen radiating from the site of DNA delivery and internal electrode placement (since DNA is delivered around the electrode, this makes perfect sense), and no gene expression was detected in any other lobe of the lung. The levels of gene expression are relatively high and similar to those seen in the mouse lung on a per gram wet weight comparison. While electroporation of 100 μg of plasmid gave 10 ng luciferase per gram wet weight of lung in the mouse [3], electroporation of 50 mg of plasmid using the bronchoscope and an external electrode gave approximately 2 ng luciferase per gram wet weight of lung in the pig. Since the sizes of the lungs are so different, this corresponds to 2 ng of total gene expression per mouse and almost 400 ng of total expression in the pig.

Safety

As in all in vivo applications of electroporation, at the appropriate field strengths, pulmonary electroporation is safe and well tolerated. However, at much higher fields, the technique can cause significant morbidity and mortality. We have found that high levels of gene transfer can be obtained with minimal, if any, tissue damage by application of eight 10 ms pulses at 200 V/cm across the chest of the animal. In the mouse and rat, this results in no damage to the skin and no discernable damage to the lung upon histology between 1 h and 2 days after electroporation [3, 5, 15, 18, 19]. However, when the field is applied directly to the lungs using a thoracotomy approach, much higher levels of tissue damage are seen directly under the areas of the electrodes, perhaps due to the intense electric field at this point [4]. Indeed, we have noted that a transient skin burn develops immediately after pulsing in the pig when surface electrodes are placed on the chest. This only develops when greater than 1,000 V are applied to the chest for durations of greater than 0.1 ms (since the chest is about 15 cm across, this would correspond to a field of roughly 70 V/cm). However, the "burn" dissipates and disappears by 30 min, and upon histology at 2 days, faint signs of tissue damage are noted that resemble a mild sunburn.

A number of criteria have been used to evaluate the degree, or lack thereof, of potential injury in the lung following transthoracic electroporation. Histological analysis at either 1 or 24 h postelectroporation failed to notice any differences in hemorrhage, infiltrating lymphocytes or other cells, pulmonary edema, or alveolar wall thickening between control, unelectroporated lungs, or those receiving a field (200 V/cm) [3]. There was also no increase in IL-6 or IFN-γ levels in the BALF of animals electroporated with or without DNA compared to control animals or those receiving DNA only and only a slight increase in TNF-α levels in electroporated mice compared to DNA only mice

[3, 19]. This is somewhat surprising given the wealth of literature demonstrating that bacterial DNA with its unmethylated CpG motifs interacts with Toll-like receptor (TLR) 9 to initiate the innate immune response [20, 21]. Since TLR9 is located within the endosomal/lysosomal compartment, the electroporation-mediated delivery of DNA directly into the cytoplasm across the plasma membrane seems to bypass the activation of TLR9 and the innate immune response [19]. Indeed, when plasmids were electroporated into TLR9-expressing or TLR9-null cells, IL-8 (a downstream TLR9-activated gene) expression was not increased compared to controls. By contrast, when cells were transfected with the same plasmid using liposomal complexes, a significant induction of IL-8 was measured in TLR9-expressing cells, but not in the TLR9-null cells.

Perhaps the most common argument against transthoracic electroporation is that the application of an electric field across the chest will likely lead to cardiac arrhythmias and dysfunction. In the mouse and rat, application of a 200 V/cm field with 10 ms pulses delivers roughly 0.1 J of energy. This is very low and insufficient to alter cardiac electrical function. However, if the technique is to be scaled up for human application, the resulting energy would be much higher. We measured this in the pig and found that while the energy delivered is indeed much higher, it is still well within safe levels. Since the chest of a 40 kg pig is roughly 15 cm across, 3,000 V must be delivered to generate a 200 V/cm field. Because the pulse generator that we were using could not deliver pulses longer than 150 μs at this voltage, we delivered eight 150 μs pulses at 3,000 V and measured a resistance of 15 Å and an energy of just over 4 J. This is well below the 200–360 J routinely used for defibrillation. Moreover, at these fields, no changes in EKG were noted, and out of eight initial pigs exposed to this field strength, only one died; at lower field strengths (100–150 V/cm), we have had no deaths but still good gene transfer. Thus, the approach appears well tolerated and scalable.

Therapeutic Applications

While this approach for gene transfer to the lung is still in its infancy, a number of groups have used these approaches for therapeutic or biological means and have seen very positive outcomes. The first nonreporter gene to be transferred to the lung using electroporation was the β subunit of the Na^+, K^+-ATPase [5]. While minimizing pulmonary edema is known to improve outcomes in acute lung injury and the acute respiratory distress syndrome, current methods using pharmacologic interventions are suboptimal in both efficacy and side effects. Gene therapy may offer a novel and useful treatment option. It had been demonstrated that transfer of the β1 or α2 subunit of the Na^+, K^+-ATPase using recombinant adenoviruses can result in increased alveolar fluid clearance [22, 23]. A drawback to using adenovirus is that the effects on alveolar fluid clearance could only be experimentally measured 7 days after gene delivery because of the induction of inflammatory responses by the viral vector. As such, the timing of this response is not early enough to elicit meaningful effects on the injured lung. When the gene for the β2 subunit was transferred to the lungs of healthy rats, a fivefold increase in the levels of the β2 protein was detected in the lungs [5]. Moreover, alveolar fluid clearance increased twofold over that seen in control rats or those receiving β2 plasmid alone, electroporation alone, or an empty plasmid that was electroporated. This twofold increase in alveolar fluid clearance was identical to that seen using recombinant adenoviruses, the gold standard for gene transfer [22]. More importantly, the increased fluid clearance seen using electroporation was evident just 2 days after gene transfer and was not associated with any procedure-induced inflammation or injury. Therefore, these results suggest that this is a much better approach for treating the injured lung.

While transfer of genes that increase pulmonary edema clearance to the healthy lung is intriguing, it does not address whether this is a viable approach to treat the injured lung. Thus, a follow-up study demonstrated that electroporation-mediated transfer of either the α1 subunit, the β1 subunit, or a combination of the two subunits for the Na^+, K^+-ATPase provided protection from subsequent lipopolysaccharide (LPS)-induced lung injury [18]. Addition of LPS to the lungs of mice results in a significant inflammatory response and formation of pulmonary edema. Transfer of subunits of the Na^+, K^+-ATPase decreased the severity of LPS-induced lung injury as measured by a number of criteria, including wet-to-dry ratios, BALF cellularity and protein content, and lung resistance. Although this is a promising result, this is clinically irrelevant: no one would treat a patient before he/she develops acute lung injury since it is impossible to predict who will develop the disease (which is usually the result of some form of trauma or sepsis). A more meaningful experiment would be to ask whether electroporation of these genes could have any effect on the previously injured lung. Thus, we determined whether the same approach could be used to reverse previously induced lung injury by electroporating the Na^+, K^+-ATPase subunit genes into LPS-injured lungs [18]. As such, lungs were injured by administration of LPS (4 mg/kg) and, 24 h later, plasmids expressing the $\alpha1$ or the $\beta1$ subunit of the Na^+, K^+-ATPase were electroporated into the lungs either individually or in combination. As predicted, transfer of these genes increased alveolar fluid clearance in the LPS-injured lungs, reduced pulmonary edema, and reduced the cellularity and protein content of BALF. More intriguing was the fact that by histological analysis, less inflammation was noted in the lungs of LPS-injured mice that later received the combination of both subunits of the Na^+, K^+-ATPase. Perhaps most exciting about these results was that this was the first time that gene therapy was used to treat a previously injured lung. Taken together, these results suggest that electroporation of these genes may be a viable treatment for the acutely injured lung.

Schmid and colleagues have used electroporation to deliver genes to reduce the severity of bleomycin-induced pulmonary fibrosis [17]. Pulmonary fibrosis is characterized by excessive collagen deposition in the lung, impaired gas exchange, hypoxia, and high morbidity and mortality. A number of studies have suggested that damage to the alveolar epithelium and aberrant repair contribute to the development of this disease [24]. Thus, this group asked whether delivery of the gene for hepatocyte growth factor (HGF), a potent mitogenic factor for pulmonary epithelial cells, could modulate development of pulmonary fibrosis. One reason that gene delivery is attractive for this is that the half-life of the HGF protein is very low, preventing use of a protein therapeutic [25]. Alveolar epithelial cell injury, inflammation, and fibrosis were induced by intratracheal instillation of bleomycin. Seven days later, lungs were exposed by thoracotomy, and plasmids expressing HGF or empty control plasmids were transferred to the lungs of mice using electroporation with electrodes placed directly on the lungs. After, the chest was closed and the mice were allowed to recover. Transfer of HGF plasmids prevented bleomycin-induced loss of body weight in the mice and reduced fibrosis measured by collagen content and histology. Further, transfer of the HGF plasmids caused increased proliferation of alveolar epithelial cells and a decrease in the apoptosis of these cells. Finally, TGF-$\beta1$ levels, which are tightly linked to development of pulmonary fibrosis, were reduced in HGF plasmid electroporated lungs, suggesting that TGF- $\beta1$ may be involved in the HGF-induced reduction of bleomycin-induced lung fibrosis.

More recently, another group has used electroporation to transfer the gene for keratinocyte growth factor (KGF) to lungs following pulmonary resection to aid in repair [26]. It is well documented that the lung undergoes compensatory growth after lung injury or surgical resection in a number of animal models, and that levels of KGF are increased during this proliferation. However, the exact mechanisms governing this regrowth are unknown. It has been shown that KGF is a mesenchymal cell-derived factor that is an epithelial cell mitogen, and addition of KGF protein can enhance alveolar proliferation and compensatory lung growth after pneumonectomy in adult rats [27]. Three of the four right lobes of the rat lung were removed and plasmid expressing either FLAG-tagged KGF or the empty FLAG vector was injected into the remaining fourth lobe and electroporated by placing electrodes directly on the surface of the lung. Increased proliferation of cells and increased PCNA staining (a marker of proliferation) were detected in the lungs of animals receiving the KGF vector, but not in animals electroporated with the empty vector. Although levels of FLAG-tagged KGF were not measured in the lungs of these animals, these increases in measures that are controlled by KGF suggest that KGF levels were indeed increased.

A final example of electroporation-mediated transfer, expression, and use of a nonreporter gene is using a physiological gene as a novel reporter. Mizgerd and colleagues were interested in elucidating the mechanisms of neutrophil recruitment in the lung following *Streptococcus pneumoniae* infection [28]. As with infection with many microbes, TNF-α and IL-1 are rapidly induced upon infection. When knockout mice for either of these two cytokines were infected with *S. pneumoniae*, neutrophil recruitment was inhibited as was pulmonary expression of KC and MIP-2. Since all of these cytokines are controlled by NF-κB activation, the authors wanted to evaluate NF-κB activity directly in mouse lungs in response to *S. pneumoniae* infection. To do this, wild-type and TNF receptor/IL-1 receptor knockout mouse lungs were electroporated with NF-κB transcription reporter plasmids [28]. These plasmids contain 4 tandem NF-κB-binding sites upstream of a minimal promoter driving luciferase expression so that increased NF-κB levels induce increased luciferase expression. In essence, they created a conditional transgenic NF-κB reporter mouse, not by breeding that would take months, but rather instillation of plasmid and electroporation which takes minutes and can be done in any strain background. Using this approach, they were able to demonstrate that both TNF and IL-1 receptor pathways are needed for *S. pneumoniae* activation of NF-κB.

Conclusion

These studies demonstrate that electroporation can be used effectively to deliver DNA to the lungs of living animals, both small and large. The techniques are rapid, easy to perform, and reproducible. They mediate the highly efficient delivery of DNA (and most likely oligonucleotides) to the lung and result in levels of gene expression that approach and even surpass those achieved with the best viral and nonviral means. In contrast to all other techniques developed to date, electroporation promotes gene transfer to multiple cell layers and cell types within the lung without the need to damage the pulmonary epithelium itself. Moreover, the technique is safe at the appropriate field strengths. Thus, based on the ease, efficiency, and nontraumatic nature of these electroporation methods for pulmonary gene transfer, its use may be of great experimental and clinical potential.

References

1. West J, Rodman DM. Gene therapy for pulmonary diseases. Chest. 2001;119(2):613–17.
2. Weiss D. Delivery of gene transfer vectors to lung: obstacles and the role of adjunct techniques for airway administration. Mol Ther. 2002;6(2):148–52.
3. Dean DA et al. Electroporation as a method for high-level non-viral gene transfer to the lung. Gene Ther. 2003;10(18):1608–15.
4. Pringle IA et al. Electroporation enhances reporter gene expression following delivery of naked plasmid DNA to the lung. J Gene Med. 2007;9(5):369–80.
5. Machado-Aranda D et al. Gene transfer of the Na+, K+-ATPase b1 subunit using electroporation increases lung liquid clearance in rats. Am J Respir Crit Care Med. 2005;171:204–11.
6. Gautam A et al. Enhanced gene expression in mouse lung after PEI–DNA aerosol delivery. Mol Ther. 2000;2:63–70.
7. Li S, Huang L. *In vivo* gene transfer via intravenous administration of cationic lipid- protamine-DNA (LPD) complexes. Gene Ther. 1997;4(9):891–900.
8. Aihara H, Miyazaki J. Gene transfer into muscle by electroporation *in vivo*. Nat Biotechnol. 1998;16(9):867–70.
9. Mathiesen I. Electropermeabilization of skeletal muscle enhances gene transfer *in vivo*. Gene Ther. 1999;6:508–14.

10. Mir LM et al. High-efficiency gene transfer into skeletal muscle mediated by electric pulses. Proc Natl Acad Sci USA. 1999;96:4262–7.
11. Blair-Parks K, Weston BC, Dean DA. Gene delivery to the cornea by plasmid injection and electroporation. J Gene Med. 2002;4:92–100.
12. Martin JB et al. Gene transfer to intact mesenteric arteries by electroporation. J Vasc Res. 2000;37(5):372–80.
13. Wolff JA et al. Long-term persistence of plasmid DNA and foreign gene expression in mouse muscle. Hum Mol Genet. 1992;1:363–9.
14. Gill DR et al. Increased persistence of lung gene expression using plasmids containing the ubiquitin C or elongation factor 1alpha promoter. Gene Ther. 2001;8(20):1539–46.
15. Gazdhar A et al. *In vivo* electroporation and ubiquitin promoter – a protocol for sustained gene expression in the lung. J Gene Med. 2006;8(7):910–18.
16. Degiulio JV, Kaufman CD, Dean DA. The SP-C promoter facilitates alveolar type II epithelial cell-specific plasmid nuclear import and gene expression. Gene Ther. 2010;17(4):541–9.
17. Gazdhar A et al. Gene transfer of hepatocyte growth factor by electroporation reduces bleomycin-induced lung fibrosis. Am J Physiol Lung Cell Mol Physiol. 2007;292(2):L529–36.
18. Mutlu GM et al. Electroporation-mediated gene transfer of the Na+, K+-ATPase rescues endotoxin-induced lung injury. Am J Respir Crit Care Med. 2007;176(6):582–90.
19. Zhou R et al. Electroporation-mediated transfer of plasmids to the lung results in reduced TLR9 signaling and inflammation. Gene Ther. 2007;14(9):775–80.
20. Kaisho T, Akira S. Toll-like receptor function and signaling. J Allergy Clin Immunol. 2006;117(5):979–87; quiz 988.
21. Hemmi H et al. A Toll-like receptor recognizes bacterial DNA. Nature. 2000;408(6813):740–5.
22. Factor P et al. Augmentation of lung liquid clearance via adenovirus-mediated transfer of a Na, K-ATPase beta1 subunit gene. J Clin Invest. 1998;102(7):1421–30.
23. Adir Y et al. Na, K-ATPase gene transfer increases liquid clearance during ventilation-induced lung injury. Am J Respir Crit Care Med. 2003;168(12):1445–8.
24. Selman M, King TE, Pardo A. Idiopathic pulmonary fibrosis: prevailing and evolving hypotheses about its pathogenesis and implications for therapy. Ann Intern Med. 2001;134(2):136–51.
25. Dohi M et al. Hepatocyte growth factor attenuates collagen accumulation in a murine model of pulmonary fibrosis. Am J Respir Crit Care Med. 2000;162(6):2302–7.
26. Matsumoto K et al. Keratinocyte growth factor accelerates compensatory growth in the remaining lung after trilobectomy in rats. J Thorac Cardiovasc Surg. 2009;137(6):1499–507.
27. Kaza AK et al. Keratinocyte growth factor enhances post-pneumonectomy lung growth by alveolar proliferation. Circulation. 2002;106(12 Suppl 1):I120–4.
28. Jones MR et al. Lung NF-kappaB activation and neutrophil recruitment require IL-1 and TNF receptor signaling during pneumococcal pneumonia. J Immunol. 2005;175(11):7530–5.

Chapter 16
Gene Electrotransfer to Muscle Tissue: Moving into Clinical Use

Pernille Hojman

Abstract Electrotransfer has been proven as a unique method for gene delivery into tissues. Muscle tissue has been an attractive target due to high efficiency, long-term transgenic expression, and simplicity of the procedure. Gene transfer to muscle is interesting both for vaccination purposes, production of systemic proteins, as well as local correction of myopathies. During the last decade, a large volume of knowledge from rodent studies has accumulated. Presently, the field is moving towards experiments in larger animals and humans where seven clinical trials have been initiated so far. The present review will focus on the knowledge obtained from the preclinical and clinical studies, including the mechanisms and practical considerations when performing muscle electrotransfer both in animals and humans. In addition, the therapeutic applications of muscle electrotransfer will be reviewed.

Keywords Electroporation • Skeletal muscle • Gene therapy • Systemic secretion

Introduction

Gene therapy is a promising tool for the treatment of numerous diseases, and currently more than 1,500 clinical trials on gene therapy have been initiated worldwide [1]. The main obstacle for gene therapy has been the delivery of genes to the target tissue. However, gene transfer by electroporation (DNA electrotransfer) has overcome this barrier and offers high transfection efficiency and improved safety. The clinical perspective of electrotransfer was proven with trials on electrochemotherapy [2], and currently several clinical trials with DNA electrotransfer to muscle tissue are being conducted.

DNA electrotransfer was first reported by Neumann and colleagues in 1982, where they showed that electric pulses could be used for the introduction of plasmid DNA into cells [3]. In 1998, four independent groups consistently demonstrated high transfection levels in vivo using trains of long pulses: Aihara and Miyazaki, and Mir and colleagues in skeletal muscles [4, 5], Rols and colleagues in tumors [6], and Suzuki and colleagues in liver [7]. Since these original studies, a large body of evidence has shown that DNA electrotransfer is efficient in essentially all tissues and in all species (reviewed in [8]).

P. Hojman (✉)
Center of Inflammation and Metabolism at Department of Infectious Diseases, Rigshospitalet, University of Copenhagen, Blegdamsvej 9, 2100 Copenhagen, Denmark
e-mail: pehm@heh.regionh.dk

S.T. Kee et al. (eds.), *Clinical Aspects of Electroporation*,
DOI 10.1007/978-1-4419-8363-3_16,

DNA electrotransfer is a multistep process, involving (1) electrophoretic migration of DNA towards the plasma membrane, (2) DNA accumulation and interaction with the plasma membrane, (3) intracellular trafficking of the DNA to the nucleus, and (4) gene expression [9]. Steps 1 and 2 are effectively dependent on the electric pulses and the efficiency of these two steps can be controlled through the regulation of the electric parameters. The question of intracellular transport has received much less attention, yet Dean and colleagues have shown that plasmid DNA utilizes the microtubular network for transport from the plasma membrane to the nucleus [10]. Furthermore, the efficacy of gene expression depends on the target cell and the promoter strength of the transgene. Muscle fibers are generally postmitotic long-lived cells, and numerous studies have shown long-term persistent expression in muscles [11, 12].

Skeletal muscles are attractive targets for DNA electrotransfer due to their intrinsic physiological properties such as:

1. Skeletal muscles constitute about 30–40% of normal adult body mass, meaning that the muscle tissue is a large and easily accessible target organ.
2. Skeletal muscle fibers are terminally differentiated; thus individual fibers are designated to persist for a long time, allowing long-term stable transgene expression.
3. Skeletal muscles function as a protein factory, producing large amounts of protein both for maintenance of the contractile apparatus and secretion of myokines (Fig. 16.1).
4. Skeletal muscles have abundant blood supply with an extensive capillary network enfolding the fibers and providing an efficient transport system for carriage of secreted proteins into the circulation.

Nevertheless, muscle tissue is a favorable tissue for DNA electrotransfer as reflected by the large number of publications on muscle electrotransfer. With 27% of all in vivo DNA electrotransfer papers focusing on muscle electrotransfer, muscle tissue is the second most exploited tissue after tumors [9]. That is because DNA electrotransfer to muscle tissue is highly efficient with 200-fold increase in gene expression compared to naked DNA injection [11, 13]. Persistent gene expression with transgene production has been detected for more than a year [11, 12]. In addition, DNA electrotransfer ensures low variability in the level of expression and precise delineation of the transfected tissue by placement of the electrodes [14]. One point, which is noteworthy, is that muscle fibers may produce a different carboxylation and phosphorylation pattern than endogenous production

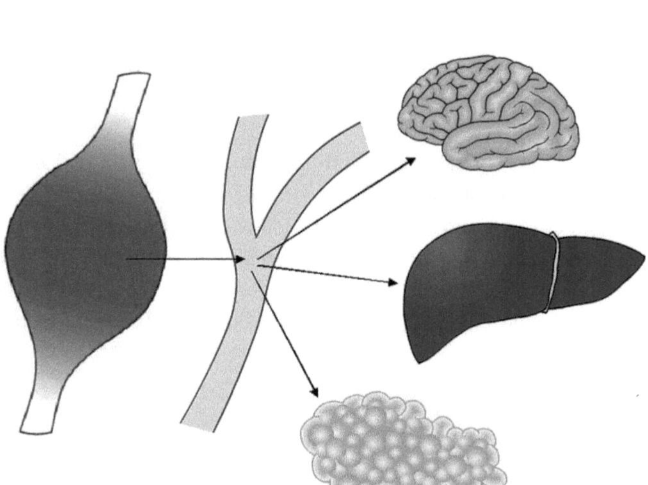

Fig. 16.1 Muscle as an endocrine organ. The muscle has an innate ability to secrete proteins, and the extensive capillary network enfolding the muscle fibers provides an efficient transport system for carrying the produced proteins from the muscle to the whole body including the brain, liver, and adipose tissue

sites, resulting in transgenic produced proteins that are slightly different from endogenous produced proteins [15]. Yet, no functional disturbances have so far been reported for transgenic proteins produced after DNA electrotransfer.

Mechanism of Action

The principles of electroporation are reviewed in the previous chapters, and will not be discussed in details here. However, it should be noted that membrane permeabilization results from position-dependent changes in the transmembrane potential, caused by the external electric field. The changes are described by Schwann's equation ($\Delta V = f\,g(\lambda) r\,E\,cos\,\theta$), which shows that the induced transmembrane potential is proportional to the external electric field (*E*) and the cell radius (*r*). The last parameter is quite important for muscle transfection, as muscle fibers are long multinucleated cylinders, indicating that relatively low electric fields are needed for muscle fiber permeabilization. In continuation, satellite cells will not be permeabilized by the same electric parameters as muscle fibers as these cells are considerably smaller in size.

Permeabilization in Muscles

Studies using the inert molecule ^{51}Cr-EDTA have been performed in mice to determine the permeabilization threshold in skeletal muscles. Using eight pulses of 100 μs at 1 Hz resulted in a permeabilization threshold of 530 V/cm, while longer pulses (eight pulses of 20 ms) resulted in a threshold of 100 V/cm. With longer pulses (250 V/cm), the irreversible permeabilization threshold was reached and cells were no longer able to reseal [14, 16]. The studies also showed that in vivo resealing was complete within 9 min. These studies were performed with plate electrodes placed transcutaneuosly where the results demonstrated that as the first cell became irreversible permeabilized, the transfection efficiency dropped dramatically [17].

Rodent muscles have been shown to have higher impedance than muscles in larger species e.g., rabbit, monkey, and pig [18, 19]. This implies that the optimized electric parameters for rodent muscles cannot be directly translated into clinical use; however they may serve as guidelines for selecting pulse parameters.

Pulses for DNA Electrotransfer of Muscles

Large efforts have been put into optimizing and describing the role of the electric pulses. For in vivo studies, square wave pulse generators are generally used as these offer independent control of both amplitude and length of the delivered electric pulses. Most rodent studies have concentrated on electrotransfer with long pulses of ms duration as one of the first muscle papers proved these to be superior in direct comparison with short (100 μs) high voltage pulses [20]. The electric pulses have been shown to act both on the permeabilization of the plasma membrane and on the electrophoretic displacement of the DNA [21, 22]. Permeabilization can be obtained with both short and long electric pulses, given that they are above permeabilization threshold, while the electrophoretic displacement of the DNA requires ms pulses, which can be both above and below permeabilization threshold. This has led to two pulse regiments: trains of ms pulses at 150–200 V/cm or combinations of one short (100 μs) high voltage pulse, followed by long (>100 ms) pulse(s) of low voltage pulses [23].

Monitoring of Tissue Permeabilization in Real Time

The most noticeable, measurable change in tissues undergoing electric pulsing is an increase in tissue conductivity and decrease in tissue resistance due to membrane permeabilization. This changes the electric field distribution and the corresponding current as predicted by Ohm's law *(R (resistance) = V (voltage)/I (current))*. Thus if the resistance drops, while the voltage is maintained constant, the current (flow of electric charge) through the tissue will increase (Fig. 16.2). In larger animals, where the muscle impedance is lower, this current increase is augmented. The current is important for the generation of heat (watt) as predicted by the following equation: W *(watt)* = $I^2 * R * t$ *(time)*. If the increase in current is not controlled, it might lead to tissue heating with subsequently tissue damage and pain [24].

Regulation of Expression

Intrinsic in the DNA electrotransfer method lies the possibility to control gene expression as it offers several ways of reaching target concentrations in vivo. These include (1) plasmid amount, (2) area of transfection, (3) promoter systems, and/or (4) retransfection [25].

Many studies have shown a clear dose-dependency between the amount of injected plasmid and the level of gene expression. However, as the efficiency of the transcription depends on promoter strength, target cell, and species, no general recommendations of plasmid concentration can be proposed. Nevertheless, plasmid concentrations ranging from 0.05 to 2 μg/μL have typically been used for muscle tissue. It should be noted that excessive plasmid DNA can lead to decreased gene expression probably due to toxic effects of the DNA [25].

A particular feature of DNA electrotransfer is the selective target of the area encompassed by the electrodes, thus electrode placement can be used as a restrictor of the anatomical extent of the transfected muscle tissue. With the current electrode configurations, this area maximally covers 1 cm^3. As much more muscle tissue is available, transfection at multiple sites can increase the total level of transgenic expression. It should be noted that the transgenic product probably is distributed throughout the transfected cells, which for the muscle fibers can be many centimeters.

Inducible promoter systems are available where the level of gene expression can be controlled by adjusting the administered dose of a given inducer drug e.g., doxycycline [25, 26]. These systems have proven to give good control in rodents and monkeys, yet the adverse effects of the inducer drug discourage their clinical use.

a b

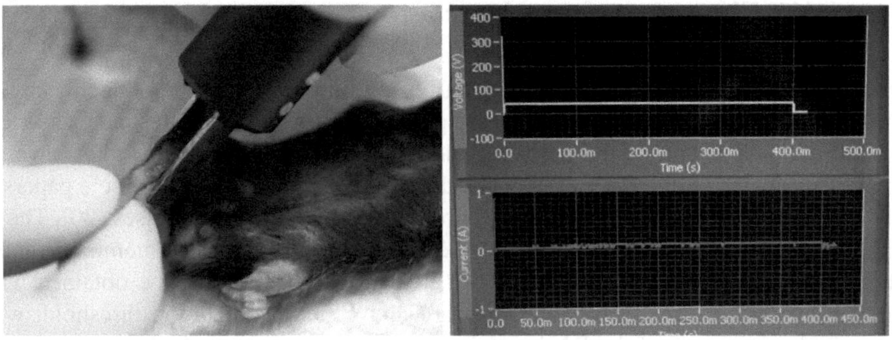

Fig. 16.2 Pulse application to mouse muscle and a representative current trace. (**a**) Application of electric pulses to the tibialis cranialis muscle of a C57Black/C mouse using plate electrodes. (**b**) A representative current trace measured during the application of HV + LV pulses as depicted in (**a**)). The upper curve represents the applied voltage, while the lower curve shows the current measured during pulse application

Finally, DNA electrotransfer shows no immunogenicity towards the vector, meaning that the delivery can be repeated without risk of inducing an immunological reaction. Several studies have shown that retransfer to muscles results in secondary increases in transgenic expression [26–28].

Practical Considerations for DNA Electrotransfer to Muscle

DNA electrotransfer to muscle tissue is basically injection of an isotonic plasmid solution into the muscle, followed by the application of electric pulses by means of electrodes, which are placed around the injection site. Although simple, several points must be considered for successful transfection.

Plasmid Composition

Generally, the plasmid must be composed of a promoter, signal sequences, gene-of-interest, and trafficking signals. Most rodent studies have been conducted using the constitutive active CMV or CAGGS promoters. Experience with larger animal studies suggests that these viral/bacterial promoters are not as efficient in larger animals as seen in rodents. Instead, natural or synthetic muscle-specific promoters including the ubiquitin promoters have been used [29]. Inducible promoter systems are also available, however these rely on administration of an inducer drug e.g., doxycycline to turn on gene expression [30]. Signal sequences helps direct the product to the correct cellular compartment e.g., the secretory pathway [31]. Currently, all studies in larger animals including humans utilize codon optimization to maximize gene expression in the given species. Finally, intracellular trafficking signals including the SV40 enhancer site can facilitate translocation to the nucleus and increase gene expression [32].

Intramuscular Injection

For small animals, the injection volume should be adjusted to the holding capacity of the muscle. Preferentially, the plasmid solution should be injected along the muscle fibers to ensure good distribution along the fibers. For smaller muscles, multiple injections are not recommended as the plasmid might seep out of the previous injection sites.

Electrodes

Application of the electric field results from the voltage applied between two electrodes, thus the electrode design is important for the electric field distribution and in turn, the transfection efficacy. Various electrode designs are available, but electrodes are generally divided into needle or plate electrodes (see also Chap. 5). Plate electrodes can be used to treat superficial tissues and rodent muscles, while needle electrodes can target deeper lying tissues e.g., muscles in larger animals.

For DNA electrotransfer to muscles in small mammals, the most practical way of delivering the electric pulses is by placing plate electrodes around the leg. This prevents surgical interventions and ensures delivery of a homogenous field. Yet good contact between leg and electrodes must be ensured by depilation and application of electrode gel.

For clinical use, needle electrodes of various designs are generally used. Models include a six-needle circular electrode, a hexagonal electrode, and an electrode with two opposing arrays of needles [33]. At least two patented solutions for integrated plasmid injection and needle electrodes exist: Trigrid (Ichor) and Elgen (Inovio) (See Chap. 5). These systems are used in ongoing clinical trials for muscle electrotransfer.

Application of Electric Pulses to Muscles In Vivo

Application of electric pulses to muscles must consider muscle fiber geometry. Placement of the electrodes parallel to the muscle fibers ensures a homogenous field and even transfection in the central region between the two electrodes. In contrast, placement of the electrodes perpendicular to the muscle fibers results in a skewed field distribution with high field strengths near the electrodes and low field strengths in the body of the muscle. In fact, one of the first studies on muscle transfection delivered the electric pulses perpendicular to the muscle fibers, resulting in cell death near the electrodes, transfection in an area, and no changes in the middle of the muscles [13].

Toxicity

The first clinical muscle vaccination studies showed that electrotransfer is well tolerated with no severe side effects and all patients completed the treatment [34]. Applying electric pulses in muscles always results in muscle contraction, even in anesthetized subjects. Also, the frequency of the pulses determines how many muscle contractions are experienced. In the first clinical trials with electrotransfer to the deltoid muscle, the electric pulses were applied without analgesia. In these studies, the patients reported pain for the procedure to be one for needle insertion and four for the electric pulse application on the visual analog pain scale (scale 0–10, with 10 being worst pain imaginable) [35]. The pain subsided within minutes. At 48 h after treatment, 97% of the patients reported no more pain. No systemic increases in markers of muscle damage, i.e., creatine kinase (CK) or lactate dehydrogenase (LDH), were observed, and lymphocyte and neutrophil counts remained unchanged throughout the study. All subjects were willing to undergo the procedure again.

Rodent studies have investigated the physiological effect of electrotransfer on muscles. These studies have shown a transient exchange of ions across the sarcolemma, loss of ATP, and a drop in the contractile force immediately after pulse application [36]. These changes are largely dependent on the pulse parameters, as muscle damage and regeneration were only observed for the more rigid high voltage pulse regiments. Likewise, differential gene expression profiles have been investigated after electrotransfer, showing modest changes in gene expression, mainly in genes involved in cytoskeleton and intracellular transport [37]. Regardless of pulse parameters, all studies have shown full muscle recovery after 1–2 weeks, where increased transgenic expression persists.

Therapeutic Use of DNA Electrotransfer to Muscle Tissue

Therapeutic use of DNA electrotransfer to muscle tissue involves vaccination purposes, systemic delivery of therapeutic proteins and local intramuscular expression. The clinical advances have so far been made within DNA vaccines to muscle, where a large preclinical literature exists exploring systemic release of therapeutic proteins after DNA electrotransfer to muscle tissue. The ongoing clinical trials are summarized in Table 16.1, while examples of different therapeutic applications of muscle electrotransfer are discussed below.

Table 16.1 Ongoing clinical trials using muscle electrotransfer

Condition	Status as of August 2009	Enrolled	Primary outcome	Intervention	Clinical Trial.gov identifier	Sponsor
Prostate cancer	Open		A phase I/II trial of DNA vaccine with a PSMA27/pDom fusion gene given through intramuscular injection in HLA A2+ patients with prostate carcinomas with or without electroporation	Biological: prostate specific membrane antigen (PSMA)/pdom fusion gene Device: Medpulser DDS device	UK-112	Inovio biomedical corporation
Papillomavirus infections	Open	24	Safety and tolerability of escalating doses of VGX-3100, administered by IM injection with EP to adult female subjects postsurgical or ablative treatment of grade 2 or 3 CIN as adjuvant treatment	Biological: VGX-3100, E6 and E7 proteins of HPV subtypes 16 and 18 Device: CELLECTRA constant current device	NCT00685412	VGX pharmaceuticals, Inc.
Chronic hepatitis C virus infections	Open	12	Safety and tolerability of electroporation mediated IM delivery of CHRONVAC-C® in chronically HCV infected, treatment naive patients with low viral load	Biological: CHRONVAC-C® Device: Medpulser DDS device	NCT00563173	Tripep AB
Malignant melanoma	Open	25	Safety and feasibility of electroporation mediated intramuscular delivery of a mouse tyrosinase plasmid DNA vaccine in patients with stage IIB, IIC, III, or IV melanoma	Biological: xenogeneic tyrosinase DNA vaccine Device: TriGrid delivery system	NCT00471133	Ichor medical systems incorporated
HIV Infections	Open, accrual completed	40	Safety of an intramuscular prime and boost injection of the ADVAX DNA-based HIV vaccine via TriGrid™ electroporation at three dosing levels	Biological: ADVAX HIV DNA vaccine Device: TriGrid™ delivery system	NCT00545987	Rockefeller university
Healthy adults	Completed	24	Assessment of the tolerability of the MedPulser DDS device	Biological: V930 Device: Medpulser DDS device	NCT00721461	Merck

DNA Vaccination

DNA vaccination by electrotransfer is extensively reviewed in Chap. 18, and the results of the different studies will therefore not be covered in this chapter. However, it is noteworthy that the role of the electric pulses has additional roles in DNA vaccination compared to transfection studies. The role of the electric pulses are both to increase the number of transfected cells and induce mild tissue damage with local inflammation, and increased recruitment of antigen-presenting cells and the activation of danger signals. Thus, electric parameters are typically more rigid than those used for regular DNA electrotransfer.

Systemic Delivery of Therapeutic Proteins

A potentially large benefit of muscle electrotransfer is systemic secretion of therapeutic proteins. Muscles produce and secrete endocrine factors such as interleukin-6, interleukin-8, and leukemia inhibitory factor (LIF) during exercise, proving their potential as exogenous protein factories [38]. Typical examples of potential therapeutic proteins, which have been electrotransferred to muscle tissue, include anticancer agents, hematopoietic growth factors, and metabolic proteins.

One molecule, which is close to clinical testing for systemic release, is GHRH. GHRH stimulates the growth hormone axis. Overexpression of GHRH in muscles has been shown to ensure maintenance of the pulsatile release of GH and respond to endogenous feedback regulation. A number of studies have investigated the role of GHRH in anemia and cachexia associated with cancer and renal failure. In these studies with cancer-bearing or old dogs, long-term expression of transgenic GHRH is associated with increased weight, restoration of activity levels and exercise tolerance, and improvement in hematological factors, proving a role for GHRH in treatment of the catabolic process associated with aging and cancer.

The single most studied molecule for muscle electrotransfer is erythropoietin (EPO) probably due to its easy detection and high efficiency [28, 39–42]. A small amount of EPO is enough to generate physiological effects. In fact, transferring as little as 0.5 μg of plasmid into one muscle results in large increases in the hemoglobin levels in mice and 20-fold increases in circulating EPO [25, 26]. The clinical potential of EPO electrotransfer has been proven in beta-thalessemic mice, where EPO electrotransfer results in both increases in hemoglobin levels and correction of erythrocytes phenotype with increased erythrocyte lifespan [27].

Other potential hematopoietic candidates include factor VIII [43] and IX [44], which have been tested for correction of hemophilia A and B, respectively in mice and dogs. In these studies, as little as 0.5–2% of normal protein levels were enough to reverse the clinical phenotype. This has made these diseases attractive for gene therapy and trials with other delivery methods that have been going on for years, while electrotransfer could be a possible alternative.

A large focus has been on generating muscle-secreted anticancer agents such as interleukins (IL-12) [20, 45, 46], interferons (IFN-α) [47–49], and antiangiogenic factors (metargidin) [50, 51]. All these agents have shown efficient antitumor effect in rodent studies with regression of transplanted tumor and suppression of metastases with foreseen clinical advances.

In addition to the above-mentioned candidates, a large number of molecules have been electrotransferred to study their potential in treatment of disorders like diabetes, ischemia, atherosclerosis, neuropathy, and autoimmune diseases. These have been reviewed in detail in [52] and [53].

DNA Electrotransfer of Genes with Local Effect

Among muscle-specific diseases, the myopathies, e.g., Duchenne muscular dystrophy, are the most pronounced. The most severe dystrophies are characterized by defects in the dystrophin gene, which encodes a cellular scaffolding protein. Several preclinical studies have electrotransferred full-length dystrophin (>17 kb) or shorter versions of the gene, minidystrophin or microdystrophin, into the dystrophic muscles, and found dystrophin formation at the plasma membrane increased muscle fiber strength and improved motor function [54–56]. A different approach to treatment is electrotransfer of oligonucleotides, which can introduce exon shipping and alternative splicing, resulting in a functional dystrophin protein [57]. These studies have also found dystrophin formation at the plasma membrane, and increase muscle fiber robustness and strength.

In the last couple of years, many groups have taken up DNA electrotransfer as a research tool for studying the biological effects of proteins in muscles. Examples include electrotransfer of IGF-1 [58–63] and myogenin [64] for studying muscle regeneration after injury. Other examples of muscle processes, which have been studied by overexpression of mediator molecules, include glucose uptake [65, 66], lipid metabolism [67–69], muscle fiber composition [70, 71], and muscle hypertrophy [72].

Conclusion

Muscle electrotransfer is the nonviral transfer of genes into muscle with high efficiency. It has the advantages of being fast, easy to perform, cost-efficient, and nonimmunological. In this chapter, the mechanisms for muscle electrotransfer and practical considerations when transfecting both animals and humans have been covered in details, showing the large amount of knowledge on muscle electrotransfer, which has been generated during the last decade. The therapeutic perspectives of muscle electrotransfer ranges from the already initiated clinical trials on DNA vaccination to trials utilizing the muscle's potential to act as an endocrine organ, secreting proteins at therapeutic concentrations for treatment of e.g., anemia, inflammatory diseases, and cancer.

References

1. Gene Therapy Clinical Trials Worldwide. http://www.wiley.co.uk/wileychi/genmed/clinical/. 16th September 2009.
2. Belehradek M, Domenge C, Luboinski B, Orlowski S, Belehradek Jr J, Mir LM. Electrochemotherapy, a new antitumor treatment. First clinical phase I-II trial. Cancer. 1993;72(12):3694–700.
3. Neumann E, Schaefer-Ridder M, Wang Y, Hofschneider H. Gene transfer into mouse lyoma cells by electroporation in high electric fields. EMBO J. 1982;1(7):841–5.
4. Aihara H, Miyazaki J. Gene transfer into muscle by electroporation *in vivo*. Nat Biotechnol. 1998;16:867–70.
5. Mir LM, Bureau MF, Rangara R, Schwartz B, Scherman D. Long term, high level *in vivo* gene expression after electric pulse-mediated gene transfer into skeletal muscle. C R Acad Sci Paris. 1998;321:893–9.
6. Rols MP, Delteil C, Golzio M, Dumond P, Cros S, Teissie J. *In vivo* electrically mediated protein and gene transfer in murine melanoma. Nat Biotechnol. 1998;16:168–71.
7. Suzuki T, Shin B, Fujikura K, Matsuaki T, Takata K. Direct gene transfer into rat liver cells by *in vivo* electroporation. FEBS Lett. 1998;425:436–40.
8. Mir LM, Moller PH, Andre F, Gehl J. Electric pulse-mediated gene delivery to various animal tissues. Adv Genet. 2005;54:83–114.
9. Favard C, Dean DS, Rols MP. Electrotransfer as a non viral method of gene delivery. Curr Gene Ther. 2007;7(1):67–77.

10. Vaughan EE, Dean DA. Intracellular trafficking of plasmids during transfection is mediated by microtubules. Mol Ther. 2005;13(2):422–8.
11. Mir LM, Bureau MF, Gehl J, Rangara R, Rouy D, Caillaud JM, et al. High-efficiency gene transfer into skeletal muscle mediated by electric pulses. Proc Natl Acad Sci USA. 1999;96(8):4262–7.
12. Muramatsu T, Arakawa S, Fukazawa K, Fujiwara Y, Yishida T, Sasaki R, et al. *In vivo* gene electroporation in skeletal muscle with special reference to the duration of gene expression. Int J Mol Med. 2001;7(1):37–42.
13. Mathiesen I. Electropermeabilisation of skeletal muscle enhances gene transfer *in vivo*. Gene Ther. 1999;6:508–14.
14. Gehl J, Sorensen TH, Nielsen K, Raskmark P, Nielsen SL, Skovsgaard T, et al. *In vivo* electroporation of skeletal muscle: threshold, efficacy and relation to electric field distribution. Biochim Biophys Acta. 1999;1428(2–3):233–40.
15. Lu QL, Bou-Gharios G, Partridge TA. Non-viral gene delivery in skeletal muscle: a protein factory. Gene Ther. 2003;10:131–42.
16. Gehl J, Mir LM. Determination of optimal parameters for *in vivo* gene transfer by electroporation, using a rapid *in vivo* test for cell permeabilization. Biochem Biophys Res Com. 1999;261(2):377–80.
17. Gehl J, Skovsgaard T, Mir LM. Vascular reactions to *in vivo* electroporation: characterization and consequences for drug and gene delivery. Biochim Biophys Acta. 2002;1569(1–3):51–8.
18. Khan AS, Pope MA, Draghia-Akli R. Highly efficient constant-current electroporation increases *in vivo* plasmid expression. DNA Cell Biol. 2005;24(12):810–8.
19. Zampaglione I, Arcuri M, Cappelletti M, Ciliberto G, Perretta G, Nicosia A, et al. *In vivo* DNA gene electrotransfer: a systematic analysis of different electrical parameters. J Gene Med. 2005;7(11):1475–81.
20. Lucas ML, Heller R. Immunomodulation by electrically enhanced delivery of plasmid DNA encoding IL-12 to murine skeletal muscle. Mol Ther. 2001;3:47–53.
21. Satkauskas S, Bureau MF, Puc M, Mahfoudi A, Scherman D, Miklavcic D, et al. Mechanisms of *in vivo* DNA electrotransfer: respective contributions of cell electropermeabilisation and DNA electrophoresis. Mol Ther. 2002;5(2):133–40.
22. Zaharoff DA, Barr RC, Li CY, Yaun F. Electromobility of plasmid DNA in tumor tissues during electric field-mediated gene delivery. Gene Ther. 2002;9:1286–90.
23. Andre F, Gehl J, Sersa G, Preat V, Hojman P, Eriksen J, et al. Efficiency of high and low voltage pulse combinations for gene electrotransfer in muscle, liver, tumor and skin. Hum Gene Ther. 2008;19(11):1261–71.
24. Pliquett U. Joule heating during solid tissue electroporation. Med Biol Eng Comput. 2003;41(2):215–9.
25. Hojman P, Gissel H, Gehl J. Sensitive and precise regulation of haemoglobin after gene transfer of erythropoietin to muscle tissue using electroporation. Gene Ther. 2007;14(12):950–9.
26. Rizzuto G, Cappelletti M, Maione D, Savino R, Lazzaro D, Costa P, et al. Efficient and regulated erythropoietin production by naked DNA injection and muscle electroporation. Proc Natl Acad Sci USA. 1999;96:6417–22.
27. Payen E, Bettan M, Rouyer-Fessard P, Beuzard Y, Scherman D. Improvement of mouse [beta]-thalassemia by electrotransfer of erythropoietin cDNA. Exp Hematol. 2001;29(3):295–300.
28. Maruyama H, Sugawa M, Moriguchi Y, Imazeki I, Ishikawa Y, Ataka K, et al. Continuous erythropoietin delivery by muscle-targeted gene transfer using *in vivo* electroporation. Hum Gene Ther. 2000;11(3):429–37.
29. Li X, Eastman EM, Schwartz RJ, Draghia-Akli R. Synthetic muscle promoters: activities exceeding naturally occurring regulatory sequences. Nat Biotechnol. 1999;17(3):241–5.
30. Gossen M, Bujard H. Tight control of gene expression in mammalian cells by tetracycline-responsive promoters. Proc Natl Acad Sci USA. 1992;89:5547–51.
31. Draghia-Akli R, Pope MA, Brown PA, Khan AS. Plasmid-based expression technology using growth hormone releasing hormone: a novel method for physiologically stimulating long-term growth hormone secretion. Comb Chem High Throughput Screen. 2006;9:181–5.
32. Gasiorowski JZ, Dean DA. Intranuclear trafficking of episomal DNA is transcription-dependent. Mol Ther. 2007;15(12):2132–9.
33. Gehl J. Electroporation for drug and gene delivery: doctors go electric. Methods Mol Biol. 2008;423:351-9.
34. Sallberg M, Frelin L, Diepolder HM, Jung MC, Mathiesen I, Kjeken R, et al. Activation of T cell responses and reductions in the viral load following therapeutic vaccination using naked DNA delivered by *in vivo* electroporation in patients with chronic hepatitis C. Mol Ther. 2009;17(1):S15.
35. Low L, Mander A, McCann KJ, Dearnaley D, Tjelle TE, Mathiesen I, et al. DNA vaccination with electroporation induces increased antibody responses in patients with prostate cancer. Hum Gene Ther. 2009;20(11):1269–78.
36. Hojman P, Gissel H, Andre F, Cournil-Henrionnet C, Eriksen J, Gehl J, et al. Physiological effects of high and low voltage pulse combinations for gene electrotransfer in muscle. Hum Gene Ther. 2008;19(11):1249–61.
37. Hojman P, Zibert J, Gissel H, Eriksen J, Gehl J. Gene expression profiles in skeletal muscle after gene electrotransfer. BMC Mol Biol. 2007;8(1):56.
38. Pedersen BK, Febbraio MA. Muscle as an endocrine organ: focus on muscle-derived interleukin-6. Physiol Rev. 2008;88(4):1379–406.

39. Ataka K, Maruyama H, Neichi T, Miyazaki J, Gejko F. Effects of erythropoietin-gene electrotransfer in rats with adenine-induced renal failure. Am J Nephrol. 2003;23:315–23.
40. Kreiss P, Bettan M, Crouzet J, Scherman D. Erythropoietin secretion and physiological effect in mouse after intramuscular plasmid DNA electrotransfer. J Gene Med. 1999;1(4):245–50.
41. Rizzuto G, Cappelletti M, Mennuni C, Wiznerowicz M, DeMartis A, Maione D, et al. Gene electrotransfer results in a high-level transduction of rat skeletal muscle and corrects anemia of renal failure. Hum Gene Ther. 2000;11(13):1891–900.
42. Samakoglu S, Fattori E, Lamartina S, Toniatti C, Stockholm D, Heard JM, et al. betaMinor-globin messenger RNA accumulation in reticulocytes governs improved erythropoiesis in beta thalassemic mice after erythropoietin complementary DNA electrotransfer in muscles. Blood. 2001;97(8):2213–20.
43. Long YC, Jaichandran S, Ho LP, Tien SL, Tan SY, Kon OL. FVIII gene delivery by muscle electroporation corrects murine hemophilia A. J Gene Med. 2006;7:494–505.
44. Fewell JG, MacLaughlin F, Mehta V, Gondo M, Nicol F, Wilson E, et al. Gene therapy for the treatment of hemophilia B using PINC-formulated plasmid delivered to muscle with electroporation. Mol Ther. 2001;3(4):574–83.
45. Lee SC, Wu CJ, Wu PY, Huang YL, Wu CW, Tao MH. Inhibition of established subcutaneous and metastatic murine tumors by intramuscular electroporation of the interleukin-12 gene. J Biomed Sci. 2003;10(1):73–86.
46. Lucas ML, Heller L, Coppola D, Heller R. IL-12 plasmid delivery by *in vivo* electroporation for the successful treatment of established subcutaneous B16.F10 melanoma. Mol Ther. 2002;5(6):668–75.
47. Li S, Zhang X, Xia X, Zhou L, Breau R, Suen J, et al. Intramuscular electroporation delivery of IFN-alpha gene therapy for inhibition of tumor growth located at a distant site. Gene Ther. 2001;8(5):400–7.
48. Zhang GH, Tan XF, Shen D, Zhao SY, Shi YL, Jin CK, et al. Gene expression and antitumor effect following im electroporation delivery of human interferon alpha 2 gene. Acta Pharmacol Sin. 2003;24(9):891–6.
49. Aurisicchio L, Ceccacci A, La Monica N, Palombo F, Traboni C. Tamarin alpha-interferon is active in mouse liver upon intramuscular gene delivery. J Gene Med. 2001;3(4):394–402.
50. Martel-Renoir D, Trochon-Joseph V, Galaup A, Bouquet C, Griscelli F, Opolon P, et al. Coelectrotransfer to skeletal muscle of three plasmids coding for antiangiogenic factors and regulatory factors of the tetracycline-inducible system: tightly regulated expression, inhibition of transplanted tumor growth, and antimetastatic effect. Mol Ther. 2003;8(3):425–33.
51. Trochon-Joseph V, Martel-Renoir D, Mir LM, Thomaidis A, Opolon P, Connault E, et al. Evidence of antiangiogenic and antimetastatic activities of the recombinant disintegrin domain of metargidin. Cancer Res. 2004;64(6):2062–9.
52. Trollet C, Bloquel C, Scherman D, Bigey P. Electrotransfer into skeletal muscle for protein expression. Curr Gene Ther. 2006;6(5):561–78.
53. Prud'homme GJ, Glinka Y, Khan AS, Draghia-Akli R. Electroporation-enhanced nonviral gene transfer for the prevention or treatment of immunological, endocrine and neoplastic diseases. Curr Gene Ther. 2006;6(2):243–73.
54. Murakami T, Nishi T, Kimura E, Goto T, Maeda Y, Ushio Y, et al. Full-length dystrophin cDNA transfer into skeletal muscle of adult mdx mice by electroporation. Muscle Nerve. 2003;27(2):237–41.
55. Vilquin JT, Kennel PF, Paturneau-Jouas M, Chapdelaine P, Boissel N, Delaère P, et al. Electrotransfer of naked DNA in the skeletal muscles of animal models of muscular dystrophies. Gene Ther. 2001;8:1097–107.
56. Gollins H, McMahon J, Wells KE, Wells DJ. High-efficiency plasmid gene transfer into dystrophic muscle. Gene Ther. 2003;10:504–12.
57. Wells KE, Fletcher S, Mann CJ, Wilton SD, Wells DJ. Enhanced *in vivo* delivery of antisense oligonucleotides to restore dystrophin expression in adult mdx mouse muscle. FEBS Lett. 2003;552(2–3):145–9.
58. Takahashi T, Ishida K, Itoh K, Konishi Y, Yagyu K, Tominaga A, et al. IGF-I gene transfer by electroporation promotes regeneration in a muscle injury model. Genesis. 2003;10:612–20.
59. Rabinovsky ED, Draghia-Akli R. Insulin-like growth factor I plasmid therapy promotes *in vivo* angiogenesis. Mol Ther. 2004;9(1):46–55.
60. Schertzer JD, Plant DR, Lynch GS. Optimizing plasmid-based gene transfer for investigating skeletal muscle structure and function. Mol Ther. 2006;13(4):795–803.
61. Sacco A, Doyonnas R, LaBarge MA, Hammer MM, Kraft P, Blau HM. IGF-I increases bone marrow contribution to adult skeletal muscle and enhances the fusion of myelomonocytic precursors. J Cell Biol. 2005;171(3):483–92.
62. Schakman O, Gilson H, de Coninck V, Lause P, Verniers J, Havaux X, et al. Insulin-like growth factor-I gene transfer by electroporation prevents skeletal muscle atrophy in glucocorticoid-treated rats. Endocrinology. 2005;146(4):1789–97.
63. Alzghoul MB, Gerrard D, Watkins BA, Hannon K. Ectopic expression of IGF-I and Shh by skeletal muscle inhibits disuse-mediated skeletal muscle atrophy and bone osteopenia *in vivo*. FASEB J. 2003;18(1):221–3.
64. Ekmark M, Gronevik E, Schjerling P, Gundersen K. Myogenin induces higher oxidative capacity in pre-existing mouse muscle fibres after somatic DNA transfer. J Physiol (Lond). 2003;548(1):259–69.

65. Kramer HF, Witczak CA, Taylor EB, Fujii N, Hirshman MF, Goodyear LJ. AS160 regulates insulin- and contraction-stimulated glucose uptake in mouse skeletal muscle. J Biol Chem. 2006;281(42):31478–85.
66. Cleasby ME, Davey JR, Reinten TA, Graham MW, James DE, Kraegen EW, et al. Acute bidirectional manipulation of muscle glucose uptake by *in vivo* electrotransfer of constructs targeting glucose transporter genes. Diabetes. 2005;54(9):2702–11.
67. Bruce CR, Brolin C, Turner N, Cleasby ME, van der Leij FR, Cooeny GJ, et al. Overexpression of carnitine palmitoyltransferase I in skeletal muscle *in vivo* increases fatty acid oxidation and reduces triacylglycerol esterification. Am J Physiol Endocrinol Metab. 2007;292:E1231–7.
68. Roorda BD, Hesselink MKC, Schaart G, Moonen-Kornips E, Martinez-Martinez P, Losen M, et al. DGAT1 overexpression in muscle by *in vivo* DNA electroporation increases intramyocellular lipid content. J Lipid Res. 2005;46(2):230–6.
69. Ban A, Yamanouchi K, Matsuwaki T, Nishihara M. *In vivo* gene transfer of PPARγ is insufficient to induce adipogenesis in skeletal muscle. J Vet Med Sci. 2008;70(8):761–7.
70. Shi H, Scheffler JM, Pleitner JM, Zeng C, Park S, Hannon KM, et al. Modulation of skeletal muscle fiber type by mitogen-activated protein kinase signaling. FASEB J. 2008;22(8):2990–3000.
71. Ekmark M, Gronevik E, Schjerling P, Gundersen K. Myogenin induces higher oxidative capacity in pre-existing mouse muscle fibres after somatic DNA transfer. J Physiol Online. 2003;548(1):259–69.
72. Nielsen AR, Hojman P, Erikstrup C, Fischer CP, Plomgaard P, Mounier R, et al. Association between IL-15 and obesity: IL-15 as a potential regulator of fat mass. J Clin Endocrinol Metab. 2008;98:4486–93.

Chapter 17
Gene Electrotransfer to Skin

Anita Gothelf and Julie Gehl

Abstract Gene electrotransfer to skin is achieving increasing interest and is likely to gain considerable clinical application due to the ease with which it is performed and the safety of the procedure. There is a potential use of gene electrotransfer to skin in e.g., DNA vaccinations, local production of therapeutic molecules as well as production of molecules for systemic therapy.

More than 30 preclinical studies concerning gene electrotransfer to skin have been reported in the literature and this chapter aims at creating an overview of plasmids injected, electrical parameters used, and duration and level of transgene expression.

Keywords Skin • Gene electrotransfer • Electroporation

Introduction

The skin holds a number of advantages which can be very convenient in gene transfection: it is accessible and can be easily evaluated, not only clinically but also histologically.

The diversity of cells in the skin displays another quality which theoretically can be useful in gene transfection. Different approaches with different genes can give a variety of responses depending on the purpose of the transfection (Fig. 17.1). Additionally, skin has the capability of producing therapeutic molecules, which can not only act locally or systemically, but can also create an immunological response when antigen-presenting cells are targeted.

This chapter describes gene electrotransfer to skin in terms of efficacy of the transfer procedure. Electrotransfer is also frequently used in vaccination trials and a separate chapter is devoted to this (see Chap. 18).

The first study with gene electrotransfer to skin was performed in 1991 by Titomirov et al. [1]. Newborn mice were transfected with a plasmid coding for a neomycin resistance gene. Fibroblasts from the treated skin area were cultured 24–168 h after the transfection and the number of neomycin resistant clones was observed. They found that fibroblasts from the transfected mice yielded neomycin resistant clones whereas the controls did not. Since then, a number of studies with different genes have been completed and have stated that gene electrotransfer to skin is feasible, efficient, and comparable to other tissues [2].

A. Gothelf (✉)
Center for Experimental Drug and Gene Electrotransfer (C*EDGE), Department of Oncology 54B1, Copenhagen University Hospital Herlev, 75 Herlev Ringvej, 2730 Herlev, Denmark
e-mail: anbigo01@heh.regionh.dk

S.T. Kee et al. (eds.), *Clinical Aspects of Electroporation*,
DOI 10.1007/978-1-4419-8363-3_17,

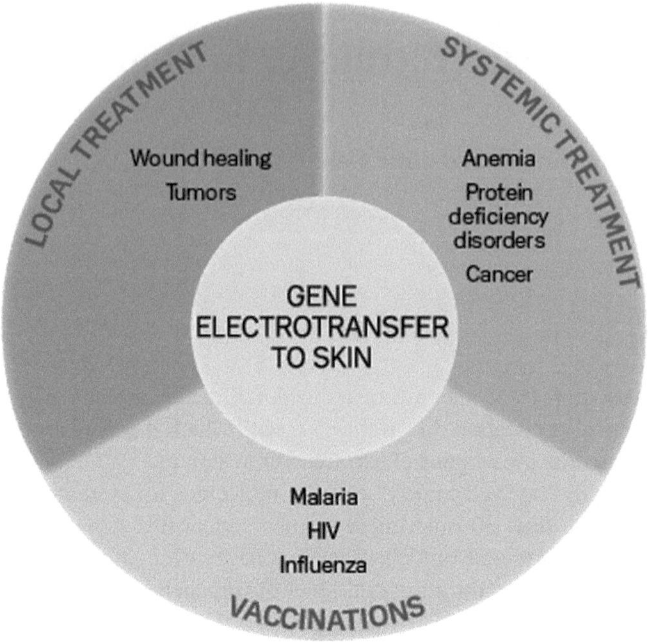

Fig. 17.1 Different objectives for gene electrotransfer to skin. Gene electrotransfer to skin has perspectives in "systemic treatment," "local treatment," and in "DNA vaccinations"

Skin and Electroporation

The purpose of the skin is to provide protection against exogenous stimuli and to secure the homeostasis of fluid and temperature. It is the biggest organ in the body and has neurological and immunological properties.

The skin is divided in three layers with the epidermis being the most superficial. The epidermis contains mainly layers of keratinocytes which is developed from stem cells on the basal membrane. Melanocytes and Langerhans cells are also present in this layer. The keratinocytes move from the basal layer to the surface of the skin, losing the properties of a cell and ending up being flat keratin-rich membrane shells creating the cornified layer (stratum corneum).

Below the basal membrane is the dermis which contains connective tissue with the antigen-presenting cells (Langerhans cells, dendritic cells, mast cells, and macrophages). Finally, there is the subcutaneous layer which consists of connective and fatty tissue. The appendages of the skin, which are hair follicles and glands, are located both in the dermis and the subcutaneous layer.

Since the purpose of the skin is to protect the body, one can speculate that transferring DNA across the skin is not the easiest task to perform. The stratum corneum creates an insulating layer, which must be overcome with appropriate electric pulses in order to electroporate the underlying cells (Fig. 17.2).

Needle electrodes which penetrate the skin can, to some extent, circumvent this issue [3], but tape stripping, which is the repeated application and removal of adhesive tape on the skin in order to remove the layer of dead cells, has also been explored [4, 5].

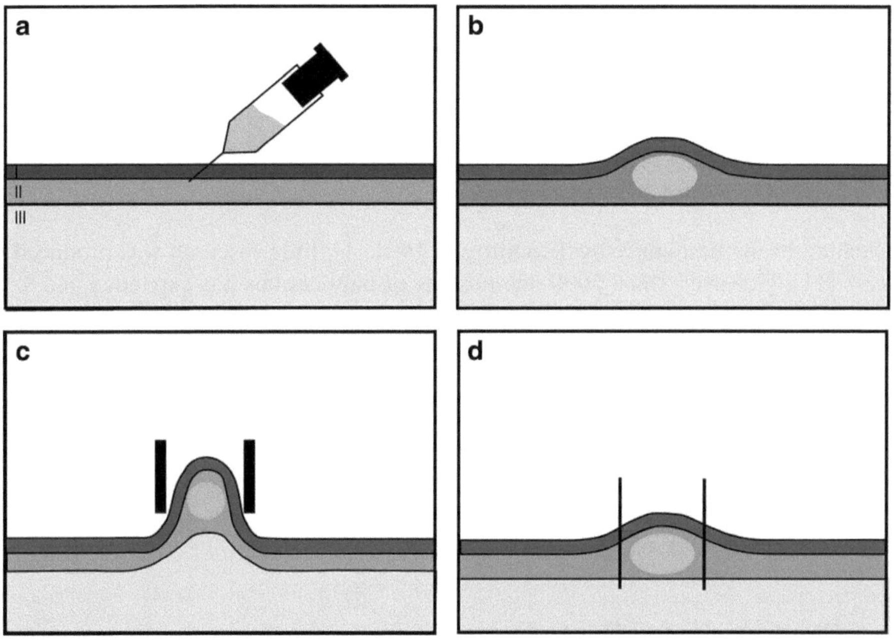

Fig. 17.2 Noninvasive vs. invasive electrodes. (**a**) Cartoon showing the injection of plasmid in the epidermis (I) and dermis (II). Layer III designates the subcutaneous layer. (**b**) Due to the epidermis being only few μm deep, the injected volume is predominantly situated in the dermis. (**c**) Electroporation with plate electrodes; the skin fold containing the injected volume is located between the plates. (**d**) Electroporation with needle electrodes; the needles penetrate the skin and enclose the injected volume

Moreover, it has been shown in vitro that keratinocytes are able and willing to produce a transgene and excrete it into the environment [6] and in vivo this process may be facilitated by the extensive blood supply that exists in the skin.

Although the histological structure of skin is the same in the animal models and in every part of the body, differences exist in regards to the size and thickness, which must be considered when working with gene electrotransfer to skin. The difference in thickness is often dependent on the thickness of the dermis (where thick skin such as the palms of the hands and soles on the feet in humans are discounted).

Likewise, skin that has been heavily sun exposed, been previously irradiated, or aged represent issues that must be taken into account in gene electrotransfer to skin during clinical trials.

Rodents such as mice and rats are the animal models most frequently used in gene transfection studies, but porcine skin is also investigated due to the similarity to human skin [3, 7–10]. In humans, the epidermis is 75–150 μm thick and the dermis is up to 4 mm thick, but is generally between 2 and 3 mm. It is similar in pigs but in rodents, especially in mice, the epidermis and dermis are much thinner.

From animal studies, we know that with different pulses and injection techniques it is possible to target different layers of the skin [11], which can be of value depending which type of transfection is wanted.

Also, the age of the skin can have some importance where studies have shown a tendency towards a higher degree of transfection in younger mice compared to older ones [12]. It is probably due to a larger amount of dividing cells or a larger mitotic activity. Even with the injection of naked plasmid alone, the younger skin gives a higher level of expression than older skin [12].

In Vivo Studies

After publication of the first study by Titomirov in 1991 [1], little research was produced over the next 10 years [11]. However, since 2000, the number of publications has expanded and to this date at least 30 in vivo studies regarding gene electrotransfer to skin have been published. The identified studies are listed in Table 17.1 and a great variety in terms of plasmids transfected, electrode configurations, and pulses delivered are displayed.

Up to now, no clinical studies concerning gene electrotransfer to normal skin have been published; the only reported study belonging to metastatic melanoma [13], but the preclinical trials confirm it is feasible and safe to transfect genes to skin, and clinical trials with DNA vaccines are ongoing (can be found at Clinicaltrials.gov).

The Gene Electrotransfer Procedure

Electrodes

Electrodes for gene electrotransfer to skin can be divided into *noninvasive electrodes*, namely different kinds of plates and patches, and *invasive electrodes*, which are needle configurations (Fig. 17.2). A more detailed description of electrodes is presented in Chap. 5.

Noninvasive electrodes consist often of two plates with either fixed or adjustable distance. The distance lies between 1 and 6 mm depending on the type of skin and injected volume. The plates are placed on the skin with the injected volume between the plates. The electric pulses are delivered either with fixed polarity or with reversal of polarity after a number of pulses. Commercially available plate electrodes are manufactured (described in Chap. 5) and are used in the clinical setting in electrochemotherapy. Heller et al. have made an electrode termed 4PE [14], which is made of four plates creating a quadratic field where the electric pulses first are delivered in one direction and afterwards in the direction perpendicular to the first.

Other types of noninvasive electrodes are contact wires placed on the skin with the injected volume between two wires [15–17] or a flat patch electrode [9, 18], which is placed directly on the injected volume. For topical delivery a custom built electrode has been developed by Preat et al. [4], which consists of two chambers with the plasmid in the one facing the cathode and the two plates encompassing the chambers.

Invasive electrodes consist of needles which penetrate into the skin and are also commercially available for the treatment of tumors or vaccinations (described in Chap. 5). The needles can be arranged in an array, e.g., two rows with four needles in each, or in a circular or triangular pattern. The length and diameter of the needles varies from type to type. The needles are inserted into the skin preferably around the injected volume to prevent leakage of the plasmid and the electric pulses are delivered.

Similar to the contact wires which are placed on the surface of the skin, Maruyama et al. used two penetrating needles that were inserted into the skin parallel to the surface [19]. They also combined this electrode with a plate placed superficially on the skin, and termed this "fork-and-plate electrode."

Table 17.1 Preclinical studies encompassing gene electrotransfer to skin

Reference	Plasmid	Dose (μg)	Animal	Voltage		Duration	Number
Noninvasive electrodes							
Plate electrode – adjustable or fixed distance							
Titomirov et al. [1]	NeoR	2–12,5	Mouse	400–600	V/cm	100–300 μs	2
Zhang et al. [11]	LacZ	40	Mouse	120	V	10–20 ms	3
Drabick et al. [8]	GFP	50–300	Pig	1,750	V/cm	100 μs	6
	Luc						
Heller et al. [15]	Luc	50–100	Mouse	100	V/cm	20 ms	8
	IL-12			1,500	V/cm	100 μs	8
Lucas et al. [28]	Luc	100	Mouse	100	V/cm	20 ms	8
				1,500	V/cm	100 μs	8
				750+14+EEP	V/cm	50 μs+20 ms+20 ms	2+4+1
Maruyama et al. [19]	EPO	200–1,600	Rat	12–24	V	50 ms	8
Chesnoy and Huang [12]	GFP	20	Mouse	200–400	V/cm	20 ms	10
	Luc						
Zhang et al. [18]	LacZ	2–100	Mouse	50–100	V	15–30 ms	3–30
	Luc		Human skin graft	75	V	20 ms	1–12
				100	V	2 ms	60
Lee et al. [32]	Luc	40	Mouse	200–400	V/cm	20 ms	6
Medi et al. [26]	LacZ	50	Rabbit	50	V	30 ms	10
				100	V	10–30 ms	5
				100–300	V	10 ms	5
Pavselj and Preat [20]	GFP	30–50	Rat	200	V/cm	400 ms	1
	Luc		Mouse	250	V/cm	20 ms	6
	Ova			1,000	V/cm	100 μs	1
				1,750	V/cm	100 μs	6
				1,000+140–200	V/cm	100 μs+400 ms	1+1
				700+200	V/cm	100 μs+400 ms	1+1
Thanaketpaisarn et al. [2]	LacZ	20	Mouse	50–1,000	V/cm	5 ms	12
	Luc						
Heller et al. [14]	GFP	100	Mouse	800	V/cm	2 ms	8
	Luc						

(continued)

Table 17.1 (continued)

Reference	Plasmid	Dose (μg)	Animal	Voltage		Duration	Number
Noninvasive electrodes							
Vandermeulen et al. [36]	Luc	12–50	Mouse	700+200	V/cm	100 μs+400 ms	1+1
Andre et al. [22]	Luc	50	Rat	1,000+80–200	V/cm	100 μs+400 ms	1+1
Vandermeulen et al. [5, 23]	Luc	0.5–50	Mouse	700+200	V/cm	100 μs+400 ms	1+1
Gothelf et al. [24, 27]	EPO	50–150	Mouse	1,000+100	V/cm	100 μs+400 ms	1+1
	Katushka						
	Luc						
Gothelf [3]	Luc	100	Pig	1,000+80–160	V/cm	100 μs+400 ms	1+1
Wires on skin – custom built clips – flat patches – 4PE							
Dujardin et al. [4]	GFP	50	Rat	335	V	0.5 ms	10
				335	V	5 ms	
				1,000	V	100 μs	
Heller et al. [15]	IL-12	50	Mouse	1,500	V/cm	100 μs	8
Zhang et al. [18]	Luc	2–100	Mouse	75	V	25 ms	6
Babiuk et al. [9]	GFP	100	Pig	60–80	V	60 ms	6
	Luc						
Heller et al.[a] [14]	GFP	10–200	Mouse	10–1,500	V/cm	0.1–2,000 ms	8
	Luc						
Pedron-Mazoyer et al. [16]	DsRed	50–70	Mouse	60–240	V	20 ms	8
	VEGF						
Heller et al. [25]	Luc	100	Mouse	100	V/cm	150 ms	8
Invasive electrodes							
Needle electrodes – needle arrays							
Glasspool-Malone et al. [7]	GFP	100	Pig	1,750	V/cm	100 μs	6
	Luc						
Drabick et al. [8]	GFP	50–300	Mouse	1,500	V/cm	100 μs	2–6
	Luc		Pig	1,750	V/cm	100 μs	2–6
				2,000	V/cm	100 μs	2–6
Byrnes et al. [40]	Luc	0.1–50	Mouse	200–400	V/cm	20 ms	6
				400–1,800	V/cm	20 ms	6
				1,750	V/cm	100 μs	6–18
Marti et al. [30]	KGF	25–100	Mouse	1,800	V/cm	100 μs	6

Lin et al. [31]	KGF	100	Rat	1,800	V/cm	100 μs	6
	Luc						
Roos et al. [34]	Luc	10	Mouse	200	V/cm	100 μs	6
	PSA			275	V/cm	10 ms	8
				1,125	V/cm	50 μs	2
				1,750	V/cm	100 μs	6
				1,125+275	V/cm	50 μs+10 ms	2+8
Hirao et al. [10]	GFP	50–200	Pig	0.1–0.4	A[b]	20–52 ms	2–3
	SEAP						
Kang et al. [21]	Luc	5	Mouse	50–250	V/cm	100 ms	6
Liu et al. [33]	Hif-1α	50–200	Mouse	200–1,800	V/cm	20 ms	10
	Luc						
Ferraro et al. [29]	VEGF	8–100	Rat skin	200	V/cm	20 ms	8
Roos et al. [35]	Luc	10–20	Mouse	1,125+275	V/cm	50 μs+10 ms	2+8
	PSA						
Gothelf [3]	Luc	100	Pig	1,000+80–140	V/cm	100 μs+400 ms	1+1
Needles parallel to skin surface – syringes – plate and fork electrodes							
Maruyama et al. [19]	EPO	100–1,600	Rat	12–50	V	50 ms	8
	LacZ						
Lee et al. [32]	Luc	30–40	Mouse	50–200	V/cm	20 ms	6
	TGF						

For simplicity, doses of plasmid are reported as an overall range for all plasmids used in the studies. For details about doses of single plasmids, please see the original paper. *Note* [a]numerous electrical parameters tested, [b]reported in Ampere and not Volt or Volt per cm (V/cm) Reasons for papers not included in the list: studies with gene electrotransfer to skin concerning primarily DNA vaccinations: [37–39, 41]. Papers reporting the gene electrotransfer procedures and the results have been reported elsewhere: [42–45] Papers regarding numerical models or field calculations: [17, 46]

Electric Pulses

Probably all possible pulse combinations have been explored in the effort of transfecting genes into skin by electroporation. The variation goes from very low voltages and long pulse lengths to high-voltage (HV) pulses with a very short duration and also combinations of high and low-voltage (LV) pulses.

The border between HV pulses and LV pulses are arbitrary, but there is a tendency towards pulses below 400 V/cm being in the millisecond range (typically 10–400 ms) and pulses above 400 V/cm being in the microsecond range (typically 50–100 μs).

Nevertheless, some studies have performed a thorough analysis of different pulse amplitudes and pulse durations [14, 20], while others focused on whether the use of electric pulses were more efficient in transfecting genes into skin than the injection of naked plasmid alone [21].

The optimal pulse conditions reported depend on the type of skin transfected, type of electrode, and possibly also the type of DNA. Some groups prefer a combination pulse with one short HV pulse and one or several longer LV pulses [20, 22–24]. Others prefer several HV pulses, but transfection has also been achieved with LV pulses alone [25].

In spite of the many different pulse combinations, many authors agree that a certain threshold has to be overcome in order to transfect cells and with higher voltages; a plateau is reached where cell damage will be evident [26]. Efficient protocols for gene electrotransfer are combination pulses (1 HV 1,000 V/cm, 100 μs + 1 LV 100 V/cm, 400 ms) [24, 27], several short HV pulses (6 HV 1,750 V/cm, 100 μs) [8], and several long LV pulses (8 LV 100 V/cm, 150 ms) [25].

Nearly all studies were carried out using square wave pulses for electroporation. Only Zhang et al. from 1996 [11] used exponential pulses. Lucas et al. [28] used a pulse combination with high and LV pulses and an exponentially enhanced pulse (EEP) as well, and found this pulse configuration efficient.

Plasmids

The most frequently used plasmids have been reporter genes such as luciferase, green fluorescent protein (GFP), and LacZ (betagalactosidase) (Table 17.1), and with these it is possible to visualize and quantify the extent and amount of expression.

Studies have been performed in order to find the optimal dose, especially for luciferase, and the overall conclusion is the more plasmid, the more gene expression although often the expression seems to reach a plateau. Also, the dose injected depends on the type of plasmid but for reporter genes, 10–100 μg are often used with a concentration of 0.5–2.0 μg/μL.

Of the therapeutically relevant plasmids used for gene electrotransfer to skin the growth factors such as vascular endothelial growth factor (VEGF) [29], keratinocyte growth factor (KGF) [30, 31], and transforming growth factor (TGF) [32] dominate the list, but also erythropoietin (EPO) [19, 24] and interleukin-12 (IL-12) [15] have been investigated.

The growth factors have a potential in increasing wound healing and hypoxia inducible factor-1α (Hif-1α) has been studied in animal models with diabetic mice [33].

EPO is a hormone released from the kidney as a response to hypoxia and is a well tested compound, also in gene electrotransfer (i.e., to muscle). Its function is to increase the hemoglobin level and is of importance in treating patients with kidney failure and chronic anemia. Preclinical studies have shown that it is feasible to transfect skin with EPO and achieve significant systemic levels of this hormone resulting in increased production of hemoglobin [24].

IL-12 has the potential in treating malignant melanoma and the work by Daud et al. regarding gene electrotransfer to tumor describes the first published clinical trial [13].

Other studies have encompassed genes such as prostate-specific antigen, PSA (cancer vaccine) [34, 35], secreted embryonic alkaline phosphatase, SEAP (marker/reporter gene) [10], and other reporter genes such as DsRed [16, 17] and Katushka [27].

Injection

If gene electrotransfer to skin is the goal, the injection technique becomes very important since different types of cells would be targeted with a subcutaneous injection than with an intradermal injection.

Babiuk et al. [9] tried a BioJect device which pressed the plasmid into the tissue by a jet stream and subsequently electroporated the area with a flat patch electrode. They compared it to conventional injection and found that the distribution of injected dye was broader with BioJect, but there was no statistical difference in luciferase expression between the two injection types.

DNA Promoters and Adjuvants

There is no doubt that the electric field is crucial for the degree of electroporation and expression, but the plasmid and the promoters are also important.

In most studies, the promoters used for gene electrotransfer to skin are ubiquitous promoters such as CMV or CAG, but studies have been performed on tissue specific promoters as well [23].

A number of studies have added different kinds of physical alterations or chemical adjuvants to the plasmid to increase the expression such as adding hyaluronidase [5, 36], aurintricarboxylic acid ATA [7], or liposomes [25] and increasing the ionic strength of the solution [12]. However, the effect is not clear and has to be validated with further studies.

Detection and Evaluation of the Result

A number of techniques are available to detect the result of gene electrotransfer to skin: either direct analysis of the treated area or indirect analysis by measuring different substances in the blood. The direct analysis can either be detection of the transgene in skin samples or in vivo visualization like bioimaging. In either case detection of the result is not always as easy as it seems. Furthermore, when excising biopsies from the animal, utmost care must be taken in order to remove the correct area since it is not always enough to mark the skin superficially. Tattooing with ink in small dots on the skin has proven to be more efficient and durable.

Luciferase Detection

After gene transfection with luciferase to skin or other tissues, it is possible to quantify the amount of expression. A number of kits are available for the laboratory and in principle, they work the same way. The skin samples are homogenized, a luciferin substrate is added to the supernatant and if luciferase is present, light is emitted. This is normally measured in relative light units (RLU's) and can be converted to pg luciferase per sample or per weight by a standard curve.

The drawback with luciferase is that it has a very high variance, often of several logs, on the results, which has been shown in a number of studies [3, 20]. This makes it very difficult to compare studies, even if they are performed with the same setup.

GFP Detection

GFP is unfortunately not very suitable for transfection to skin. It can be visualized in vivo by scanning the whole animal or in a fluorescent microscope either as a whole skin sample or in frozen sections, but due to very high level of autofluorescence in skin, it is very difficult to distinguish between a transfected cell and normal conditions. A number of studies have presented results regarding gene electrotransfer with GFP to skin.

For macroscopic detection of the expression, gene electrotransfer with luciferase and subsequent bioimaging could be an alternative to GFP, since this technique is better at distinguishing between transfected and nontransfected areas.

Histological analysis with immunohistochemistry is a possibility for evaluating the extent of transfection with GFP to skin microscopically, although up to this day it has not yet been reported in literature.

Betagalactosidase

Another reporter gene used in gene electrotransfer to skin is plasmid coding for betagalactosidase. Once inside the cell, an enzyme is produced which converts a colorless substrate (X-gal) into a blue product. This can be visualized microscopically either directly in frozen sections, on fixated tissue or with immunohistochemistry.

Maruyama et al. [19] found expression in the epidermal layer 1 day after transfection and in the subcutaneous muscle layer after 7 days when rat skin was transfected using the "plate and fork" electrode, while others found expression of betagalactosidase activity in the dermal layer after 1 day [18], 2 [26], or 3 days [11] after the transfection.

Other plasmids such as EPO, IL-12, and various growth factors can be evaluated either directly, as with measurement of serum EPO, or indirectly with blood samples of e.g., hemoglobin [24] or interferon-γ [15].

Duration and Level of Expression

Few studies have been conducted with the focus on duration and level of transgene expression and luciferase has most often been the subject of investigation [14, 18, 20]. After gene electrotransfer with luciferase to skin, a peak in the level of expression is obtained after 2–3 days and the expression remained elevated compared to controls 2 weeks after the transfection [14]. Our studies with gene electrotransfer with luciferase to murine skin validated that a peak in the level of transgene expression was reached after 3 days, but with gene electrotransfer with Katushka to skin, evaluated with continuous monitoring of fluorescence, we found a peak in the level of transgene expression 9 days after the transfection [27]. Studies with gene electrotransfer to skin with EPO showed a peak in transgene expression after 2 weeks and had slightly prolonged duration of expression compared to Katushka; 4 vs. 3 weeks [24, 27].

Since the peak of transgene expression for Katushka and EPO occurs later than the peak of luciferase expression and since duration of transgene expression seems longer than previously thought, luciferase may not be the most optimal choice for investigating the kinetics after gene transfection.

Vaccination Studies to Skin

The skin is a part of the body's immune surveillance and contains antigen-presenting cells such as dendritic cells, Langerhans cells, and mononuclear cells. The thought of using skin for the vaccination of infectious diseases is not new, and with electroporation, there is now a possibility of using DNA vaccines.

Different infectious diseases have been studied in animal studies with gene electrotransfer to skin. Hepatitis B has been investigated the most [8, 9, 26, 37] but studies have also been performed with vaccines against malaria [38], HIV [10], and smallpox [39]. The efficacy of the vaccination is usually validated by the measurement of the immunological response in the blood. See Chap. 18 for a more thorough presentation of DNA vaccinations and electroporation.

Discussion and Perspectives

Almost 20 years after the first study with gene electrotransfer to skin, there is no doubt that this technique is efficient. A large variety of plasmids have been injected with an even larger variety of electric pulses applied, so we must conclude that no consensus regarding gene electrotransfer to skin exists in the literature. But there is no need for the definition of one particular set of parameters. There is a wide spectrum of electrical parameters which can be effective in transferring genes into skin, between the threshold for electroporation and the onset of tissue damage. One could speculate that the type or concentration of plasmid and type or age of skin has a large influence on the procedure and that this may infer important changes in the electrical parameters to be used.

Theoretically there can be different optimal pulses for delivering genes that have a local effect, genes with a systemic effect and for DNA vaccinations (Fig. 17.1).

It is possible that different cell types are transfected with different genes, and even more so, that different cell types are transfected with different electrical parameters. The pulses needed to permeabilize a cell membrane depend on the shape of the cell (see Chap. 3 for more detail) and since the skin consists of many different cell types, a difference in transfection efficacy is theoretically possible. Still, it is very important to establish which types of cells are transfected in order to utilize this knowledge in future work with gene electrotransfer to skin.

Furthermore, the duration of expression in the skin is approximately 3–4 weeks and is short compared to gene transfection to muscles, but that can be an advantage in cases where a long-term expression is not warranted.

Additionally, the perspective with gene electrotransfer to skin lies in enabling the skin to produce relevant drugs or vaccines, which can act locally or systemically. Serious conditions such as cancer, protein deficiency disorders and infectious diseases are candidates for gene electrotransfer to skin with relevant therapeutic compounds as well as chronic wounds and skin diseases.

Gene electrotransfer to skin is likely to gain considerable clinical use due to the ease with which it is performed, the safety of the procedure and the potential use for e.g., DNA vaccination, local production of therapeutic molecules as well as production of molecules for systemic therapy.

References

1. Titomirov AV, Sukharev S, Kistanova E. *In vivo* electroporation and stable transformation of skin cells of newborn mice by plasmid DNA. Biochim Biophys Acta. 1991;1088(1):131–4.
2. Thanaketpaisarn O, Nishikawa M, Yamashita F, Hashida M. Tissue-specific characteristics of *in vivo* electric gene: transfer by tissue and intravenous injection of plasmid DNA. Pharm Res. 2005;22(6):883–91.
3. Gothelf A, Mahmood F, Dagnaes-Hansen F, Gehl J. Importance of electrode choice on gene electrotransfer to skin; evaluated by efficacy of transgene expression and electric field calculation in a porcine model. Manuscript submitted for publication 2011.
4. Dujardin N, Van Der SP, Preat V. Topical gene transfer into rat skin using electroporation. Pharm Res. 2001;18(1):61–6.
5. Vandermeulen G, Daugimont L, Richiardi H, Vanderhaeghen ML, Lecouturier N, Ucakar B, et al. Effect of tape stripping and adjuvants on immune response after intradermal DNA electroporation. Pharm Res. 2009;26(7):1745–51.
6. Christensen R, Kolvraa S, Blaese RM, Jensen TG. Development of a skin-based metabolic sink for phenylalanine by overexpression of phenylalanine hydroxylase and GTP cyclohydrolase in primary human keratinocytes. Gene Ther. 2000;7(23):1971–8.
7. Glasspool-Malone J, Somiari S, Drabick JJ, Malone RW. Efficient nonviral cutaneous transfection. Mol Ther. 2000;2(2):140–6.
8. Drabick JJ, Glasspool-Malone J, King A, Malone RW. Cutaneous transfection and immune responses to intradermal nucleic acid vaccination are significantly enhanced by *in vivo* electropermeabilization. Mol Ther. 2001;3(2):249–55.
9. Babiuk S, Baca-Estrada ME, Foldvari M, Baizer L, Stout R, Storms M, et al. Needle-free topical electroporation improves gene expression from plasmids administered in porcine skin. Mol Ther. 2003;8(6):992–8.
10. Hirao LA, Wu L, Khan AS, Satishchandran A, Draghia-Akli R, Weiner DB. Intradermal/subcutaneous immunization by electroporation improves plasmid vaccine delivery and potency in pigs and rhesus macaques. Vaccine. 2008;26(3):440–8.
11. Zhang L, Li L, Hoffmann GA, Hoffman RM. Depth-targeted efficient gene delivery and expression in the skin by pulsed electric fields: an approach to gene therapy of skin aging and other diseases. Biochem Biophys Res Commun. 1996;220(3):633–6.
12. Chesnoy S, Huang L. Enhanced cutaneous gene delivery following intradermal injection of naked DNA in a high ionic strength solution. Mol Ther. 2002;5(1):57–62.
13. Daud AI, DeConti RC, Andrews S, Urbas P, Riker AI, Sondak VK, et al. Phase I trial of interleukin-12 plasmid electroporation in patients with metastatic melanoma. J Clin Oncol. 2008;26(36):5896–903.
14. Heller LC, Jaroszeski MJ, Coppola D, McCray AN, Hickey J, Heller R. Optimization of cutaneous electrically mediated plasmid DNA delivery using novel electrode. Gene Ther. 2007;14(3):275–80.
15. Heller R, Schultz J, Lucas ML, Jaroszeski MJ, Heller LC, Gilbert RA, et al. Intradermal delivery of interleukin-12 plasmid DNA by *in vivo* electroporation. DNA Cell Biol. 2001;20(1):21–6.
16. Pedron-Mazoyer S, Plouet J, Hellaudais L, Teissie J, Golzio M. New anti angiogenesis developments through electro-immunization: optimization by *in vivo* optical imaging of intradermal electro gene transfer. Biochim Biophys Acta. 2007;1770(1):137–42.
17. Mazeres S, Sel D, Golzio M, Pucihar G, Tamzali Y, Miklavcic D, et al. Non invasive contact electrodes for *in vivo* localized cutaneous electropulsation and associated drug and nucleic acid delivery. J Control Release. 2009;134(2): 125–31.
18. Zhang L, Nolan E, Kreitschitz S, Rabussay DP. Enhanced delivery of naked DNA to the skin by non-invasive *in vivo* electroporation. Biochim Biophys Acta. 2002;1572(1):1–9.
19. Maruyama H, Ataka K, Higuchi N, Sakamoto F, Gejyo F, Miyazaki J. Skin-targeted gene transfer using in vivo electroporation. Gene Ther. 2001;8(23):1808–12.
20. Pavselj N, Preat V. DNA electrotransfer into the skin using a combination of one high- and one low-voltage pulse. J Control Release. 2005;106(3):407–15.
21. Kang JH, Toita R, Niidome T, Katayama Y. Effective delivery of DNA into tumor cells and tissues by electroporation of polymer-DNA complex. Cancer Lett. 2008;265(2):281–8.
22. Andre FM, Gehl J, Sersa G, Preat V, Hojman P, Eriksen J, et al. Efficiency of high- and low-voltage pulse combinations for gene electrotransfer in muscle, liver, tumor, and skin. Human Gene Therapy. 2008;19(11):1261–72.
23. Vandermeulen G, Richiardi H, Escriou V, Ni J, Fournier P, Schirrmacher V, et al. Skin-specific promoters for genetic immunisation by DNA electroporation. Vaccine. 2009;27(32):4272–7.
24. Gothelf A, Hojman P, Gehl J. Therapeutic levels of erythropoietin (EPO) achieved after gene electrotransfer to skin in mice. Gene Ther. 2010;17(9):1077–84.

25. Heller LC, Jaroszeski MJ, Coppola D, Heller R. Comparison of electrically mediated and liposome-complexed plasmid DNA delivery to the skin. Genet Vaccines Ther. 2008;6:16.
26. Medi BM, Hoselton S, Marepalli RB, Singh J. Skin targeted DNA vaccine delivery using electroporation in rabbits. I: efficacy. Int J Pharm. 2005;294(1–2):53–63.
27. Gothelf A, Eriksen J, Hojman P, Gehl J. Duration and level of transgene expression after gene electrotransfer to skin in mice. Gene Ther. 2010;17(7):839–45.
28. Lucas ML, Jaroszeski MJ, Gilbert R, Heller R. *In vivo* electroporation using an exponentially enhanced pulse: a new waveform. DNA Cell Biol. 2001;20(3):183–8.
29. Ferraro B, Cruz YL, Coppola D, Heller R. Intradermal delivery of plasmid VEGF(165) by electroporation promotes wound healing. Mol Ther. 2009;17(4):651–7.
30. Marti G, Ferguson M, Wang J, Byrnes C, Dieb R, Qaiser R, et al. Electroporative transfection with KGF-1 DNA improves wound healing in a diabetic mouse model. Gene Ther. 2004;11(24):1780–5.
31. Lin MP, Marti GP, Dieb R, Wang J, Ferguson M, Qaiser R, et al. Delivery of plasmid DNA expression vector for keratinocyte growth factor-1 using electroporation to improve cutaneous wound healing in a septic rat model. Wound Repair Regen. 2006;14(5):618–24.
32. Lee PY, Chesnoy S, Huang L. Electroporatic delivery of TGF-beta1 gene works synergistically with electric therapy to enhance diabetic wound healing in db/db mice. J Invest Dermatol. 2004;123(4):791–8.
33. Liu L, Marti GP, Wei X, Zhang X, Zhang H, Liu YV, et al. Age-dependent impairment of HIF-1alpha expression in diabetic mice: correction with electroporation-facilitated gene therapy increases wound healing, angiogenesis, and circulating angiogenic cells. J Cell Physiol. 2008;217:319–27.
34. Roos AK, Moreno S, Leder C, Pavlenko M, King A, Pisa P. Enhancement of cellular immune response to a prostate cancer DNA vaccine by intradermal electroporation. Mol Ther. 2006;13(2):320–7.
35. Roos AK, Eriksson F, Walters DC, Pisa P, King AD. Optimization of skin electroporation in mice to increase tolerability of DNA vaccine delivery to patients. Mol Ther. 2009;17(9):1637–42.
36. Vandermeulen G, Staes E, Vanderhaeghen ML, Bureau MF, Scherman D, Preat V. Optimisation of intradermal DNA electrotransfer for immunisation. J Control Release. 2007;124(1–2):81–7.
37. Zhang L, Widera G, Rabussay D. Enhancement of the effectiveness of electroporation-augmented cutaneous DNA vaccination by a particulate adjuvant. Bioelectrochemistry. 2004;63(1–2):369–73.
38. Dobano C, Widera G, Rabussay D, Doolan DL. Enhancement of antibody and cellular immune responses to malaria DNA vaccines by *in vivo* electroporation. Vaccine. 2007;25(36):6635–45.
39. Hooper JW, Golden JW, Ferro AM, King AD. Smallpox DNA vaccine delivered by novel skin electroporation device protects mice against intranasal poxvirus challenge. Vaccine. 2007;25(10):1814–23.
40. Byrnes CK, Malone RW, Akhter N, Nass PH, Wetterwald A, Cecchini MG, et al. Electroporation enhances transfection efficiency in murine cutaneous wounds. Wound Repair Regen. 2004;12(4):397–403.
41. Nomura M, Nakata Y, Inoue T, Uzawa A, Itamura S, Nerome K, et al. *In vivo* induction of cytotoxic T lymphocytes specific for a single epitope introduced into an unrelated molecule. J Immunol Methods. 1996;193(1):41–9.
42. Maruyama H, Miyazaki J, Gejyo F. Epidermis-targeted gene transfer using *in vivo* electroporation. Methods Mol Biol. 2005;289:431–6.
43. Roos AK, King A, Pisa P. DNA vaccination for prostate cancer. Methods Mol Biol. 2008;423:463–72.
44. Marti GP, Mohebi P, Liu L, Wang J, Miyashita T, Harmon JW. KGF-1 for wound healing in animal models. Methods Mol Biol. 2008;423:383–91.
45. Medi BM, Singh J. Delivery of DNA into skin via electroporation. Methods Mol Biol. 2008;423:225–32.
46. Pavselj N, Preat V, Miklavcic D. A numerical model of skin electropermeabilization based on *in vivo* experiments. Ann Biomed Eng. 2007;35(12):2138–44.

Chapter 18
Electroporation-Mediated DNA Vaccination

Paolo Fagone, Devon J. Shedlock, Stephen Kemmerer, Dietmar Rabussay, and David B. Weiner

Abstract There are many positive attributes to DNA vaccination that make it a conceptually desirable platform. In clinical studies, however, standard DNA injection alone generally induces low levels of transgene-specific immunity when compared to other vaccine approaches. In order to boost the immunogenicity of this platform, next-generation DNA vaccines require additional techniques such as the administration of electroporation. This new method involves the generation of a brief electric field in tissue around a local injection site that results in the transient poration, or permeabilization, of the cellular membranes. As a result, antigen-specific immune responses are greatly enhanced and are likely due to increased DNA uptake and antigen expression. Thus, electroporation-mediated DNA vaccination represents a promising new strategy for the elicitation of strong immune responses directed against the expressed antigen(s) and not the vector, and ongoing studies are currently underway to optimize the working parameters of this technique. Here, we review the uses of this technology in conjunction with vaccination and suggest future directions for its further exploration.

Keywords DNA vaccination • Electroporation • Electropermeabilization • Plasmid

Abbreviations

Hbs Ag	Hepatitis B surface antigen
HBV	Hepatitis B virus
HCV	Hepatitis C virus
IFN	Type I interferons
pDNA	Plasmid DNA
TBK1	TANK-binding kinase I
TLR	Toll-like receptors

D.B. Weiner (✉)
Department of Pathology and Laboratory Medicine, University of Pennsylvania School of Medicine, 422 Curie Blvd, 505 Stellar-Chance Laboratories, Philadelphia, PA 19104, USA
e-mail: dbweiner@mail.med.upenn.edu

S.T. Kee et al. (eds.), *Clinical Aspects of Electroporation*,
DOI 10.1007/978-1-4419-8363-3_18,

Introduction

The discouraging results from the recent human HIV trial performed by Merck and collaborators, named "STEP," raises serious questions about current vaccine approaches using replication-defective viral vectors [1]. This study was an international phase II "test of concept" trial in uninfected volunteers at high risk for acquiring HIV infection which showed that vaccination using a recombinant adenovirus serotype 5 vector was ineffective at preventing virus infection and even increased the rate of transmission in individuals exhibiting prior immunity to the viral vector. While this vaccine was safe and immunogenic in both humans and nonhuman primates, eliciting long-lasting and multifunctional $CD8^+$ T cell responses that were partially protective in rhesus macaques, the discovery that the vaccine could possibly heighten HIV infection was both unexpected and alarming, resulting in the immediate discontinuation of vaccinations as recommended by the independent Data Safety Monitoring Board for STEP. Since preexisting immunity against a vaccine vector may compromise its efficacy in humans, future vaccine approaches should aim to utilize vectors that exhibit minimal or no reactivity in immunocompetent vaccines.

DNA vaccination consists of the administration of genetic material encoding a desired antigen that when expressed in the vaccine, is capable of eliciting an immune response. Compared with other approaches, the advantages of DNA vaccination are many [2]; no infectious agents are involved and vaccines are unable to revert into virulent form like live vaccines. They can prime both cytotoxic [3] and humoral responses [4], and DNA vectors are easily manipulated, can be tested rapidly, produced at high yield in bacteria, and are readily isolated. They are also more temperature-stable than conventional vaccines, easily stored and transported, and do not require a cold chain. Furthermore, DNA vaccines could potentially induce immunity in newborns in situations that usually neutralize conventional vaccines via the presence of high levels of maternal antibodies [5]. The introduction of exogenous DNA into cells or tissue can be achieved using DNA conjugates [6–10], virus-derived vectors [11], or naked plasmid DNA (pDNA) [12]. Naked pDNA shows variable and low transfection efficacy when administered by conventional means, such as needle injection or topical application. However, several strategies aimed to improve pDNA vaccine immunogenicity have been developed, including codon optimization [13], mRNA optimization [14], addition of leader sequences [15], and construction of consensus immunogens [16]. While these strategies help to boost the overall immunogenicity of a DNA vaccine, they may not be applicable to all antigens. Recently, electroporation, or electropermeabilization, has gained great interest in multiple research areas including gene therapy and vaccinology [17]. Although the precise mechanism of action has not yet been well defined, it is hypothesized that cell membranes in host tissue receiving electroporation, normally impermeable to charged molecules, form pores or functionally equivalent structural changes upon application of an external electric field which facilitate the influx of macromolecules. Thus, higher transfection efficacy of naked pDNA as a result of electroporation is thought to be the major contributor to the increased immunogenicity of electroporation-mediated DNA vaccination. In addition, it has been shown that electroporation increases vaccine potency by activating antigen-presenting cells (APCs) via danger signals and local inflammation [18] and by recruiting immune cells to the site of DNA administration [19, 20]. Furthermore, direct transfection of APCs could also be facilitated by electroporation. Currently, intensive investigation is focused upon utilizing electroporation of muscle and skin as an effective method for DNA vaccine delivery to small and large animals, and in humans. The safety and feasibility of electroporation in humans has recently been demonstrated, but not finally proven [21]. Thus, the paramount question for DNA vaccines at this time is whether a sufficient level of efficacy can be reached with the present methodology, or if further improvements or breakthroughs in vaccine design and/or electroporation delivery will be necessary.

In Vivo Transgene Expression After Gene Electrotransfer

In 1990, the first transgene expression detected in skeletal muscle after injection of naked mRNA or pDNA raised the possibility of using this method for certain gene therapies and DNA vaccinations [22]. Subsequently, transgene expression was also obtained in the same way in a wide variety of other tissues, but transgene expression was generally too low and variable to be useful for the envisioned purposes [12]. Attempts to sufficiently enhance pDNA uptake, and thus transgene expression, with cationic lipids or the gene gun have also proven unsuccessful to date. The first publications on a substantial increase in transgene expression (about 100-fold) when electroporation was applied in vivo after pDNA injection appeared as late as 1996 [23], although electroporation had been used for in vitro cell transfections since 1982 [24]. In addition, as pointed out by Bettan et al. [25], when using gene electrotransfer, a higher interindividual reproducibility in gene transduction can be observed.

Skeletal muscle (Fig. 18.1) has been the most frequently targeted tissue in both gene therapy and DNA vaccine studies, either with or without electroporation. Some reasons why muscle cells (also known as myocytes) and muscle tissues continue to be attractive targets for transgene expression include: muscle tissue is easily accessible, plentiful, and well vascularized; the latter facilitates circulation of the antigens produced by the transfected muscle cells. More discussion of gene electrotransfer to muscle can be found in Chap. 16.

Electroporation and Plasmid DNA Vaccine Immunogenicity

In vivo electroporation has been used to deliver DNA vaccine encoding antigens from numerous infectious agents, summarized in Table 18.1. Enhanced immune responses to electroporation-mediated DNA vaccination have been observed both in small and large animals such as mice [26], pigs [27], and monkeys [28]. Widera et al. [26] demonstrated in mice that upon electroporative treatment, the delivery of a weakly immunogenic hepatitis B virus (HBV) surface antigen (Hbs Ag) DNA vaccine resulted in an increased humoral immune response, characterized by rapid onset and higher titers of anti-Hbs Ag antibodies. In addition, the authors observed in the same study that the potency of an HIV *gag* pDNA vaccine was increased as shown by the lower dosage of DNA required to induce higher antigen-specific antibody levels and increased $CD8^+$ T cell responses. Similarly, in a study carried out with a bovine herpes virus-1 truncated glycoprotein D DNA vaccine, Tsang et al. [29] showed that the onset of the primary humoral response was earlier in the group treated with DNA followed by electroporation, and that this group produced higher antibody levels than those in the group receiving i.m. DNA immunization or a recombinant protein vaccine only; similar results were obtained earlier with

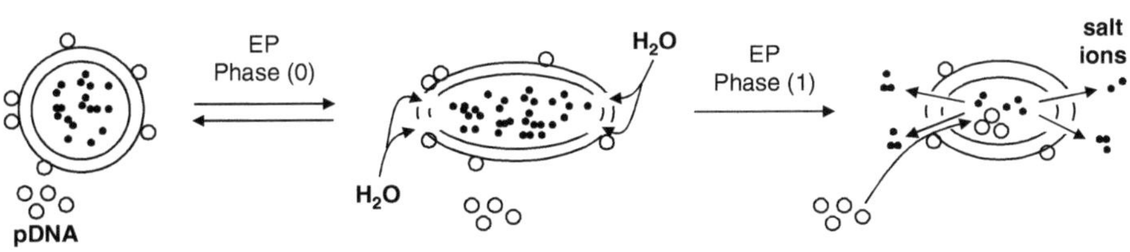

Fig. 18.1 Cellular targets of electroporation-mediated DNA vaccination. Current electroporation approaches following i.d. and i.m. DNA vaccination target skin cells (keratinocytes), muscle cells, and APCs (including Langerhans cells) by direct transfection (DT). Application of electroporation at a local immunization site induces the formation of transient complexes between the DNA and the lipids in the pore edges of the hydrophilic pore zones [62] which facilitate the translocation of pDNA into the cell cytoplasm. Once in the cytosol, pDNA may gain access to the nucleus where transgene expression may occur

Table 18.1 Antigens encoded by DNA vaccines used in combination with electroporation

Infectious agent	Encoded antigen(s)	Model	Delivery route	References
HIV	Gag	Rhesus macaques	i.m.	[63]
	Gag and Env + IL-12	Rhesus macaques		[36]
	Env	Mice		[20]
	Gag and Env + IL-12	Rhesus macaques	Skin	[36]
	Env + gp120 protein	Macaques and rabbits	i.m.	[64]
	Gag and Env	Rhesus macaques		[65]
	Gag and Env	Mice	i.m.	[26]
	gp140Env, GagPol, and TatRevNef plasmids	Rhesus macaques		[66]
H5N1 virus	HA	Rabbits and mice	i.m.	[67]
H1N1 virus	NA; HA	Mice	i.m.	[68, 69]
Avian influenza H9N2 virus	HA and NA	Mice	i.m.	[70]
HBV	preS2-S + -2 and IFN-γ	Rhesus macaques	i.m.	[71]
	preS(2)-S			[72]
	Hbs Ag	Mice		[73]
	Hbs Ag	Sheep		[74]
	Hbs Ag	Rabbits	Skin	[75]
HCV	NS3/4A		i.m.	[42]
	E2	Mice	i.m.	[76]
	NS3 to NS5B	Mice and rhesus macaques		[31]
(SARS)-CoV	N1, N2 and N3	Mice	i.m.	[77]
	Spike + IL-2	Mice	i.m.	[78, 79]
	Spike	Mice		
HDV	L-HDAg; Hbs Ag	Mice	i.m.	[80]
Coxsackievirus 3	VP1 or VP3; VP1-1 or VP1-2	Mice		[81]
Japanese encephalitis virus	Env		i.m.	[82]
Herpes virus	pgD	Pigs		[27]
Foot-and-mouth disease virus (FMDV)	cVP1, sVP1, mVP1 or P1	Mice	i.m.	[83]
	VP1	Mice		[84]
Chikungunya virus	Capsid E1 and E2	Mice	i.m.	[85]
Anthrax	Anthrax toxin protective Ag	Mice, rats, rabbits	i.m.	[86]
Smallpox		Mice	Skin	[87]
Mycobacterium tuberculosis	Ag85A	Mice	i.m.	[37, 88]
	Ag85A and ESAT-6 + proteins	Mice and rhesus macaques	i.m.	[89]
	Ag85B	Mice	i.m.	[90]
Pseudomonas aeruginosa	OprF/OprI	Mice	i.m.	[91]
Malaria	Pfs25		i.m.	[92]
	PyCSP and PyHEP17	Mice	i.m., skin	[93]
Haemonchus contortus	NPA	Sheep	i.m.	[94, 95]

an otherwise inert microparticulate adjuvant [30]. Interestingly, the efficiency of transfection by electroporation was not increased by doubling the dose of DNA administered; however, the duration of the antigen-specific antibody response was increased at a higher rate in comparison to the immunization with the same dose of plasmid without electroporation. Moreover, electroporation increased the degree of consistency among the individuals in the DNA-plus-electroporation group as seen in the 5 weeks of follow-up. Finally, a high correlation between the duration of the primary immune response and the magnitude of the secondary antibody response was observed, implying that electroporation could represent an effective approach to elicit a longer memory antibody response.

Capone et al. [31] have demonstrated that gene electrotransfer efficiently increased the cellular immune response both in mice and rhesus macaques vaccinated with a plasmid encoding a nonstructural region of hepatitis C virus (HCV). In particular, they showed by ex vivo interferon (IFN)-γ ELISPOT assay that electroporation in mice induced a fivefold more potent T cell response than DNA administration alone, and that the elicited response was directed against all six of the antigen pools spanning the HCV NS3-NS5B region. To assess whether electroporation treatment elicited similar responses in a nonhuman primate model, they immunized rhesus macaques three times with the vaccine and collected peripheral blood mononuclear cells at periodic intervals to test the T cell effector function. The immune responses observed in the electroporation-treated group showed a faster kinetic, with all the animals responding after the second challenge and reaching a peak after the third. Moreover, all animals treated with electroporation showed both $CD4^+$ and $CD8^+$ T cell responses, in comparison to the naked DNA group which showed a weaker $CD8^+$ response and no $CD4^+$ response. Finally, gene electrotransfer-immunized macaques maintained anti-HCV effector T cells for the entire observation period of 6 months, indicating that the gene electrotransfer efficiently elicited a strong memory T cell response.

DNA vaccination in association with electroporation represents an effective strategy to elicit strong, broad, and long-lasting B and T cell responses. Although muscle is the most common target for DNA vaccine immunizations [32], the presence of APCs in both the skin layers makes it an attractive target for nucleic acid vaccination, since direct transfection of APCs may be important for T cell priming upon skin DNA immunization [33] (Fig. 18.2). In a murine model using a viral

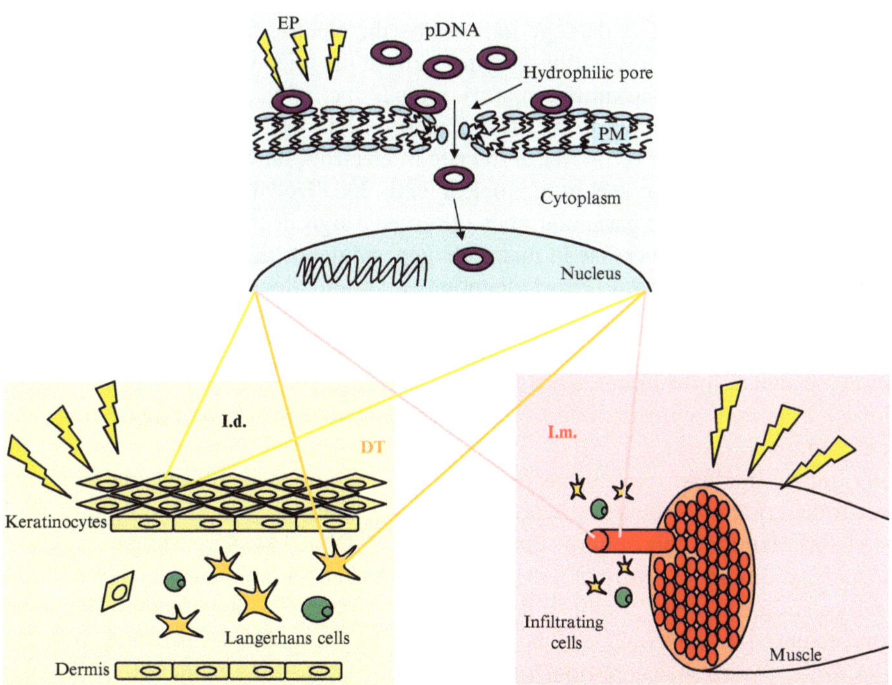

Fig. 18.2 Cellular targets of EP-mediated DNA vaccination. Current EP approaches following i.d. and i.m. DNA vaccination target skin cells (keratinocytes), muscle cells, and APC (including Langerhans cells) by direct transfection (DT). Application of EP at a local immunization site induces the formation of transient complexes between the DNA and the lipids in the pore edges of the hydrophilic pore zones [51] which facilitate the translocation of plasmid DNA (pDNA) into the cell cytoplasm. Once in the cytosol, pDNA may gain access to the nucleus where transgene expression may occur

challenge, Raz et al. [34] have demonstrated that a single intradermal (i.d.) injection (without electroporation) of naked DNA encoding the influenza nucleoprotein gene is sufficient to induce production of antigen-specific antibodies and cytotoxic T lymphocytes that persist for at least 68 weeks and are protective against a lethal challenge with a heterologous strain of influenza virus. Furthermore, immune responses to i.d. DNA vaccination have been recorded to be significantly enhanced by in vivo electroporation [35]; analysis of the antibody response to an Hbs Ag-encoding plasmid delivered i.d. upon electroporation in mice has revealed a strong enhancement of the T_h1 response, which is mainly characterized by a strong cell-mediated response, compared to that elicited by protein immunization, which showed an exclusively T_h2 pattern, characterized by a dominant humoral responses. Also, in a nonhuman primate model study carried out in rhesus macaques [36], the i.d.-plus-electroporation group developed 50% more IFN-γ-producing cells and twice more memory T cells than the group not treated with electroporation. Higher antibody responses were recorded in the i.d.-plus-electroporation group when compared to the i.m.-plus-electroporation group. Altogether, these results support the idea that electroporation following DNA injection, both in muscle and skin, represents an effective approach to large animal immunization.

Electroporation-Mediated Local Inflammation

Several authors have hypothesized that inflammation caused by electroporation is important to prime the immune response to DNA vaccination [19, 37, 38]. Local inflammation was previously proposed to augment immune responses in studies where pDNA was coinjected with bupivicaine-HCl [39–41]. The localized tissue damage induced by the electric field is thought to recruit $CD3^+$ cells, increasing the number of infiltrating immune cells at the injection site [42]. Indeed, electroporation caused the activation of proinflammatory signals including the expression of chemokines such as MIP-1α, MIP-1β, MIP-1γ, IP-10, MCP-2, and XCL1 [18]. Liu et al. [20] characterized the extent and nature of the cellular infiltrates at the site of electroporative vaccine delivery in mice and found both polymorphonuclear and mononuclear cells localized in the perivascular spaces and throughout the muscle tissue. In particular, they observed a significant increase in B cells, $CD4^+$ and $CD8^+$ T cells, and a dramatic increase in macrophages and dendritic cells compared to vaccination alone. No difference, however, was recorded among cell populations of blood, spleen, and draining lymph nodes of the mice treated with or without electroporation, suggesting that only local factors are involved in the augmentation of immune responses following electroporation. Also, these authors observed that cell infiltrates were transient and resolved within 2 weeks. Thus, improved antigen presentation may represent one of the mechanisms by which electroporation may elicit a more potent immune response.

Typically, innate immune recognition of the adjuvant component of vaccine formulations has been shown to be critical for their immunogenicity [43]. Many adjuvants are ligands for Toll-like receptors (TLRs), like monophosphoryl lipid A and CpG DNA [44, 45], while some conventional adjuvants, such as aluminum hydroxide and incomplete Freud's adjuvant are free of TLR ligands [46]. Therefore, these examples demonstrate that multiple innate immune recognition and signaling pathways are required for adjuvants to function [44]. In the case of DNA vaccines, it has been controversial as to the main vaccine component contributing most to the induction of both innate and adaptive immune responses; while CpG motifs expressed within the plasmid backbone can stimulate innate immunity through TLR 9, the induction of adaptive immune responses were unaffected in the absence of this innate receptor [47, 48]. However, it has recently been shown that the double-stranded structure of DNA, independently of CpG sequences, possesses immunomodulatory effects when administered intracellularly [44], which can trigger TLR-independent, TANK-binding kinase I

(TBK1)- and INF regulatory factor 3-dependent innate activation of both immune and nonimmune cells to produce type I INFs and their inducible genes [49, 50]. Recently, Ishii et al. [51] have reported that the enhancement of DNA vaccine immunogenicity achieved by electroporation may be due to increased transfection rates resulting from this technique, which better contributes to local inflammation by activating cells to produce IFN through the TBK1-dependent signaling pathway. These data suggest that TBK1 is a key signaling molecule for DNA vaccination immunogenicity by regulating innate immune signaling, which is critical for the induction of adaptive immune responses, and that the enhanced immunogenicity of pDNA by electroporation may be a result of more pDNA interacting with intracellular TBK1.

In accordance with this hypothesis, Peng et al. [18] postulated that local inflammation is more important than the actual quantity of expressed transgene in determining the magnitude of the immune response, demonstrated by higher antibody titers and $CD4^+$ T cell proliferation rates observed by applying electric pulses 3–7 days prior to i.m. DNA immunization. In this case, it can be postulated that both increased cross-presentation and direct transfection of infiltrating APCs resulting from increased local inflammation may contribute to the augmented immune response in electroporation-mediated DNA vaccination. It appears that the mechanisms by which electroporation enhance the responses to naked plasmid vaccination is by an increase in DNA transfection and possibly include local inflammation, which may be augmented by the magnitude or duration of transgene expression. Indeed, Babiuk et al. [19] observed that the highest level of lymphocytic infiltration was only in muscle tissue treated with electroporation, which elicited higher levels of transgene expression, as was expected considering that antigen production is critical for the retention of the cellular infiltrates at sites of local inflammation.

Electroporation-Mediated DNA Vaccination in Humans

Although two DNA vaccines have been recently approved in the USA and Canada for the vaccination of horses against West Nile virus [52] and salmon against infectious hematopoietic necrosis virus [53], no DNA vaccine has been approved for use in humans. However, encouraging results from preclinical trials using electroporation technology with DNA vaccination in large animal models has prompted much interest in the technique and its safety. Currently, tolerability in humans has been demonstrated in healthy volunteers [54], anti-DNA antibodies have not been detected in patients electroporated after muscle DNA injection, and the integration of pDNA into host chromosomes following electroporation-mediated delivery has not been observed [55]. Together, these results have been sufficient for the regulatory approval of several clinical trials [56]. As reported on clinicaltrials.gov, seven electrotransfer DNA vaccine trials for cancer and three clinical trials using DNA vaccine against infectious agents in association with electroporation are currently open. Ongoing clinical studies using electroporation-mediated DNA vaccination against infectious agents include three phase I studies involving muscle electroporation. The first will test safety and immunological effects of PENNVAX™-B, an HIV vaccine encoding Gag, Pol, and Env, in HIV-infected individuals (VGX Pharmaceuticals, Inc.); the second will assess safety, tolerability, and immunogenicity of human papillomavirus (HPV) DNA Plasmid (VGX-3100™) delivered by electroporation in adult females postsurgical or ablative treatment of Grade 2 or 3 Cervical Intraepithelial Neoplasia (VGX Pharmaceuticals, Inc.); the third one, a Phase I/II trial is testing tolerability and efficacy of i.m.-administered CHRONVAC-C™ in combination with electroporation in chronic HCV genotype 1 infected and naïve patients with low viral load (Tripep AB).

The amount of pain and distress associated with electroporation in humans has been of a tolerable level for the anticipated benefit [57]. To date, electroporation-mediated DNA vaccination in humans is performed administrating an injection volume of 0.2–0.5 mL followed by short (10–60 ms), low electric field strength (60–250 V/cm) pulses (2–10 pulses). Given that these conditions are efficient for the DNA vaccination of large animals, such as nonhuman primates, they should be sufficient in humans. Electroporation results in a sharp, but quick pain that is comparable to receiving a short electrical shock. While this sensation is transient, administration of short-acting sedative drugs or painkillers before treatment has been considered. Accordingly, as reported by Daud et al. [57], in a clinical trial using an interleukin-12-encoding plasmid delivered by electroporation in patients with metastatic melanoma, in order to limit patients' discomfort, lidocaine was either administered topically or injected around each tumor site, and intravenous analgesic and/or anxiolytic drugs were offered to the patients before electroporation. Notably, previous studies have shown that pain is not a limiting factor as patient discomfort is limited to the period of electrical stimulation, and subjects have usually returned for repeated treatments without asking for sedation. Also, after muscle electroporation, like muscle injection, a mild ache may be experienced at the site of electroporation for some days, and similar to that following a strenuous workout. Several factors determine the strength of pain associated with electroporation, although there is a high interindividual variability in the perception of pain. Among these factors are the number, length, spacing, and thickness of the electrode needles, but primarily the electric pulse parameters dictate the pain threshold [58].

Exclusion criteria for electroporation treatment may include the presence of metal implants near the site of electrical delivery, the presence of a pacemaker, and in the case of muscle electroporation, obesity, since treatment efficacy may be decreased if muscle tissue is not reached for vaccine and/or electric pulse delivery.

Electrical Parameters and Electroporation Equipment

Electroporation-mediated DNA vaccine delivery requires a pulse generator that controls the parameters of individual pulses or pulse trains (amplitude, duration, number, polarity, wave form, frequency), and electrodes usually integrated into an applicator. Electrodes are in direct contact with the subject to be treated and it is their geometry (shape, size, and distance from each other) that ultimately determines the shape and strength of the electric field and the electrical currents in the target tissue (Fig. 18.3). Thus, both the properties of the pulse(s) and the electrodes are responsible for the desired enhancement of DNA delivery as well as undesirable side effects. Proper design of pulses and electrodes will maximize the effectiveness of a given DNA vaccine and minimize unwanted side effects, such as long-lasting histological changes, pain, and muscle contractions. Further discussion of electroporation parameters and equipment can be found in Chaps. 4 and 5.

Skin Electroporation and Equipment

Skin is a potentially interesting target tissue for DNA vaccines because of its natural role in the immune defense of the body and its ready accessibility. Discussion of gene electrotransfer of DNA in general and to skin can be found in Chaps. 13 and 17, respectively.

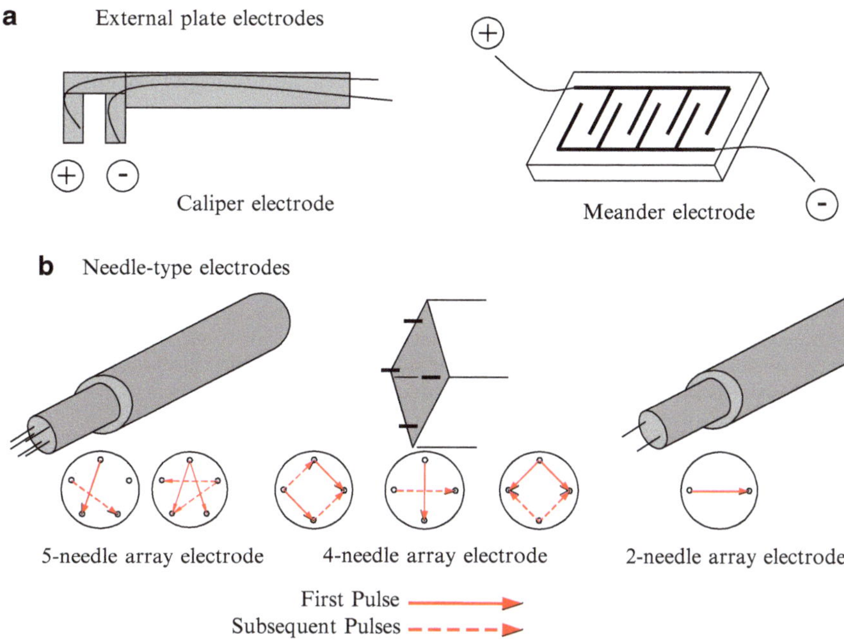

Fig. 18.3 Main types of electrodes used for EP. Examples of the two main types of electrodes used for delivering EP: Surface (**a**) and needle-type (**b**) electrodes. Surface electrodes come in the form of caliper electrodes or consist of an array of interweaving electrode fingers (meander). Needle-type electrodes consist of a variable number of (primarily) stainless steel needles arranged in different configurations. Picture depicts a 5-needle array firing rotating chord patterns, a 4-needle array fired in opposing pairs, crossing or triangular patterns, and a 2-needle array firing pin to pin

Conclusion

The goal of any vaccination strategy is to prime a broad and long-lasting immune response that is capable of robust effector responses upon antigenic restimulation [59–61] and protect against infectious agents, while minimizing toxicity of the vaccine. Since complications may arise due to the use of viral-based vectors, such as preexisting immunity regulating vaccine effectiveness and the possibility of reversion into virulence that may decrease vaccine efficacy or safety, alternative approaches should be explored for future vaccine approaches. DNA vaccination appears an even more attractive candidate for future vaccines since it is safe, immunogenic, and does not stimulate vector-specific immunity. Extensive literature supports the hypothesis that electroporation represents a valid approach to vaccine administration in that it increases the consistency and potency of vaccination, inducing higher levels of both antibody-mediated and cytotoxic T cell responses. In this way, electroporation may help augment translocation of exogenous DNA into the nucleus. Furthermore, it has been proven to be effective in enhancing immune responses to antigens regardless of the degree of transgene expression achieved. Recent evidence suggests that innate immune recognition of the adjuvant component of vaccines and the danger signals provided by the method of vaccination may be important in determining the magnitude of the resultant immune response. Electroporation may enhance local inflammation at the site of immunization by facilitating the transfection of greater amounts of pDNA, which may be more readily available to interact with intracellular signaling proteins that trigger the secretion of inflammatory cytokines and their inducible genes. While electroporation-mediated DNA vaccination is currently the topic of intensive research, more theoretical studies and practical trials are required to optimize the delivery of the vaccine into the target tissue, and the electrical parameters facilitating DNA uptake while calibrating local tissue damage and reducing pain associated with vaccine delivery through electroporation.

Acknowledgments We would like to thank Karuppiah Muthumani and Shaheed Abdulhaqq for critical review of the manuscript and members of the DBW laboratory for helpful discussion.

Competing financial interests: The laboratory of D.B.W. has grant funding and collaborations, advising, or consulting including serving on scientific review committees for commercial entities and therefore notes possible conflicts associated with this work with Pfizer, Inovio, BMS, Virxsys, Ichor, Merck, Althea, VGXI, J&J, Aldevron, and possibly others. The authors have no other relevant affiliations or financial involvement with any organization or entity with a financial interest in or financial conflict with the subject matter or materials discussed in the manuscript apart from those disclosed. No writing assistance was utilized in the production of this manuscript.

References

1. Sekaly RP. The failed HIV Merck vaccine study: a step back or a launching point for future vaccine development? J Exp Med. 2008;205:7–12.
2. Shedlock DJ, Weiner DB. DNA vaccination: antigen presentation and the induction of immunity. J Leukoc Biol. 2000;68:793–806.
3. Ulmer JB, Donnelly JJ, Parker SE, Rhodes GH, Felgner PL, Dwarki VJ, et al. Heterologous protection against influenza by injection of DNA encoding a viral protein. Science (New York, NY). 1993;259:1745–9.
4. Tang DC, DeVit M, Johnston SA. Genetic immunization is a simple method for eliciting an immune response. Nature. 1992;356:152–4.
5. Chen J, Zhang F, Fang F, Chang H, Chen Z. Vaccination with hemagglutinin or neuraminidase DNA protects BALB/c mice against influenza virus infection in presence of maternal antibody. BMC Infect Dis. 2007;7:118.
6. Nicolau C, Le Pape A, Soriano P, Fargette F, Juhel MF. *In vivo* expression of rat insulin after intravenous administration of the liposome-entrapped gene for rat insulin I. Proc Natl Acad Sci USA. 1983;80:1068–72.
7. Kaneda Y, Iwai K, Uchida T. Increased expression of DNA cointroduced with nuclear protein in adult rat liver. Science (New York, NY). 1989;243:375–8.
8. Mannino RJ, Gould-Fogerite S. Liposome mediated gene transfer. Biotechniques. 1988;6:682–90.
9. Benvenisty N, Reshef L. Direct introduction of genes into rats and expression of the genes. Proc Natl Acad Sci USA. 1986;83:9551–5.
10. Wu GY, Wu CH. Receptor-mediated gene delivery and expression *in vivo*. J Biol Chem. 1988;263:14621–4.
11. Schoenly KA, Weiner DB. Human immunodeficiency virus type 1 vaccine development: recent advances in the cytotoxic T-lymphocyte platform "spotty business". J Virol. 2008;82:3166–80.
12. Wolff JA, Budker V. The mechanism of naked DNA uptake and expression. Adv Genet. 2005;54:3–20.
13. Deml L, Bojak A, Steck S, Graf M, Wild J, Schirmbeck R, et al. Multiple effects of codon usage optimization on expression and immunogenicity of DNA candidate vaccines encoding the human immunodeficiency virus type 1 Gag protein. J Virol. 2001;75:10991–1001.
14. Schneider R, Campbell M, Nasioulas G, Felber BK, Pavlakis GN. Inactivation of the human immunodeficiency virus type 1 inhibitory elements allows Rev-independent expression of Gag and Gag/protease and particle formation. J Virol. 1997;71:4892–903.
15. Yang JS, Kim JJ, Hwang D, Choo AY, Dang K, Maguire H, et al. Induction of potent Th1-type immune responses from a novel DNA vaccine for West Nile virus New York isolate (WNV-NY1999). J Infect Dis. 2001;184:809–16.
16. Gao F, Weaver EA, Lu Z, Li Y, Liao HX, Ma B, et al. Antigenicity and immunogenicity of a synthetic human immunodeficiency virus type 1 group m consensus envelope glycoprotein. J Virol. 2005;79:1154–63.
17. Wells DJ. Gene therapy progress and prospects: electroporation and other physical methods. Gene Ther. 2004;11:1363–9.
18. Peng B, Zhao Y, Xu L, Xu Y. Electric pulses applied prior to intramuscular DNA vaccination greatly improve the vaccine immunogenicity. Vaccine. 2007;25:2064–73.
19. Babiuk S, Baca-Estrada ME, Foldvari M, Middleton DM, Rabussay D, Widera G, et al. Increased gene expression and inflammatory cell infiltration caused by electroporation are both important for improving the efficacy of DNA vaccines. J Biotechnol. 2004;110:1–10.

20. Liu J, Kjeken R, Mathiesen I, Barouch DH. Recruitment of antigen-presenting cells to the site of inoculation and augmentation of HIV-1 DNA vaccine immunogenicity by *in vivo* electroporation. J Virol. 2008;82:5643–9.
21. Gehl J. Electroporation for drug and gene delivery in the clinic: doctors go electric. Methods Mol Biol. 2008;423:351–9.
22. Wolff JA, Malone RW, Williams P, Chong W, Acsadi G, Jani A, et al. Direct gene transfer into mouse muscle *in vivo*. Science (New York, NY). 1990;247:1465–8.
23. Heller R, Jaroszeski M, Atkin A, Moradpour D, Gilbert R, Wands J, et al. *In vivo* gene electroinjection and expression in rat liver. FEBS Lett. 1996;389:225–8.
24. Neumann E, Schaefer-Ridder M, Wang Y, Hofschneider PH. Gene transfer into mouse lyoma cells by electroporation in high electric fields. EMBO J. 1982;1:841–5.
25. Bettan M, Emmanuel F, Darteil R, Caillaud JM, Soubrier F, Delaere P, et al. High-level protein secretion into blood circulation after electric pulse-mediated gene transfer into skeletal muscle. Mol Ther. 2000;2:204–10.
26. Widera G, Austin M, Rabussay D, Goldbeck C, Barnett SW, Chen M, et al. Increased DNA vaccine delivery and immunogenicity by electroporation *in vivo*. J Immunol. 2000;164:4635–40.
27. Babiuk S, Baca-Estrada ME, Foldvari M, Storms M, Rabussay D, Widera G, et al. Electroporation improves the efficacy of DNA vaccines in large animals. Vaccine. 2002;20:3399–408.
28. Zhao YG, Peng B, Deng H, Chen G, Yang F, Shao M, et al. Anti-HBV immune responses in rhesus macaques elicited by electroporation mediated DNA vaccination. Vaccine. 2006;24:897–903.
29. Tsang C, Babiuk S, van Drunen Littel-van den Hurk S, Babiuk LA, Griebel P. A single DNA immunization in combination with electroporation prolongs the primary immune response and maintains immune memory for six months. Vaccine. 2007;25:5485–94.
30. Zhang L, Widera G, Rabussay D. Enhancement of the effectiveness of electroporation-augmented cutaneous DNA vaccination by a particulate adjuvant. Bioelectrochemistry (Amsterdam, Netherlands). 2004;63:369–73.
31. Capone S, Zampaglione I, Vitelli A, Pezzanera M, Kierstead L, Burns J, et al. Modulation of the immune response induced by gene electrotransfer of a hepatitis C virus DNA vaccine in nonhuman primates. J Immunol. 2006;177:7462–71.
32. Danko I, Williams P, Herweijer H, Zhang G, Latendresse JS, Bock I, et al. High expression of naked plasmid DNA in muscles of young rodents. Hum Mol Genet. 1997;6:1435–43.
33. Porgador A, Irvine KR, Iwasaki A, Barber BH, Restifo NP, Germain RN. Predominant role for directly transfected dendritic cells in antigen presentation to CD8+ T cells after gene gun immunization. J Exp Med. 1998;188:1075–82.
34. Raz E, Carson DA, Parker SE, Parr TB, Abai AM, Aichinger G, et al. Intradermal gene immunization: the possible role of DNA uptake in the induction of cellular immunity to viruses. Proc Natl Acad Sci USA. 1994;91:9519–23.
35. Drabick JJ, Glasspool-Malone J, King A, Malone RW. Cutaneous transfection and immune responses to intradermal nucleic acid vaccination are significantly enhanced by *in vivo* electropermeabilization. Mol Ther. 2001;3:249–55.
36. Hirao LA, Wu L, Khan AS, Hokey DA, Yan J, Dai A, et al. Combined effects of IL-12 and electroporation enhances the potency of DNA vaccination in macaques. Vaccine. 2008;26:3112–20.
37. Gronevik E, Mathiesen I, Lomo T. Early events of electroporation-mediated intramuscular DNA vaccination potentiate Th1-directed immune responses. J Gene Med. 2005;7:1246–54.
38. McMahon JM, Wells KE, Bamfo JE, Cartwright MA, Wells DJ. Inflammatory responses following direct injection of plasmid DNA into skeletal muscle. Gene Ther. 1998;5:1283–90.
39. Caselli E, Betti M, Grossi MP, Balboni PG, Rossi C, Boarini C, et al. DNA immunization with HIV-1 tat mutated in the trans activation domain induces humoral and cellular immune responses against wild-type Tat. J Immunol. 1999;162:5631–8.
40. Chattergoon MA, Robinson TM, Boyer JD, Weiner DB. Specific immune induction following DNA-based immunization through *in vivo* transfection and activation of macrophages/antigen-presenting cells. J Immunol. 1998;160:5707–18.
41. Coney L, Wang B, Ugen KE, Boyer J, McCallus D, Srikantan V, et al. Facilitated DNA inoculation induces anti-HIV-1 immunity *in vivo*. Vaccine. 1994;12:1545–50.
42. Ahlen G, Soderholm J, Tjelle T, Kjeken R, Frelin L, Hoglund U, et al. *In vivo* electroporation enhances the immunogenicity of hepatitis C virus nonstructural 3/4A DNA by increased local DNA uptake, protein expression, inflammation, and infiltration of CD3+ T cells. J Immunol. 2007;179:4741–53.
43. Pulendran B, Ahmed R. Translating innate immunity into immunological memory: implications for vaccine development. Cell. 2006;124:849–63.
44. Kawai T, Akira S. Signaling to NF-kappaB by Toll-like receptors. Trends Mol Med. 2007;13:460–9.
45. Mata-Haro V, Cekic C, Martin M, Chilton PM, Casella CR, Mitchell TC. The vaccine adjuvant monophosphoryl lipid A as a TRIF-biased agonist of TLR4. Science (New York, NY). 2007;316:1628–32.
46. Gavin AL, Hoebe K, Duong B, Ota T, Martin C, Beutler B, et al. Adjuvant-enhanced antibody responses in the absence of toll-like receptor signaling. Science (New York, NY). 2006;314:1936–8.

47. Babiuk S, Mookherjee N, Pontarollo R, Griebel P, van Drunen Littel-van den Hurk S, Hecker R, et al. TLR9−/− and TLR9+/+ mice display similar immune responses to a DNA vaccine. Immunology. 2004;113:114–20.
48. Spies B, Hochrein H, Vabulas M, Huster K, Busch DH, Schmitz F, et al. Vaccination with plasmid DNA activates dendritic cells via Toll-like receptor 9 (TLR9) but functions in TLR9-deficient mice. J Immunol. 2003;171:5908–12.
49. Ishii KJ, Coban C, Kato H, Takahashi K, Torii Y, Takeshita F, et al. A Toll-like receptor-independent antiviral response induced by double-stranded B-form DNA. Nat Immunol. 2006;7:40–8.
50. Stetson DB, Medzhitov R. Recognition of cytosolic DNA activates an IRF3-dependent innate immune response. Immunity. 2006;24:93–103.
51. Ishii KJ, Kawagoe T, Koyama S, Matsui K, Kumar H, Kawai T, et al. TANK-binding kinase-1 delineates innate and adaptive immune responses to DNA vaccines. Nature. 2008;451:725–9.
52. Minke JM, Siger L, Karaca K, Austgen L, Gordy P, Bowen R, et al. Recombinant canarypoxvirus vaccine carrying the prM/E genes of West Nile virus protects horses against a West Nile virus-mosquito challenge. Arch Virol Suppl. 2004;18:221–30.
53. Garver KA, LaPatra SE, Kurath G. Efficacy of an infectious hematopoietic necrosis (IHN) virus DNA vaccine in Chinook Oncorhynchus tshawytscha and sockeye O. nerka salmon. Dis Aquat Organ. 2005;64:13–22.
54. Rune K, Torunn ET, Dag K, and Iacob M. Clinical Evaluation of Pain and Muscle Damage Induced by Electroporation of Skeletal Muscle in Humans Abstracts from the American Society of Gene Therapy 7th Annual Meeting. June 2–6, 2004, Minneapolis, Minnesota, USA. Mol Ther. 2004;9 Suppl 1:S1–435.
55. Strain AJ. The uptake and fate of exogenous cellular DNA in mammalian cells. Dev Biol (Basel). 2006;123:23–8. discussion 55–73.
56. ClinicalTrials.gov. U.S. National Institutes of Health; 2008.
57. Daud AI, DeConti RC, Andrews S, Urbas P, Riker AI, Sondak VK, et al. Phase I trial of interleukin-12 plasmid electroporation in patients with metastatic melanoma. J Clin Oncol. 2008;26:5896–903.
58. Rabussay D. Applicator and electrode design for *in vivo* DNA delivery by electroporation. Methods Mol Biol. 2008;423:35–59.
59. Janssen EM, Lemmens EE, Wolfe T, Christen U, von Herrath MG, Schoenberger SP. CD4+ T cells are required for secondary expansion and memory in CD8+ T lymphocytes. Nature. 2003;421:852–6.
60. Shedlock DJ, Shen H. Requirement for CD4 T cell help in generating functional CD8 T cell memory. Science (New York, NY). 2003;300:337–9.
61. Sun JC, Bevan MJ. Defective CD8 T cell memory following acute infection without CD4 T cell help. Science (New York, NY). 2003;300:339–42.
62. Hristova NI, Tsoneva I, Neumann E. Sphingosine-mediated electroporative DNA transfer through lipid bilayers. FEBS Lett. 1997;415:81–6.
63. Rosati M, Valentin A, Jalah R, Patel V, von Gegerfelt A, Bergamaschi C, et al. Increased immune responses in rhesus macaques by DNA vaccination combined with electroporation. Vaccine. 2008;26:5223–9.
64. Cristillo AD, Weiss D, Hudacik L, Restrepo S, Galmin L, Suschak J, et al. Persistent antibody and T cell responses induced by HIV-1 DNA vaccine delivered by electroporation. Biochem Biophys Res Commun. 2008;366:29–35.
65. Otten G, Schaefer M, Doe B, Liu H, Srivastava I, zur Megede J, et al. Enhancement of DNA vaccine potency in rhesus macaques by electroporation. Vaccine. 2004;22:2489–93.
66. zur Megede J, Sanders-Beer B, Silvera P, Golightly D, Bowlsbey A, Hebblewaite D, et al. A therapeutic SIV DNA vaccine elicits T-cell immune responses, but no sustained control of viremia in SIVmac239-infected rhesus macaques. AIDS Res Hum Retroviruses. 2008;24:1103–16.
67. Wang S, Zhang C, Zhang L, Li J, Huang Z, Lu S. The relative immunogenicity of DNA vaccines delivered by the intramuscular needle injection, electroporation and gene gun methods. Vaccine. 2008;26:2100–10.
68. Chen J, Fang F, Li X, Chang H, Chen Z. Protection against influenza virus infection in BALB/c mice immunized with a single dose of neuraminidase-expressing DNAs by electroporation. Vaccine. 2005;23:4322–8.
69. Kadowaki S, Chen Z, Asanuma H, Aizawa C, Kurata T, Tamura S. Protection against influenza virus infection in mice immunized by administration of hemagglutinin-expressing DNAs with electroporation. Vaccine. 2000;18:2779–88.
70. Qiu M, Fang F, Chen Y, Wang H, Chen Q, Chang H, et al. Protection against avian influenza H9N2 virus challenge by immunization with hemagglutinin- or neuraminidase-expressing DNA in BALB/c mice. Biochem Biophys Res Commun. 2006;343:1124–31.
71. Zhao YG, Xu Y. Electroporation-mediated HBV DNA vaccination in primate models. Methods Mol Biol. 2008;423:487–95.
72. Peng JL, Zhao YG, Mai JH, Pang WK, Guo W, Chen GM, et al. Non-cytolytic antigen clearance in DNA-vaccinated mice with electroporation. Acta Pharmacol Sin. 2007;28:1024–30.
73. Babiuk S, Tsang C, van Drunen Littel-van den Hurk S, Babiuk LA, Griebel PJ. A single HBsAg DNA vaccination in combination with electroporation elicits long-term antibody responses in sheep. Bioelectrochemistry (Amsterdam, Netherlands). 2007;70:269–74.

74. Luxembourg A, Hannaman D, Ellefsen B, Nakamura G, Bernard R. Enhancement of immune responses to an HBV DNA vaccine by electroporation. Vaccine. 2006;24:4490–3.
75. Medi BM, Hoselton S, Marepalli RB, Singh J. Skin targeted DNA vaccine delivery using electroporation in rabbits. I: efficacy. Int J Pharm. 2005;294:53–63.
76. Zucchelli S, Capone S, Fattori E, Folgori A, Di Marco A, Casimiro D, et al. Enhancing B- and T-cell immune response to a hepatitis C virus E2 DNA vaccine by intramuscular electrical gene transfer. J Virol. 2000;74:11598–607.
77. Dutta NK, Mazumdar K, Lee BH, Baek MW, Kim DJ, Na YR, et al. Search for potential target site of nucleocapsid gene for the design of an epitope-based SARS DNA vaccine. Immunol Lett. 2008;118:65–71.
78. He H, Tang Y, Qin X, Xu W, Wang Y, Liu X, et al. Construction of a eukaryotic expression plasmid encoding partial S gene fragments of the SARS-CoV and its potential utility as a DNA vaccine. DNA Cell Biol. 2005;24:516–20.
79. Hu H, Lu X, Tao L, Bai B, Zhang Z, Chen Y, et al. Induction of specific immune responses by severe acute respiratory syndrome coronavirus spike DNA vaccine with or without interleukin-2 immunization using different vaccination routes in mice. Clin Vaccine Immunol. 2007;14:894–901.
80. Shiau YT, Huang YH, Wu JC, Tao MH, Syu Jr W, Chang FY, et al. Analysis of humoral immunity of hepatitis D virus DNA vaccine generated in mice by using different dosage, gene gun immunization, and *in vivo* electroporation. J Chin Med Assoc. 2006;69:7–13.
81. Kim JY, Jeon ES, Lim BK, Kim SM, Chung SK, Kim JM, et al. Immunogenicity of a DNA vaccine for coxsackievirus B3 in mice: protective effects of capsid proteins against viral challenge. Vaccine. 2005;23:1672–9.
82. Wu CJ, Lee SC, Huang HW, Tao MH. *In vivo* electroporation of skeletal muscles increases the efficacy of Japanese encephalitis virus DNA vaccine. Vaccine. 2004;22:1457–64.
83. Kim SA, Liang CM, Cheng IC, Cheng YC, Chiao MT, Tseng CJ, et al. DNA vaccination against foot-and-mouth disease via electroporation: study of molecular approaches for enhancing VP1 antigenicity. J Gene Med. 2006;8:1182–91.
84. Yang NS, Wang JH, Lin KF, Wang CY, Kim SA, Yang YL, et al. Comparative studies of the capsid precursor polypeptide P1 and the capsid protein VP1 cDNA vectors for DNA vaccination against foot-and-mouth disease virus. J Gene Med. 2005;7:708–17.
85. Muthumani K, Lankaraman KM, Laddy DJ, Sundaram SG, Chung CW, Sako E, et al. Immunogenicity of novel consensus-based DNA vaccines against Chikungunya virus. Vaccine. 2008;26:5128–34.
86. Luxembourg A, Hannaman D, Nolan E, Ellefsen B, Nakamura G, Chau L, et al. Potentiation of an anthrax DNA vaccine with electroporation. Vaccine. 2008;26:5216–22.
87. Hooper JW, Golden JW, Ferro AM, King AD. Smallpox DNA vaccine delivered by novel skin electroporation device protects mice against intranasal poxvirus challenge. Vaccine. 2007;25:1814–23.
88. Zhang X, Divangahi M, Ngai P, Santosuosso M, Millar J, Zganiacz A, et al. Intramuscular immunization with a monogenic plasmid DNA tuberculosis vaccine: enhanced immunogenicity by electroporation and co-expression of GM-CSF transgene. Vaccine. 2007;25:1342–52.
89. Li Z, Song D, Zhang H, He W, Fan X, Zhang Y, et al. Improved humoral immunity against tuberculosis ESAT-6 antigen by chimeric DNA prime and protein boost strategy. DNA Cell Biol. 2006;25:25–30.
90. Tollefsen S, Tjelle T, Schneider J, Harboe M, Wiker H, Hewinson G, et al. Improved cellular and humoral immune responses against *Mycobacterium tuberculosis* antigens after intramuscular DNA immunisation combined with muscle electroporation. Vaccine. 2002;20:3370–8.
91. Saha S, Takeshita F, Sasaki S, Matsuda T, Tanaka T, Tozuka M, et al. Multivalent DNA vaccine protects mice against pulmonary infection caused by *Pseudomonas aeruginosa*. Vaccine. 2006;24:6240–9.
92. LeBlanc R, Vasquez Y, Hannaman D, Kumar N. Markedly enhanced immunogenicity of a Pfs25 DNA-based malaria transmission-blocking vaccine by *in vivo* electroporation. Vaccine. 2008;26:185–92.
93. Dobano C, Doolan DL. Identification of minimal CD8+ and CD4+ T cell epitopes in the *Plasmodium yoelii* hepatocyte erythrocyte protein 17kDa. Mol Immunol. 2007;44:3037–48.
94. Yen HH, Scheerlinck JP. Co-delivery of plasmid-encoded cytokines modulates the immune response to a DNA vaccine delivered by *in vivo* electroporation. Vaccine. 2007;25:2575–82.
95. Scheerlinck JP, Karlis J, Tjelle TE, Presidente PJ, Mathiesen I, Newton SE. *In vivo* electroporation improves immune responses to DNA vaccination in sheep. Vaccine. 2004;22:1820–5.

Part IV
Irreversible Electroporation

Chapter 19
Irreversible Electroporation (IRE) on Liver Tumor Ablation: A Summary of Preclinical Translational Research

Edward W. Lee, Daphne Wong, and Stephen T. Kee

Abstract In the recent years the topic of irreversible electroporation has created an excitement in the ablation community due to its advantageous characteristics. In this chapter, we will explore these advantages such as complete cell death, demarcated ablation zones, quick procedure time, feasibility with real time imaging, and the lack of the "heat sink" effect that is affecting currently used ablation techniques such as radiofrequency ablation (RFA). Additionally, we will explore in depth the mechanism of IRE, preliminary research and our in vivo studies in a swine liver, and rabbit VX2 tumor model.

Keywords Irreversible electroporation • Electroporation • VX2 • Swine animal model • Rabbit animal model • Liver tumor • Hepatocellular carcinoma • Image-guided ablation

Introduction

The application of short and intense electric fields across a cell membrane has the ability to permeabilize the cell membrane through a process known as "electroporation" [1]. This permeabilization of the cell membrane leads to complete disruption of cellular homeostasis between the intra- and extracellular compartments. The way by which the cell membrane is permeabilized is not yet fully understood, though it is thought to be related to the formation of nanoscale pores in the cell membrane. Permeabilization of a the cell membrane may be transient, after which the cells survive as the nanopores reverse and seal themselves [2]. This process is known as "reversible electroporation." Permeabilization of a cell membrane may, however, be permanent, thereby irreversibly causing cell death in a process known as "irreversible electroporation" [3].

During the last 20 years, the field of electroporation has been dominated by reversible electroporation. Irreversible electroporation (IRE) was considered an undesirable result and was simply studied to determine the upper limit of the electrical parameters that could be used to safely induce reversible electroporation. Recently, however, IRE has begun to emerge as an important medical

S.T. Kee (✉)
Ronald Reagan Medical Center at UCLA, Division of Interventional Radiology, Department of Radiology, David Geffen School of Medicine at UCLA, 757 Westwood Plaza, RM2125, Los Angeles, CA 90095, USA
e-mail: Skee@mednet.ucla.edu

S.T. Kee et al. (eds.), *Clinical Aspects of Electroporation*,
DOI 10.1007/978-1-4419-8363-3_19,

ablation technology [4]. In recent studies, IRE has been used to destroy prokaryotic and eukaryotic cells in vitro, and as a method to kill microorganisms, mammalian normal cells and mammalian cancer cells in vivo [1, 5–8]. Such studies have demonstrated the ability of IRE to fully eliminate an entire population of cells without causing any thermal damage.

In this chapter, we will present some of the published and unpublished data from our group and others, summarizing the preclinical translational research data for a better understanding of IRE in liver tumor ablation.

Translational Models to Investigate Tumor Ablation

Developmental Stage of IRE Liver Ablation

The early developmental stage of IRE ablation technology was based on mathematical and computer modeling to analyze the physics, geometry, and hypothesis of IRE [9] prior to translation into a basic science bench study evaluating the electrical parameters in vitro [4]. From those fundamental basic science studies, researchers were able to derive several important facts about IRE: (1) high electrical fields create innumerable nanopores in the cell membrane which can cause abnormal communication between the intra- and extracellular compartments, (2) these electrical fields can cause the cell membrane to become permanently permeabilized, resulting in cell death, and (3) adjacent cells and structures are not affected as there is no undesirable thermal heating associated with IRE. In addition to these early findings, recent mathematical, computational, and in vitro studies have become additional tools in delineating the fundamental mechanisms of IRE. Recently, Daniels and Rubinsky demonstrated improved parameters for creating IRE ablation in the more heterogeneous geometric anatomy of the human body [10]. A combination of this work with additional findings by Neal et al. has suggested a possible role of IRE in treating breast cancer or other heterogeneous tissue containing differing morphology and density [11, 12].

With these promising results, many in vivo studies were initiated and developed into more relevant investigations to answer several important questions:

- Can IRE effectively cause liver cell death in vivo? Although many investigators have shown the effectiveness of IRE in causing in vitro hepatocyte death, this is clearly not sufficient to translate the technology into clinical settings. In addition, the effects on pericellular environments such as stromal cells, vessels, and nerves were not accounted for in these prior studies.
- How is IRE different from many already-existing locoregional treatment options such as radiofrequency ablation (RFA), cryoablation, or microwave ablation? Prior studies have suggested possible "nonthermal" ablative effects of IRE, but this must be validated and confirmed in larger animal models before translation into clinical applications. Also, what other characteristics of IRE distinguishes it from other ablative methods? How fast does it work? What side effects can occur?
- How safe and feasible is IRE in animal studies? The equipment and ablation probes used in mathematical or in vitro studies are clearly not acceptable in animal or clinical studies. In addition, no serious medical safety issues are involved when studying a new technology in mathematical or in vitro models. However, such issues become an important factor when determining whether this technology is feasible to use in patients.
- How does IRE really work? Once again, mathematical hypotheses and in vitro results can only demonstrate preliminary and nonclinical evidence of a new technology. It is difficult to convince patients and clinicians that this new tumor-ablative technology works based on findings from a computer program and the results from cells grown in a petri dish. These methods do provide useful

information, but only in large animal models or clinical research can more detailed and convincing evidence be shown in order to translate these new technologies into the clinical setting.

Preclinical Studies

Since the introduction of IRE in 2005 by Davalos et al. [13] as a novel ablation technique, many in vivo studies in animals such as mice, rats, rabbits, and pigs were performed to answer these questions. First, Edd et al. demonstrated the characterization of tissue ablation performed with IRE in vivo in the normal livers of rats (Sprague-Dawley rats) [14]. This and other studies in normal rat liver have concluded that the areas of ablation produced by IRE are clearly defined. Within the ablated zones, cell death with ischemic damage to parenchyma and massive immunological reactions were seen [14–16].

These findings from the normal rat liver studies led investigators to look into validating these findings in tumor models as well as larger animal models. One notable study was performed by Al-Sakere et al. in 2007 where the group demonstrated that IRE can be used to cause nonthermal ablation in tumor models in vivo [5]. The C57Bl/6 sarcoma xenograft model was used to evaluate the effectiveness of IRE in treating an approximately 5 mm tumor in the flank of mice. In addition, Guo et al. have shown the feasibility of IRE in treating rat hepatoma tumors formed after injection of the N1S1 HCC cell line. Follow-up was performed with MRI up to 15 days after treatment [6].

Several larger animal studies have also been performed, and the results were a significant leap in IRE technology development. The most notable nontumor study was performed in the swine model, and subsequently, a study was performed in the rabbit model, using VX2 sarcoma in the liver. In the next sections, details of these two studies, including the rationale and methods, will be discussed, and some significant results will be presented.

IRE on Swine Liver

For the swine studies, all animals were studied under the supervision of the Animal Research Committee (ARC) and Division of Laboratory Animal Medicine (DLAM). Pigs weighing an average of 40 kg were subjected to general anesthesia using a combination of intramuscular injection of ketamine hydrochloride, xylazine, and inhaled halothane. The pigs were placed in the supine position and the upper abdomen was shaved and sterilized in the usual fashion. At this point, preablation ultrasound (US) was performed to visualize areas of interest. In certain animals, contrast-enhanced CT (CECT) and/or MRI were performed at this point using previously described protocols [7]. Under real-time US guidance, IRE needles were placed percutaneously either using a subcostal or subxyphoid approach, or using open laparotomy (Fig. 19.1a). Once the satisfactory placement of the needles was confirmed, IRE was performed with either a monopolar system (two or three 18-gauge electrodes, Fig. 19.1b) or a single bipolar system (a single 16-gauge electrode) using a NanoKnife generator (AngioDynamics, Queensbury, NY, Fig. 19.1c). The ablation zone was monitored in real-time, both intra- and postprocedure, as well as 24 h, 7 days, and 14 days after the procedure, using US, CT, or MRI. Postablation care was performed in compliance with ARC policy and in accordance with NIH guidelines.

At four different time periods (24 h, 72 h, 7 days, and 14 days) after IRE treatment, pigs were euthanized and tissues harvested for immunohistochemistry. For various immunohistological analyses, each of the processed and sectioned tissue samples was stained with Hematoxylin and Eosin (H&E), Von Kossa stain, and vonWillebrand factor (vWF), as well as subjected to TUNEL assay.

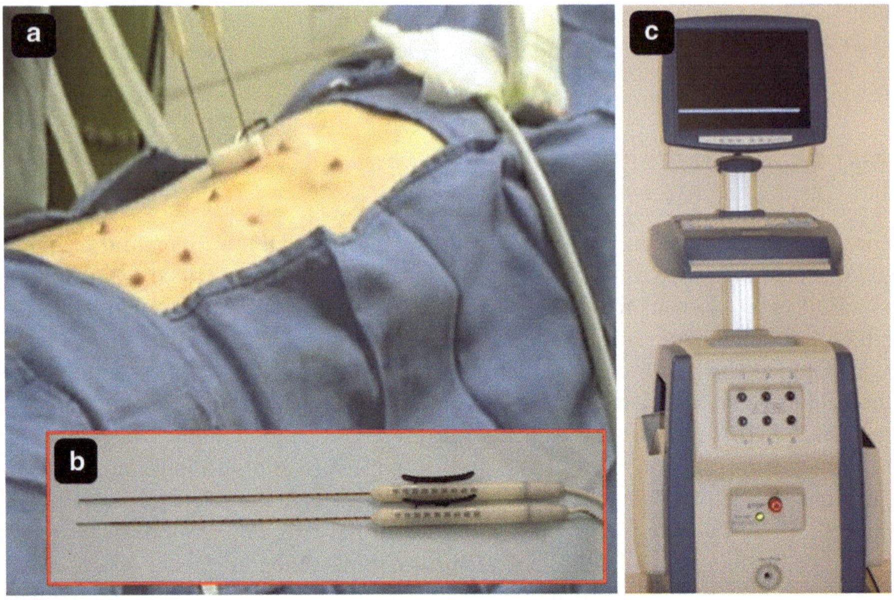

Fig. 19.1 (**a**) A photograph of percutaneous IRE ablation of swine liver using two monopolar probes. The real-time US guidance is used for probe placement, peri-ablation monitoring and postablation monitoring. (**b**) An image of IRE monopolar probes. Each probe is a 19 gauge in size with up to 4 cm tip exposure for ablation. Using two probes, various probe distance can be achieved to optimize the ablation. (**c**) A photograph of IRE generator (NanoKnife® Angiodynamics). It has three parts: monitor screen, laptop with conventional keyboard, and generator

Summary of the Swine Studies

In our swine studies, we were able to answer several very crucial questions.

Firstly, we confirmed the feasibility of performing percutaneous or laparotomy-assisted IRE in a large animal. We were able to effectively create various sizes of IRE-ablated zones (in a range of 25 × 17 to 42 × 60 mm) in normal swine hepatic parenchyma. We were able to preplan and control the various sizes of ablation zones based on the type of the needles (either bipolar or monopolar) and the distance between them (10–30 mm, Fig. 19.2) [7, 17]. This reproducible and controllable treatment with predictable ablation zones provides crucial evidence supporting translation of this protocol and parameters into human livers.

Next, our extensive immunohistochemical analyses have demonstrated that IRE can create complete cell death within the zone of ablation. We were able to reproduce this finding in both macro- and microscopic evaluation in all tissue samples we evaluated. In addition, IRE ablation provided a well-demarcated zone of ablation from nonablated normal liver parenchyma. Many of the currently available "thermal" ablation techniques suffer from the lack of completeness and distinctiveness of cell death adjacent to blood vessels due to the "heat sink" effect, and this has been shown to be a leading cause of recurrence [18]. In IRE ablation, cell death is complete within the ablation zone even up to the vascular wall, leaving no surviving cells. Hence, there is a decreased chance of recurrence or metastasis from missed foci of tumor cells.

A major advantage of IRE is the short procedure time. To ablate a lesion volume of 15 cm^3 (an oval-shaped lesion with largest diameter of 3.5 cm), IRE required an average of 7 min of procedure time from insertion of probes to the completion of the ablation [7]. The energy delivery component of the procedure, i.e., actual ablation time, takes less than a minute. We were able to significantly decrease the total procedure time to less than 10 min compared to the 30–60 min required in conventional thermal ablation methods [19, 20]. We believe that this is a critical factor in interventional

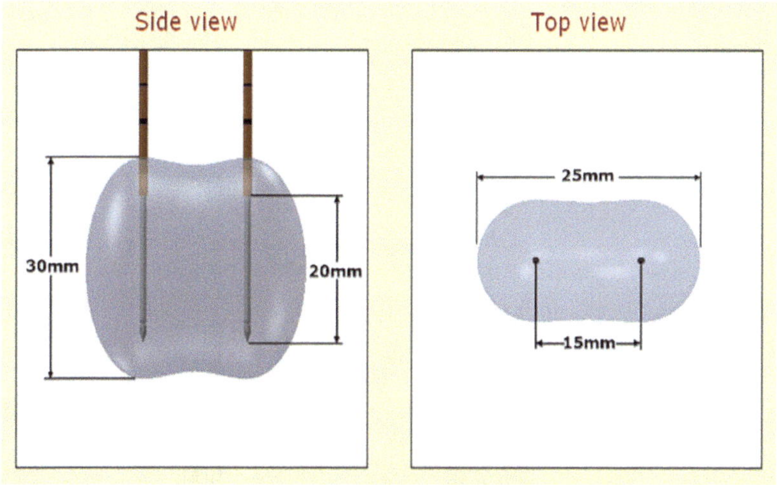

Fig. 19.2 Preplanning *side* and *top* view image of IRE. Using the IRE software, the size of IRE ablation can be accurately planned and executed. With a precise placement of probes, the accuracy of predicted size of IRE ablation is within millimeters of difference

procedures, as short procedure times can significantly reduce complication rates, postprocedure observation time, and discomfort for patients. Ultimately, short procedure times allow for additional time to be taken to create a larger size ablation zone (as big as 30–50 cm^2, an approximate volume of a lesion with largest diameter of 5 cm) with less procedure time in total minutes.

Another landmark finding of our swine studies was validation of the feasibility of using all the available imaging modalities in order to monitor the extent of the ablation and characterize the radiographic changes occurring during and immediately after the procedure using US, and within 48 h with CT and MRI (Fig. 19.3a–c). This provides a considerable advantage to IRE, as immediate imaging can monitor the completeness of ablation and allow for real-time planning of treatments. Most of the thermal ablation methods, including RFA, are unable to be monitored in real-time due to the formation of micro-bubbles creating hyperechogenicity on US images from thermally injured tissue. Also, CT and MRI are likewise very limited in their ability to characterize the ablation zone of RFA in short-term follow-up, as no distinct changes are seen shortly after conventional ablation [21]. By contrast, IRE creates a discrete and measurable spherical area of ablation during and immediately after the procedure. We have demonstrated this observation, and measurements of the treated area acquired during real-time monitoring using US and short-term follow-up imaging using CT and MRI correlated well with gross measurement of the ablation. Interestingly, diffusion-weighted imaging (DWI) images demonstrated an area of diffusion restriction within the ablation zone, which correlated well with the area of hypoechogenicity seen on US images. This phenomenon is likely due to increased intracellular water content seen as hypoechoic on US and decreased blood flow to the core of the ablation due to cell death and vascular congestion seen on DWI MRI. Several significant points about these findings can be highlighted: (1) to our knowledge, this is the first report using CT and MRI in evaluating IRE ablation in a large animal model, (2) this is the first investigation confirming the feasibility of using all three conventional imaging modalities (US, CT, and MRI) to evaluate IRE and its ablation zone for immediate follow-up for effective treatment planning, and (3) this is the first report using MRI DWI sequence to evaluate hepatic ablation. Two recent studies have been reported using DWI imaging in monitoring prostate thermal ablation [22, 23].

In summary, we were able to demonstrate several important findings regarding IRE ablation on hepatic tissue using a normal swine liver: (1) IRE ablation in swine liver is a feasible and reproducible procedure, (2) IRE causes complete cell death in a very complete and distinctive manner, (3) ultra-short

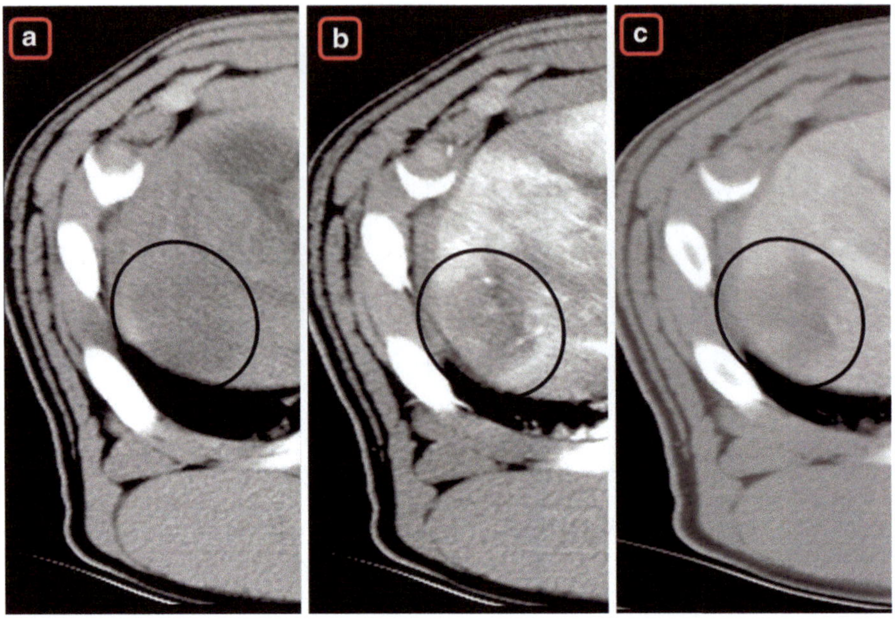

Fig. 19.3 (**a**) A noncontrast CT of the swine liver within 24 h from IRE ablation demonstrates an area of hypodensity in the poster aspect of the right lobe of the liver with very mild hyperdensity suggestive of hyperemia. (**b**) An arterial phase of the swine liver accentuates the hypodensity of ablated zone with increased peripheral enhancement. Several linear hyperdensity is noted within the ablated zone, which may correlate with the intact vessels within the ablation. (**c**) A delayed venous phase of the swine liver with a persistent hypodensity of IRE-ablated zone suggestive of successful ablation

ablation procedure time is possible, and (4) multiple imaging modalities (US, CT, and MRI) can be used to evaluate and analyze the IRE ablation zone during the procedure as a real-time monitoring tool and with short-term follow-up. Lastly, we have also performed extensive immunohistochemistry to further elucidate the basic pathophysiological background of IRE ablation in the liver.

IRE on Rabbit Liver VX2 Tumor

Following our results in swine liver ablation, several questions remained: mainly how effectively IRE would work on cancer cells. Cancer cells behave differently than normal cells in every aspect of cellular physiology, genomics, and pathology. Therefore, it was imperative to evaluate and validate the effectiveness of IRE on in vivo tumor models. The IRE studies performed on pigs had the advantages of using larger livers that allowed for the consistent creation of multiple lesions in order to define the ablation zone, pulse number and frequency, and determine the type of electrode needle required. We then shifted our focus to applying our knowledge from the swine liver IRE ablation to IRE ablation of an actual tumor tissue grown in the liver of a live animal. We determined that rabbits were the most appropriate species for this study because the rabbit VX2 liver tumor model is one of the few well-accepted large animal tumor models, since the growth of this aggressive mesenchymal tumor is comparable to that of hepatocellular carcinoma in humans. In addition, the early stages of tumor growth up to 2 weeks can be controlled and monitored to obtain a consistent tumor size. VX2 tumors grow rapidly, about 1 cm increase in diameter in 1 week within a short growth time.

Lastly, the rabbit has phylogenetically similar hepatic anatomy to that of humans and swine, so we can easily translate our findings from the swine studies into rabbit studies, and overall findings from both large animal studies can be utilized in translating the IRE ablation technology into clinical application.

Over 100 New Zealand white rabbits were studied under the supervision of the ARC and DLAM. Our experimental design was based on multiple prior studies [24, 25]. Under general anesthesia, the VX2 tumor was implanted into the hindleg of a donor rabbit and grown for about 2 weeks. Once the tumor grew to an appropriate size, the tumor was harvested, minced, and implanted into the left lobe of a recipient rabbit's liver. The rabbits were given proper care and monitored using frequent US until the VX2 tumor grew up to 1 cm in diameter (Fig. 19.4a–f).

At the time of treatment, the animals underwent general anesthesia as described above and were then placed in the supine position. The right upper quadrant was shaved and sterilized, and the VX2 tumor was located using US guidance. The IRE needle was advanced into the tumor and ablation was performed (see Section "IRE on Swine Liver" for detailed description of materials). The ablation zone was monitored in real-time, both intra- and post-procedure, as well as 24 h, 3 days, 7 days, 14 days, and 28 days after the procedure, using US and CT. Postablation care was performed in compliance with ARC policy and in accordance with NIH guidelines.

At different time periods (15 min, 30 min, 1 h, 2 h, 6 h, 12 h, 24 h, 72 h, 7 days, 14 days, and 28 days) after IRE treatment, the rabbits were euthanized. The liver tissues, including the zone of ablation, and lung tissues were harvested for both gross and microscopic pathological analysis. For various immunohistological analyses, each processed and sectioned tissue sample was then stained with H&E, vWF, P-53, Ki-67, CD30, and vascular endothelial growth factor receptor (VEGFR), as well as subjected to TUNEL assay.

On a side note, VX2 tumor can be implanted into the rabbit through either the injection of minced tumor from the hindlimb of the donor or injection of premade cell suspension. Two studies comparing the two methods concluded that injection of minced tumor from the hindlimb of the donor was far superior because it reduced tumor cell leakage (0 vs. 50% for injection) and had a

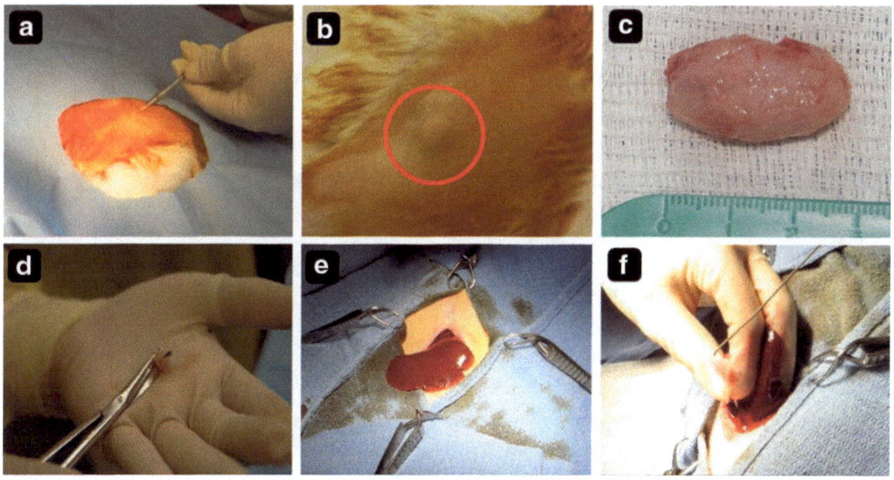

Fig. 19.4 An illustration of creating rabbit VX2 liver tumor model: (**a**) injection of VX2 tumor cells into the donor rabbit's hindleg muscle, (**b**) in 10–14 days, the VX2 tumor grows to an appropriate size, (**c**) a harvested VX2 tumor is about 2.5–3 cm in size, (**d**) the tumor is minced into millimeter size as soon as it is harvested from the hindleg, (**e**) the left lobe of the rabbit liver is exposed via midline laparotomy, and (**f**) minced VX2 tumor is implanted into the left lobe of the rabbit liver for a liver tumor growth, which usually occurs in 10–14 days

better successful inoculation (95 vs. 35% for injection) [26]. This leakage causes seeding of the tumor outside of the liver causing unnecessary pain and distress to the animal, and possibly leading to premature death. These findings were also confirmed by another recent study [27]. Therefore, we have adopted to use the method of injecting minced tumor from the donor's hindlimb.

Summary of the Rabbit Studies

The major findings include the following: (1) IRE consistently produced complete cell death in the ablated zone with a sharp margin, with both gross and histological analyses confirming the lack of any viable cells within the ablated zone, (2) IRE ablation is not affected by the heatsink effect and therefore, complete cell death of perivascular cells were achieved, (3) IRE ablation has an ultra short procedure time of under 1 min of actual IRE ablation, and (4) IRE ablation allows for real-time monitoring under US imaging and the use of CECT to monitor and evaluate ablation outcome as early as 24 h following the procedure (Fig. 19.5a, b). In addition to validating these points, IRE ablation on the rabbit VX2 tumor model studies has provided several additional key facts about IRE ablation.

One of the main findings from the rabbit studies was the effectiveness of IRE ablation in completely eradicating tumor cells in the liver of living subjects. By ablating different fractions of the tumor (e.g., ablating only half of the tumor vs. full tumor), we confirmed that complete tumor cell death was only seen within the area of ablated zone. As described above, complete cell death was seen with no residual tumor cells left within the ablated zone including perivascular tumor cells. With complete full ablation coverage of a tumor mass, no evidence of synchronous or metachronous tumors is seen within the liver or lung. This demonstrated that the IRE ablation resulted in complete remission of the tumor. We were able to stop the growth and spread of the VX2 tumor, an extremely aggressive tumor shown to have both intrahepatic and distant metastases in every rabbit in the control and sham groups. Complete ablation coverage of the tumor with a sufficient margin was possible because of several advantages of IRE ablation. We were able to evaluate and monitor the ablation zone in real-time, which allowed us to adjust the probes and ablation parameters and reablate immediately after the first ablation if needed. We were also able to perform multiple IRE ablations within a single session under the same anesthesia session as each ablation took less than a minute. Hence, a total procedure time for two or three ablations was less than 5 min. A complete

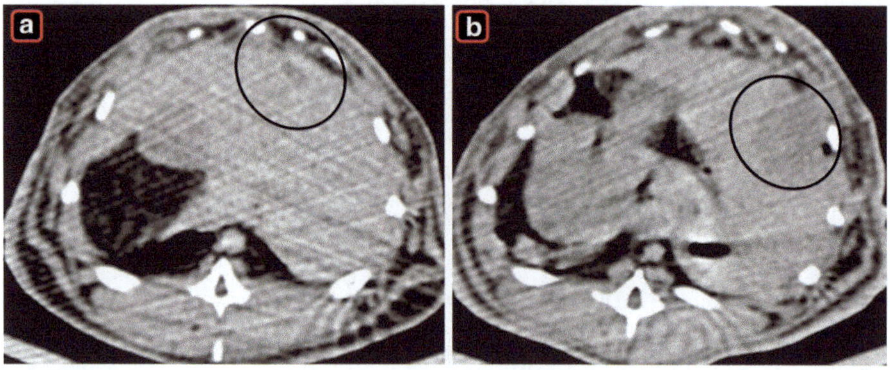

Fig. 19.5 (**a**) A contrast-enhanced CT (CECT) image of rabbit liver with an implanted VX2 tumor pre-IRE ablation demonstrates a hypodense tumor with a very mild peripheral enhancement. (**b**) 24 h post-IRE ablation CECT demonstrates a large hypodense ablation defect. This hypodense defect decreases but persists for over 3 weeks

tumor ablation is the most important feature of IRE in translating this technology into the clinical setting as many currently existing ablative technologies lack this due to the heatsink effect and inability to perform real-time monitoring.

In our rabbit studies, we also performed several additional immunohistological analyses of the IRE-ablated tissues (Fig. 19.6a–c). In addition to validating complete cell death by IRE, we investigated further into the underlying pathophysiology of how IRE produces complete cell by exploring the molecular pathways that help us understand further what IRE does to tumor cells. In both the swine normal liver study and rabbit VX2 tumor studies, we consistently found that IRE-induced cell death is intimately associated with apoptosis. During the first week post IRE ablation, apoptotic markers (e.g., BCL-2) were found to be markedly increased in the IRE-ablated zone compared to the normal liver tissues and within VX2 tumor. This method of cell death which is also known as programmed cell death occurs due to the cell's intrinsic biochemical and molecular changes [29]. Apoptosis is involved in the normal natural course of cell life such as repair after damage, allostasis to keep constancy between cell death and cell division, and during tissue development and organogenesis [30]. As apoptosis is heavily involved in many normal cellular developments, the repair of damaged tissues and regeneration of a damaged organ after apoptotic cell death is believed to be relatively faster and more efficient [29–31]. Another common method of cell death is necrosis, which is also known as traumatic cell death caused by acute cellular injury. All of the conventional thermal ablation techniques including RFA cause necrotic cell death resulting in the scarring of tissue. However, our finding regarding the relationship between IRE and apoptosis can support a theory that IRE-induced apoptotic cell death may enhance regeneration of the ablated liver by rapidly inducing tissue repair without fibrosing or scarring. This feature of IRE can be a notable clinical advantage, as quick regeneration means faster recovery for patients and faster recovery of liver function after tumor ablation.

Another clinically important finding of our rabbit VX2 tumor studies was the preservation of critical intrahepatic structures such as bile ducts and vessels. In all animal studies, the patency of hepatic arteries, hepatic veins, portal veins, and bile ducts was seen within IRE-ablated areas (Fig. 19.7). Small-vessel (less than 2 mm) vasculitis was evident; however, any vessels greater than 3 mm in diameter have shown either no structural damage or very mild narrowing. These findings were confirmed in radiographic analysis using CECT as well as both gross and microscopic analysis. We used multiple vascular wall markers, including vWF, VEGFR, and Masson's Trichrome stain, to validate architectural preservation of vessels and bile ducts. One speculation about the mild effect of IRE ablation on these structures is even though IRE eradicates every cell with intact cellular membranes within the ablated zone, the ablation preserves the thin layer of subendothelial connective tissue and elastic tissues such as internal/external elastic lamina and tunica adventitia of the vessels. These connective

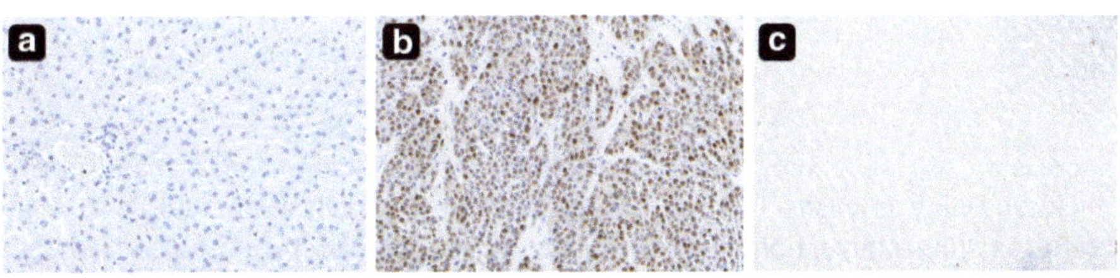

Fig. 19.6 P53 staining of (**a**) normal rabbit liver, (**b**) VX2 tumor and (**c**) IRE ablation zone. A normal liver (**a**) stains only nuclei with blue stains with essentially no P53 positive cells as P53 immunohistochemistry stains only proliferating cells. In VX2 tumor (**b**), there are innumerable P53 positive cells as demonstrating markedly proliferative nature of tumor cells. However, in IRE-ablated zone (**c**), normal hepatocytes scaffolds are seen without any nuclei or P53 positive cells consistent with complete cell death within the ablated zone. These findings are also confirmed with Ki-67 and VonKossa immunohistochemical analysis

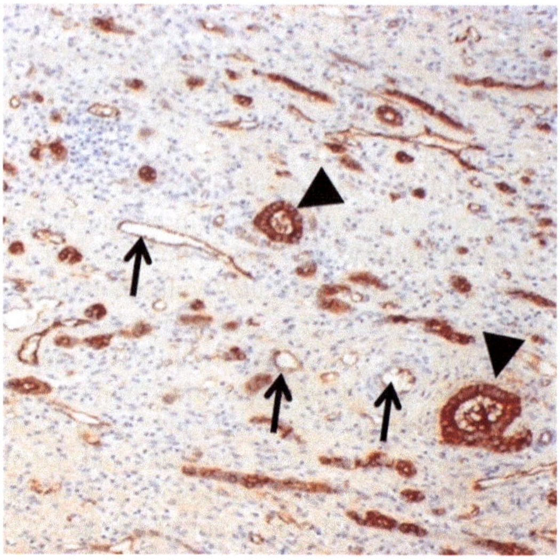

Fig. 19.7 An evaluation of small vessels and bile ducts within the IRE-ablated zone demonstrates intact vessels (*arrows*) and bile ducts (*arrowheads*) with normal microscopic morphology. Intact vascular endothelium and biliary epithelium are stained positively with VEGF receptors and vWF (not shown)

tissues are responsible for the structural integrity of the vessels; therefore, these intact connective tissues after IRE ablation are responsible for the preservation of the vessels and bile ducts. Moreover, on CECT, larger vessels appear to contain normally flowing blood in different phases (arterial, venous vs. delayed phase). This characteristic of IRE further supports our theory that IRE ablation results in tissue regeneration.

In summary, based on our swine normal liver ablation studies, we were able to develop and perform a more clinically related IRE ablation on the rabbit VX2 tumor in which we were able to validate and reproduce our findings from the swine studies. In addition, we demonstrate several crucial findings regarding IRE ablation on the hepatic tumor. We were also able to demonstrate the effectiveness of IRE ablation in eradicating hepatic tumors and were able to follow the outcome of the ablation. Furthermore, we have delineated the intricate pathophysiology of IRE-induced cell death and were able to demonstrate that IRE is capable of inducing the apoptotic pathway in the cells within the ablated zone, causing complete cell death without damaging some critical intrahepatic structures such as vessels and bile ducts. Overall, a combination of IRE-induced apoptosis and preservation of these structures may lead to rapid tissue repair and restoration of hepatic function.

Conclusion

With the increasing use of locoregional therapies for hepatic malignancies, many novel ablative methods, including high-intensity focused ultrasound (HIFU), microwave, and RFA, that complement currently existing conventional oncologic therapies have been developed and investigated [32–39]. IRE ablation is a novel technology with a promising future as it provides several advantages over other ablation methods or currently available oncologic therapies. IRE uses a nonconventional, nonthermal energy-delivering mechanism to eradicate tumors with increased efficacy, decreased procedure time, improved clinical applications with real-time monitoring, and the possibility of enhancing regeneration of ablated tissues. Overall, we believe IRE can be a powerful and safe ablation method for treating hepatic malignancies.

References

1. Neumann E, Schaefer-Ridder M, Wang Y, Hofschneider PH. Gene transfer into mouse lyoma cells by electroporation in high electric fields. EMBO J. 1982;1:841–5.
2. Chang DC, Reese TS. Changes in membrane structure induced by electroporation as revealed by rapid-freezing electron microscopy. Biophys J. 1990;58:1–12.
3. Orlowski S, Mir LM. Cell electropermeabilization: a new tool for biochemical and pharmacological studies. Biochim Biophys Acta. 1993;1154:51–63.
4. Rubinsky B. Irreversible electroporation in medicine. Technol Cancer Res Treat. 2007;6:255–60.
5. Al-Sakere B, Andre F, Bernat C, Connault E, Opolon P, Davalos RV, et al. Tumor ablation with irreversible electroporation. PLoS One. 2007;2:e1135.
6. Guo Y, Zhang Y, Klein R, Nijm GM, Sahakian AV, Omary RA, et al. Irreversible electroporation therapy in the liver: longitudinal efficacy studies in a rat model of hepatocellular carcinoma. Cancer Res. 2010;70:1555–63.
7. Lee EW, Chen C, Prieto VE, Dry SM, Loh CT, Kee ST. Advanced hepatic ablation technique for creating complete cell death: irreversible electroporation. Radiology. 2010;255:426–33.
8. Oshima T, Sato M. Bacterial sterilization and intracellular protein release by a pulsed electric field. Adv Biochem Eng Biotechnol. 2004;90:113–33.
9. Edd JF, Davalos RV. Mathematical modeling of irreversible electroporation for treatment planning. Technol Cancer Res Treat. 2007;6:275–86.
10. Daniels C, Rubinsky B. Electrical field and temperature model of nonthermal irreversible electroporation in heterogeneous tissues. J Biomech Eng. 2009;131:071006.
11. Neal II RE, Davalos RV. The feasibility of irreversible electroporation for the treatment of breast cancer and other heterogeneous systems. Ann Biomed Eng. 2009;37:2615–25.
12. Neal II RE, Singh R, Hatcher HC, Kock ND, Torti SV, Davalos RV. Treatment of breast cancer through the application of irreversible electroporation using a novel minimally invasive single needle electrode. Breast Cancer Res Treat. 2010;123:295–301.
13. Davalos RV, Mir IL, Rubinsky B. Tissue ablation with irreversible electroporation. Ann Biomed Eng. 2005;33:223–31.
14. Edd JF, Horowitz L, Davalos RV, Mir LM, Rubinsky B. *In vivo* results of a new focal tissue ablation technique: irreversible electroporation. IEEE Trans Biomed Eng. 2006;53:1409–15.
15. Ivorra A, Rubinsky B. Impedance analyzer for *in vivo* electroporation studies. Conf Proc IEEE Eng Med Biol Soc. 2006;1:5056–9.
16. Ivorra A, Rubinsky B. *In vivo* electrical impedance measurements during and after electroporation of rat liver. Bioelectrochemistry. 2007;70:287–95.
17. Lee EW, Loh CT, Kee ST. Imaging guided percutaneous irreversible electroporation: ultrasound and immunohistological correlation. Technol Cancer Res Treat. 2007;6:287–94.
18. Lu DS, Raman SS, Vodopich DJ, Wang M, Sayre J, Lassman C. Effect of vessel size on creation of hepatic radiofrequency lesions in pigs: assessment of the "heat sink" effect. AJR Am J Roentgenol. 2002;178:47–51.
19. Friedman M, Mikityansky I, Kam A, Libutti SK, Walther MM, Neeman Z, et al. Radiofrequency ablation of cancer. Cardiovasc Intervent Radiol. 2004;27:427–34.
20. Gibson TB. Radiofrequency ablation for patients with colorectal cancer and unresectable liver metastasis. Clin Colorectal Cancer. 2006;5:318–20.
21. Kim SK, Rhim H, Kim YS, Koh BH, Cho OK, Seo HS, Kim Y. Radiofrequency thermal ablation of hepatic tumors: pitfalls and challenges. Abdom Imaging. 2005;30:727–33.
22. Chen J, Daniel BL, Diederich CJ, Bouley DM, van den Bosch MA, Kinsey AM, et al. Monitoring prostate thermal therapy with diffusion-weighted MRI. Magn Reson Med. 2008;59:1365–72.
23. Kim CK, Park BK, Lee HM, Kim SS, Kim E. MRI techniques for prediction of local tumor progression after high-intensity focused ultrasonic ablation of prostate cancer. AJR Am J Roentgenol. 2008;190:1180–6.
24. Hong K, Khwaja A, Liapi E, Torbenson MS, Georgiades CS, Geschwind JF. New intra-arterial drug delivery system for the treatment of liver cancer: preclinical assessment in a rabbit model of liver cancer. Clin Cancer Res. 2006;12:2563–7.
25. Kim TJ, Moon WK, Cha JH, Goo JM, Lee KH, Kim KH, et al. VX2 carcinoma in rabbits after radiofrequency ablation: comparison of MR contrast agents for help in differentiating benign periablational enhancement from residual tumor. Radiology. 2005;234:423–30.
26. Chen JH, Lin YC, Huang YS, Chen TJ, Lin WY, Han KW. Induction of VX2 carcinoma in rabbit liver: comparison of two inoculation methods. Lab Anim. 2004;38:79–84.
27. Virmani S, Harris KR, Szolc-Kowalska B, Paunesku T, Woloschak GE, Lee FT, et al. Comparison of two different methods for inoculating VX2 tumors in rabbit livers and hind limbs. J Vasc Interv Radiol. 2008;19:931–6.

28. Rubinsky B, Onik G, Mikus P. Irreversible electroporation: a new ablation modality – clinical implications. Technol Cancer Res Treat. 2007;6:37–48.
29. Kerr JF, Wyllie AH, Currie AR. Apoptosis: a basic biological phenomenon with wide-ranging implications in tissue kinetics. Br J Cancer. 1972;26:239–57.
30. Thompson CB. Apoptosis in the pathogenesis and treatment of disease. Science. 1995;267:1456–62.
31. Susin SA, Lorenzo HK, Zamzami N, Marzo I, Snow BE, Brothers GM, et al. Molecular characterization of mitochondrial apoptosis-inducing factor. Nature. 1999;397:441–6.
32. Yan TD, Padang R, Morris DL. Longterm results and prognostic indicators after cryotherapy and hepatic arterial chemotherapy with or without resection for colorectal liver metastases in 224 patients: longterm survival can be achieved in patients with multiple bilateral liver metastases. J Am Coll Surg. 2006;202:100–11.
33. Chung MH, Ye W, Ramming KP, Bilchik AJ. Repeat hepatic cryotherapy for metastatic colorectal cancer. J Gastrointest Surg. 2001;5:287–93.
34. Daniele B, De Sio I, Izzo F, Capuano G, Andreana A, Mazzanti R, et al., CLIP Investigators. Hepatic resection and percutaneous ethanol injection as treatments of small hepatocellular carcinoma: a Cancer of the Liver Italian Program (CLIP 08) retrospective case-control study. J Clin Gastroenterol. 2003;36:63–7.
35. Oshowo A, Gillams A, Harrison E, Lees WR, Taylor I. Comparison of resection and radiofrequency ablation for treatment of solitary colorectal liver metastases. Br J Surg. 2003;90:1240–3.
36. Livraghi T, Solbiati L, Meloni MF, Gazelle GS, Halpern EF, Goldberg SN. Treatment of focal liver tumors with percutaneous radio-frequency ablation: complications encountered in a multicenter study. Radiology. 2003;226:441–51.
37. Livraghi T, Solbiati L, Meloni F, Ierace T, Goldberg SN, Gazelle GS. Percutaneous radiofrequency ablation of liver metastases in potential candidates for resection: the "test-of-time approach". Cancer. 2003;97:3027–35.
38. Satoi S, Kamiyama Y, Matsui Y, Kitade H, Kaibori M, Yamamoto H, et al. Clinical outcome of 214 liver resections using microwave tissue coagulation. Hepatogastroenterology. 2005;52:1180–5.
39. Lencioni R, Crocetti L, Cioni D, Della Pina C, Bartolozzi C. Percutaneous radiofrequency ablation of hepatic colorectal metastases: technique, indications, results, and new promises. Invest Radiol. 2004;39:689–97.

Chapter 20
Translational Research on Irreversible Electroporation: VX2 Rabbit Head and Neck

Daphne Wong, Edward W. Lee, and Stephen T. Kee

Abstract Head and neck cancers account for a small percent of new cancer cases each year in comparison to other cancers. However, the diagnosis of this disease is usually life threatening and negatively impacts the quality of the patient's life. With various treatments or therapies available for the different stages of squamous cell carcinoma of the head and neck (SCCHN), the most prominent type of head and neck cancer, significant side effects or disadvantages such as severe toxicity and lack of organ preservation sometimes outweigh the positive outcomes. Irreversible electroporation (IRE) is a novel treatment that is currently showing promise in tumor ablation without the disadvantages of other techniques. Therefore, current research is underway in order to utilize IRE against implanted VX2 rabbit tumors in the head and neck region to demonstrate its effectiveness. Through preliminary results, positive outcomes are showing great promise that IRE may be the next innovative treatment for SCCHN.

Keywords Irreversible electroporation • VX2 • Head and neck cancer • Squamous cell carcinoma of the head and neck • Chemo-radiotherapy • Epidermal growth factor receptor

Introduction

Head and neck cancer can be defined as a collection of biologically similar epithelial cancers that occur throughout the upper aerodigestive tract [1]. They have the anatomical characteristics of an infiltrative noncohesive cancer with permeation of vessels, nerves, and submucosal spread [2–4]. The majority of head and neck cancers are squamous cell carcinoma of the head and neck (SCCHN), which is considered to be the sixth most common cancer in the world [1, 5] affecting over 650,000 people worldwide and creating approximately 46,000 new cases per year in the United States, resulting in an estimated 11,260 deaths [6, 7]. Some risk factors of head and neck cancers include cigarette, cigar or pipe smoking, excessive alcohol consumption and recently, the human papilloma virus (HPV), particularly HPV type 16 [8]. SCCHN is considered one of the most difficult cancers to treat due to the growth of primary tumors that spread into adjacent tissues and lymph nodes, where primary tumor sites may include the lip, oral cavity, nasal cavity, paranasal sinuses, pharynx,

D. Wong (✉)
Division of Interventional Radiology, Department of Radiology, David Geffen School of Medicine at UCLA, 10833 Le Conte Avenue, B2-168, Los Angeles, CA 90095-1721, USA
e-mail: daphnewong@mednet.ucla.edu

S.T. Kee et al. (eds.), *Clinical Aspects of Electroporation*,
DOI 10.1007/978-1-4419-8363-3_20, © Springer Science+Business Media, LLC 2011

and larynx [1]. Unlike many other cancers, where metastases are the primary cause of death, local recurrence is the most common cause of treatment failure where approximately 50–60% of patients have recurrence within 2 years and 20–30% develop metastatic disease [1, 5, 9] having a median survival rate of no more than 6 months [10, 11]. Most head and neck cancers remain asymptomatic until late in the disease course, making them more difficult to treat and manage since it may obstruct or harm structures involved in speech, voice production, and swallowing, creating a low quality of life after dissection or other treatments [7, 12]. Therefore, it is these disabilities that fuel the need for an effective and safe treatment for SCCHN.

Head and Neck Cancer Therapies

SCCHN can be characterized into four stages: early-stage disease, locally advanced disease, recurrent and metastatic disease, and platinum-refractory disease. With each stage, different therapies are utilized to get the maximum effect. Below, current therapies for SCCHN are discussed.

Neck Dissection

Surgical management of head and neck cancers by dissection has been the primary treatment since the early 1900s [13, 14]. Currently, selective dissections are still used for stage I or II SCCHN, where nodal areas are not at risk when left undissected. Selective neck dissections are mostly applied to early-stage disease, where approximately 33% of patients have a 5-year survival rate of about 80% [1]. However, morbidity also increases with dissections when the accessory nerve is compromised during surgery, leading to shoulder disability and permanent loss of function with significant pain [13]. Therefore, dissections should be considered for SCCHN stage I or II in order to attain the best curative outcomes.

Chemo-Radiotherapy

As head and neck cancers advance to stage III or IV, single-modality treatments are no longer as effective, leading to multimodal treatments. The use of concurrent chemo-radiotherapy (CRT), which is the combination of radiotherapy with chemotherapy, has shown in both definitive and adjuvant postoperative settings a 12% reduction in mortality and an improvement of 4% in 5-year survival [15] while preserving organ function [9]. However, substantial toxicities have been observed in patients who underwent CRT [7], with acute toxicities such as mucositis, stomatitis, dermatitis, and late toxic effects that include chronic xerostomia, dysphagia, feeding-tube dependence, aspiration, and thyroid dysfunction [5]. Therefore, although CRT has advantages in organ preservation, the significant risk in toxicity may outweigh those advantages.

Molecularly Targeted Therapies with EGFR

With the prospect of severe toxicities as a result of CRT, other therapies have been studied as an alternative to treating late-stage SCCHN such as molecularly targeted therapies, with growing interest in targeting the epidermal growth factor receptor (EGFR). EGFR is part of the human epidermal receptor (HER)/Erb-B family of receptor tyrosine kinases that are responsible for transducing extracellular signals to intracellular responses [16]. It has been demonstrated that there is an overexpression of EGFR in almost all SCCHN tumors, and its overexpression is related to higher disease stage [5]; therefore, the blockage of EGFR pathways becomes a main focus as the next treatment for SCCHN. Anti-EGFR monoclonal antibodies such as cetuximab and low-molecular tyrosine kinase inhibitors such as erlotinib are currently the most developed EGFR-targeted therapies [17]. A randomized phase III trial of radiation therapy was able to demonstrate increased survival in patients with stages III to IV with the addition of cetuximab, leading to FDA approval of this agent [18].

Irreversible Electroporation

In the medical arsenal of tissue ablation, the innovative technique of irreversible electroporation (IRE) provides for the possibility of a safer, faster, and more effective means compared to other ablative methods. The uniqueness of IRE stems from its nonpharmacological and nonthermal characteristics, which separates this method from electrochemotherapy that utilizes chemical agents and may lead to problems with drug allergies, and thermal ablative methods such as radiofrequency ablation (RFA), which is temperature dependent. IRE is the process where microsecond electrical pulses are used to destabilize the electric potential of the cell membrane, causing permeabilization with nano-scale defects in the lipid bilayer, which eventually leads to cell death if a strong enough pulse is applied to inhibit the resealing of the membrane [19]. In a typical IRE protocol, electrical pulses are transmitted using two needle-like electrodes placed into and on the outer regions of the specific tissue [20]. Also, a novel feature of IRE is the ability for the electrodes to fit any tumor size, shape, and position, allowing it to accommodate any geometry [21]. A study by Maor et al. was able to demonstrate that IRE also has the ability to ablate tissues close to blood vessels without harming them even when electrical pulses were directly applied [19]. Furthermore, Onik et al. performed IRE on prostate tissues and were able to determine the unique selectivity of IRE, since it was able to destroy the cellular components of the tissue but able to keep the collagen tissue underneath intact [22]. With this finding, they were able to validate another advantage of IRE: the ability to create a distinct margin between ablated and normal tissues. A recent IRE study on swine liver also demonstrated positively the advantages of this treatment [23]. As a result, this is beneficial for tumors that are located close to large blood vessels, such as SCCHN. Overall, with further study, IRE can be considered as a novel therapy for recurrent SCCHN.

Preliminary Results of IRE on SCCHN

With the advantageous prospects of IRE on tissue ablation and our recent study on the rabbit VX2 tumor in liver, the same model was applied to demonstrate the effectiveness of IRE in the head and neck region. The rabbit was the ideal model for this study due to the successful mimicry of human head and neck tumors. The postauricular area was chosen in order to mimic this, since it follows similar lymphatic drainage to that in humans. In this study, we wanted to demonstrate IRE as an effective treatment in decreasing the rate of metastasis and lymphatic involvement of the head and neck tumor. Additionally, we wanted to evaluate the safety of this technique against adjacent vital structures such as vessels and nerves. With this study, we hoped to demonstrate, for the first time, in a scientifically controlled large animal model that in a very short treatment time under real-time image guidance, IRE can cause well-controlled and focused areas of head and neck tumor ablation, creating complete cell death while preserving adjacent vital structures.

New Zealand white rabbits were studied under the supervision of the Animal Research Committee (ARC) and Division of Laboratory Animal Medicine (DLAM). VX2 tumors were first implanted into the hind leg of a donor rabbit and were allowed to grow for approximately 14 days. Once the tumor grew to an appropriate size, it was harvested, minced, and injected into the postauricular region/muscle (in the proximal sternocleidomastoid muscle) of the recipient rabbit. The tumor was then allowed to grow to an appropriate size of 1 cm. IRE treatment was then performed using a bipolar needle electrode that was advanced into the tumor area. A square pulse of 2,500 V was applied using a pulse generator, where a total of 90 pulses were administered. The entire IRE treatment, from electrode placement to the end of pulse application, was less than 3 min. Additionally, we have found that the electric current used in IRE appears to cause muscle twitching. Therefore, we administered pancuronium before the IRE treatment in order to prevent this. After the addition of pancuronium, minimal muscle twitching was observed. Radiological imaging in the form of contrast-enhanced computed tomography (CECT) was used to evaluate tumor changes after IRE was performed. At the end of the study, the rabbits were euthanized, and the tissue around the ablation and tumor including muscle, fat, and the tumor enclosed were recovered for immunohistochemical examination.

Summary

After analyzing the results from this study, we can confirm that our attempt in presenting IRE as an effective and safe ablation technique in creating complete cell death of VX2 head and neck tumors was successful. We were able to show a decrease in the rate of metastasis and lymphatic involvement of the head and neck cancer and a distinct demarcation between the ablation site and the surrounding tissues with vital structures such as vessels (Figs. 20.1 and 20.2). Moreover, these results were detected using real-time monitoring capability through ultrasound imaging and follow-up imaging using CECT. With CECT, we were also able to identify ablations as early as 24 h after the IRE procedure; therefore validating the rapid effect of this technique (Fig. 20.3).

With faster procedure times, there is a decrease in complications and a faster recovery. Furthermore, IRE was shown not to be affected by the heat-sink effect that normally troubles RFA, demonstrating the advantage of its nonthermal characteristic. One of the most important validations is the creation of complete cell death. This can be seen in the immunohistological analyses of the IRE-ablated head and neck tissues (Figs. 20.1 and 20.2). Complete cell death was seen throughout

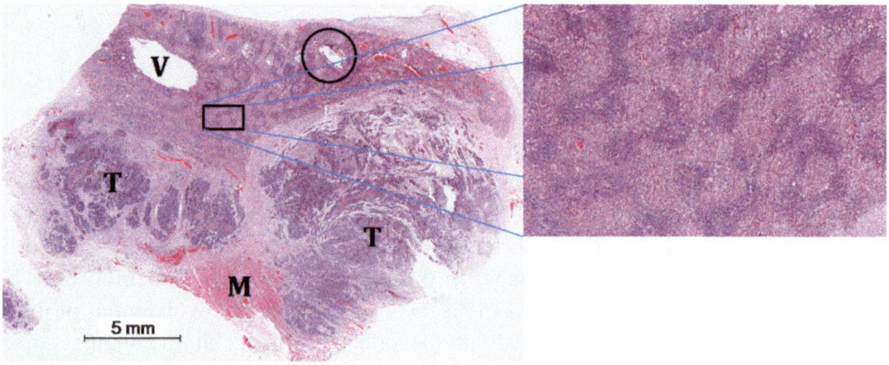

Fig. 20.1 Histological images (hematoxylin and eosin (H&E) staining) of VX2 implanted tissue in the right neck region of control rabbit including the carotid space: (T) VX2 tumor mass, (M) sternocleidomastoid muscle, (V) vessel, (*black circle*) a branch of carotid artery, and (*black box*) perivascular tumoral invasion of VX2 tumor

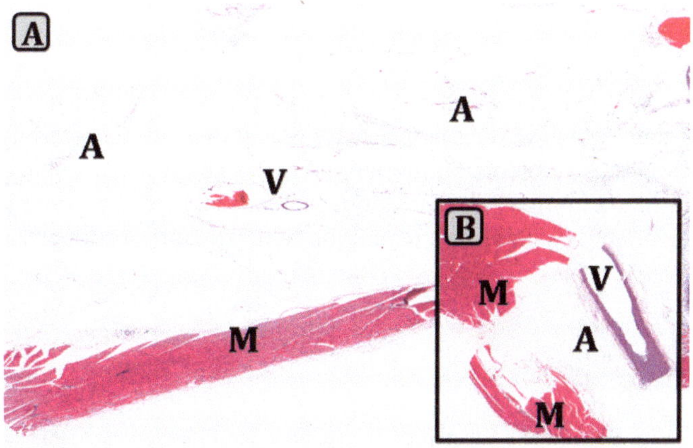

Fig. 20.2 Histological image (A, hematoxylin and eosin (H&E) staining) of IRE-treated VX2 tumor in the right neck region of rabbit including the carotid space: (A) IRE-ablated zone, (M) sternocleidomastoid muscle, (V) vessel, (B) longitudinally prepared carotid artery with intact layers

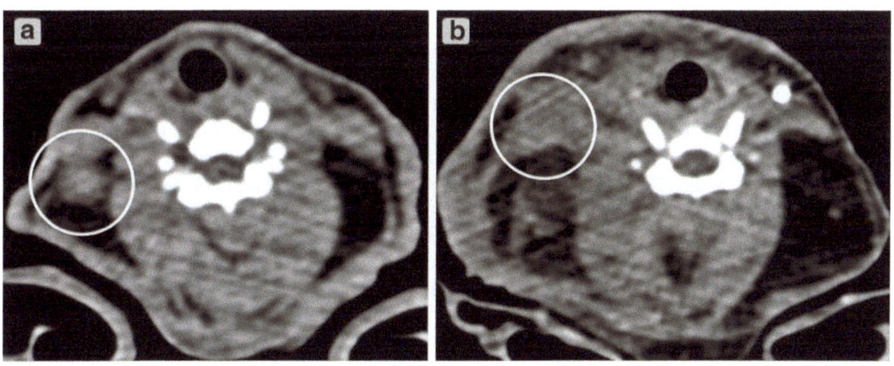

Fig. 20.3 Preablation CT image (**a**) of the VX2 tumor is observed just posterior to the right sternocleidomastoid muscle. Contrast-enhanced CT image (**b**) of IRE-ablated tumor demonstrates a hypodense mass with mildly increased contrast enhancement surrounding the ablated area

the entire ablated zone. As explained in Chap. 19 regarding the study on rabbit VX2 liver ablation with IRE, cell death was accomplished through apoptosis, which is a part of the normal course of a cell's life. By contrast, other thermal ablation techniques create cell death through ischemic insult and coagulation of vessels in the tissue or necrosis, which is caused by injury to the cell. Another finding through this study is the distinct demarcation of the ablation zone and preservation of adjacent vital structures. In concordance with the liver study, vessels within the ablation zone were seen, and vessels greater than 3 mm in diameter did not show any structural damage. This finding helps support our theory that IRE ablation may also contribute to tissue preservation, as discussed in Chap. 19.

These preliminary results provide an optimistic outlook on the future use of IRE for treatment of head and neck cancers. All in all, through this preliminary study, we can conclude that the use of IRE has had a positive outcome in the treatment of VX2 head and neck cancers in rabbits. An indepth scope of this study will probably need to be made in order to demonstrate further the feasibility of this study and its duplication in order to continue the research on IRE against head and neck cancers.

Conclusion

The incidence of head and neck cancers rises every year, and with that the need for novel treatment approaches – also in the setting of recurrent disease. As shown by the preliminary results of this study, IRE can be regarded as a potential minimally invasive ablation treatment against SCCHN. As IRE continues to gain momentum as an innovative and safe method for tumor ablation, there is no doubt that the number of studies using this technique will grow proportionally.

References

1. Gold KA, Lee HY, Kim ES. Targeted therapies in squamous cell carcinoma of the head and neck. Cancer. 2009;115(5):922–35.
2. Osaki T, Hirota J, Yoneda K, Yamamoto T, Ueta E. Distribution of surviving tumor cells after chemoradiotherapy in tongue and floor of mouth carcinomas. Head Neck. 1994;16(3):218–26.
3. Batsakis JG. Surgical excision margins: a pathologist's perspective. Adv Anat Pathol. 1999;6(3):140–8.
4. Woolgar JA. T2 carcinoma of the tongue: the histopathologist's perspective. Br J Oral Maxillofac Surg. 1999;37(3):187–93.
5. Jain P, Kumar P, Pai VR, Parikh PM. Neoadjuvant chemotherapy or chemoradiotherapy in head and neck cancer. Indian J Cancer. 2008;45(3):83–9.
6. Jemal A, Siegel R, Ward E, Murray T, Xu J, Thun MJ. Cancer statistics, 2007. CA Cancer J Clin. 2007;57(1):43–66.
7. Lango MN. Multimodal treatment for head and neck cancer. Surg Clin North Am. 2009;89(1):43–52; viii.
8. Gillison ML, Koch WM, Capone RB, Spafford M, Westra WH, Wu L, et al. Evidence for a causal association between human papillomavirus and a subset of head and neck cancers. J Natl Cancer Inst. 2000;92(9):709–20.
9. Seiwert TY, Salama JK, Vokes EE. The chemoradiation paradigm in head and neck cancer. Nat Clin Pract Oncol. 2007;4(3):156–71.
10. Kim ES, Kies M, Herbst RS. Novel therapeutics for head and neck cancer. Curr Opin Oncol. 2002;14(3):334–42.
11. Vokes EE et al. Head and neck cancer. N Engl J Med. 1993;328(3):184–94.
12. Lee JJ, Hah JH, Im SA, Kim SY, Sung MW, Kim KH, et al. Neoadjuvant chemotherapy followed by limited surgery in a mouse model of head and neck cancer. Anticancer Res. 2009;29(1):255–9.
13. Gilbert RW. Innovation in the surgical management of head and neck tumors. Hematol Oncol Clin North Am. 2008;22(6):1181–91; viii-ix.
14. Crile G. Landmark article Dec 1, 1906: excision of cancer of the head and neck. With special reference to the plan of dissection based on one hundred and thirty-two operations. By George Crile. JAMA. 1987;258(22):3286–93.
15. Pignon JP, Bourhis J, Domenge C, Designé L. Chemotherapy added to locoregional treatment for head and neck squamous-cell carcinoma: three meta-analyses of updated individual data. MACH-NC Collaborative Group. Meta-Analysis of Chemotherapy on Head and Neck Cancer. Lancet. 2000;355(9208):949–55.
16. Harari PM. Epidermal growth factor receptor inhibition strategies in oncology. Endocr Relat Cancer. 2004;11(4):689–708.
17. Karamouzis MV, Grandis JR, Argiris A. Therapies directed against epidermal growth factor receptor in aerodigestive carcinomas. JAMA. 2007;298(1):70–82.
18. Bonner JA, Harari PM, Giralt J, Azarnia N, Shin DM, Cohen RB, et al. Radiotherapy plus cetuximab for squamous-cell carcinoma of the head and neck. N Engl J Med. 2006;354(6):567–78.
19. Maor E, Ivorra A, Leor J, Rubinsky B. Irreversible electroporation attenuates neointimal formation after angioplasty. IEEE Trans Biomed Eng. 2008;55(9):2268–74.
20. Rubinsky J, Onik G, Mikus P, Rubinsky B. Optimal parameters for the destruction of prostate cancer using irreversible electroporation. J Urol. 2008;180(6):2668–74.
21. Bertacchini C, Margotti PM, Bergamini E, Lodi A, Ronchetti M, Cadossi R. Design of an irreversible electroporation system for clinical use. Technol Cancer Res Treat. 2007;6(4):313–20.
22. Onik G, Mikus P, Rubinsky B. Irreversible electroporation: implications for prostate ablation. Technol Cancer Res Treat. 2007;6(4):295–300.
23. Lee EW, Chen C, Prieto VE, Dry SM, Loh CT, Kee ST. Advanced hepatic ablation technique for creating complete cell death: irreversible electroporation. Radiology. 2010;255(2):426–33.

Chapter 21
Clinical Research on Irreversible Electroporation of the Liver

Ken Thomson and Stephen T. Kee

Abstract As part of a human clinical study regarding the safety of irreversible electroporation (IRE) using the Nanoknife™ for treatment of liver tumors, 75 liver tumor locations were treated in 29 volunteers enrolled in an IRB-approved trial. Adverse events related to the IRE of the liver were cardiac rhythm disturbance in two patients (ventricular tachycardia, atrial fibrillation), pneumothorax (one patient), and brachial plexus neuropraxia related to positioning (two patients). Except for avoidance of direct puncture, no protection was offered to major intrahepatic blood vessels, bile ducts, or adjacent structures such as diaphragm, gall bladder, stomach, or colon. CT and clinical follow-up for 3 months showed no evidence of damage to these structures. The major disadvantage of IRE compared to other ablative modalities is the need for a general anesthetic with muscle relaxants but the low incidence of morbidity related to the ablation outweighed this disadvantage. Cardiac-synchronized delivery of the IRE is necessary to avoid cardiac arrhythmia.

Keywords Abalation of liver tumors • IRE safety in humans • Liver cancer

Clinical Procedure

This clinical trial was designed as a prospective, single-center, nonrandomized cohort study and was approved by our IRB (Human Research and Ethics Committee, Alfred-Monash Research & Education Precinct). The cohort was subsequently assessed in two groups: a group of 12 patients with advanced disease where the primary initiative was to define safety without any expectation of cure and a second group of 17 patients where the tumor was confined to the liver and control of disease might be reasonably expected. In view of the possible benefit of chemotherapy in areas at the margins of the irreversible electroporation (IRE) ablation zone, where reversible electroporation may be expected to occur, cytotoxic medication was not halted prior to IRE. The AngioDynamics Nanoknife™ used for this trial was provided by AngioDynamics Inc., Queensbury, NY and is described in Chap. 5.

All procedures were performed under a general anesthetic with propofol induction, maintenance with oxygen/air/sevoflurane, and variable opioid regimes usually involving fentanyl or remifentanil.

K. Thomson (✉)
Department of Radiology, The Alfred Hospital, Monash University, Prahran, Melbourne, VIC 3181, Australia
e-mail: k.Thomson@alfred.org.au

S.T. Kee et al. (eds.), *Clinical Aspects of Electroporation*,
DOI 10.1007/978-1-4419-8363-3_21, © Springer Science+Business Media, LLC 2011

Intermediate duration nondepolarizing muscle relaxants (e.g., rocuronium) were used in all cases. Monitoring was with oximetry, noninvasive blood pressure, 5-lead electrocardiograph (ECG), temperature probe, bispectral index (BIS), and capnography. All patients had direct blood pressure monitoring, as we felt this would be helpful if we encountered arrhythmias. We also thought it prudent, at least for this trial, to be able to monitor blood gases and electrolytes as it was possible that the increased cellular permeability would cause biochemical abnormalities. Neuromuscular monitoring was recommended, as we were aware that the therapy caused intense muscle stimulation which could be modified by adequate neuromuscular blockade [1]. The majority of the patients had lower-body hot air blankets as, unlike radiofrequency ablation (RFA) where body temperature rises, these patients became cold during lengthy procedures in the CT scanning room.

Most patients were treated in the CT suite with combined CT/ultrasound guidance. A small number of patients who had tumors easily seen on ultrasound were treated in an angiography suite with ultrasound guidance. This is our usual practice with RFA of liver tumors.

Treatment parameters were supplied by AngioDynamics Inc., and were based on mathematical modeling [2] of the expected area of IRE as a function of voltage per centimeter between each electrode. Bipolar electrodes were used for small or inaccessible tumors and single electrodes for larger tumors. When single electrodes were used, three or four electrodes were used in an array. Single electrodes have a variable length of active electrode and the length (range 0.5–4.0 cm) was selected after planning the tumor treatment. Furthermore, the electrode length could be varied without removal of the electrode from the patient.

Two patients developed neuropraxia related to stretching of the brachial plexus caused by lifting the arms straight above the head under prolonged anesthesia. This complication is well recognized in surgery [3, 4]. Subsequently, liver IRE patients were positioned with their arms flexed over a large foam pad and no further cases have occurred.

Because of ventricular tachycardia in an initial patient, ECG-synchronized delivery of the IRE pulses was performed routinely. However, even with this type of delivery, one patient developed atrial fibrillation which required cardioversion. While it might seem that the distance from the heart is critical, there appeared to be no clear correlation between proximity to the heart and cardiac arrhythmia produced by IRE. It is our opinion that the patient susceptibility is probably more important. The only disadvantage of cardiac synchronization is that delivery of each pulse train takes longer, as the delivery is heart rate dependent; nevertheless, this did not significantly prolong the procedure. The rate-limiting steps in IRE, as we performed it, were the induction of anesthesia, patient positioning, and electrode positioning. We also found that programming multiple electrode parameters for an array of electrodes was not as useful, as if one sequence aborted because of excess current, the entire sequence would continue until the last programmed sequence was completed. Display of the voltage and current during the sequence was shown on completion (Fig. 21.1), but this was unsuccessful with multiple sequences because of the display limitations. Still, programming a sequence is quick and easy and provides better control of the procedure. The Nanoknife™ software aborts a portion of the sequence if current in excess of 48 A is discovered. Reasons for high current are conditions of low resistance, such as excessive electrode length, electrodes too close, necrotic tissue, overporated tissue, and placement of an electrode within a blood vessel or the extrahepatic fat.

Tumor treatment planning was performed using contrast-enhanced triple-phase CT with tumor volume estimations from axial and coronal slices. Once the volume had been estimated, the electroporation fields were calculated using the information supplied by AngioDynamics Inc. Unfortunately, it was revealed that while the Nanoknife™ had indicated satisfactory electroporation, in fact the sequences were not delivered as indicated, which may explain some cases of poor patient outcome. Even after a faulty circuit board has been replaced, uncertainty remains. Therefore, we have been investigating the use of segmentation software (Intio Inc., Denver, CO) to aid the planning and post-IRE assessment process (Fig. 21.2).

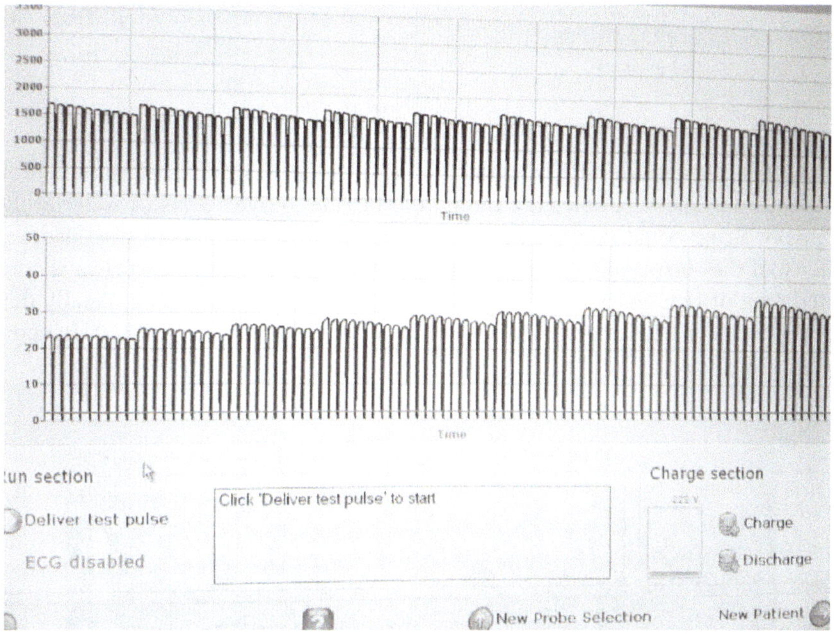

Fig. 21.1 Nanoknife™ waveform display. The unit displays voltage (*top*) and current information (*bottom*) for each sequence upon completion. This information is stored within the unit. The voltage decreases slightly because it is derived from a capacitor. The current increases as cell permeability increases and resistance falls

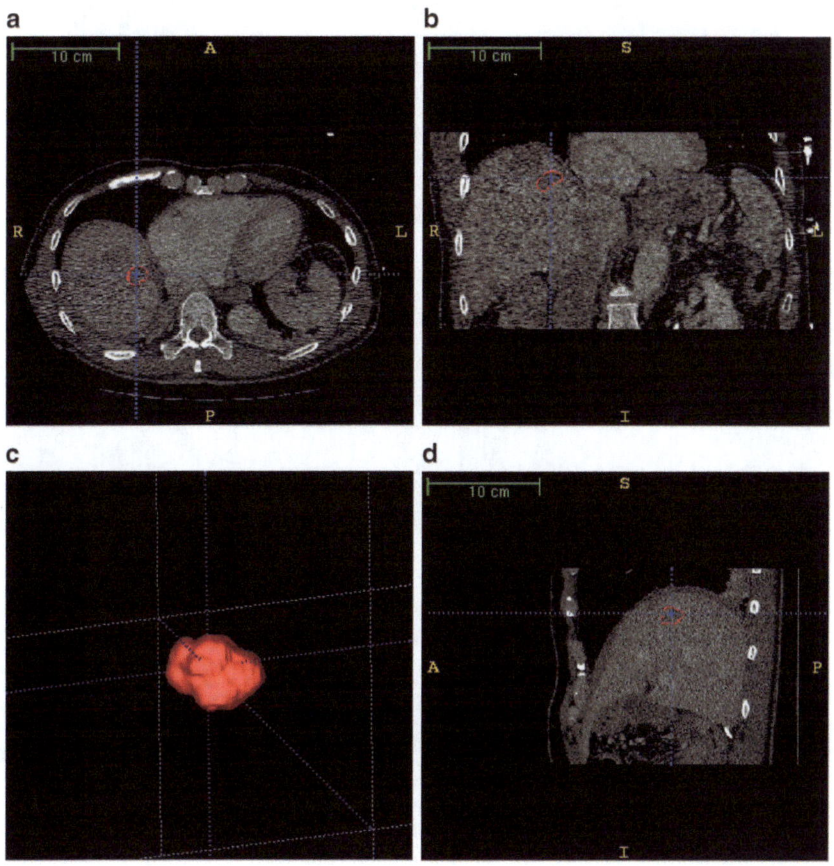

Fig. 21.2 Intio Inc., Denver, CO provided this segmentation image to aid irreversible electroporation (IRE) planning and eventually it is hoped this technology will be available in the CT suite on-line to provide confirmation of the correct area of ablation with IRE. The part figures are representative CT slices in axial (**a**), coronal (**b**) and sagittal (**d**) of a tumour outlined in a red circle of interest which is shown in (**c**) as a segmented object

Results

Ultrasound imaging during the IRE sequence revealed the development of numerous bubbles around each electrode. These bubbles are thought to be due to hydrolysis of water at the electrode surface (Rubinsky B, personal communication 2009). In most cases there was also a decrease in the echogenicity of the surrounding tissue, although this was not uniform or always corresponding to the expected area of IRE. Also, CT imaging at the end of electroporation usually demonstrated bubbles of gas within the treated area but not in a consistent fashion (Fig. 21.3). In certain tumors,

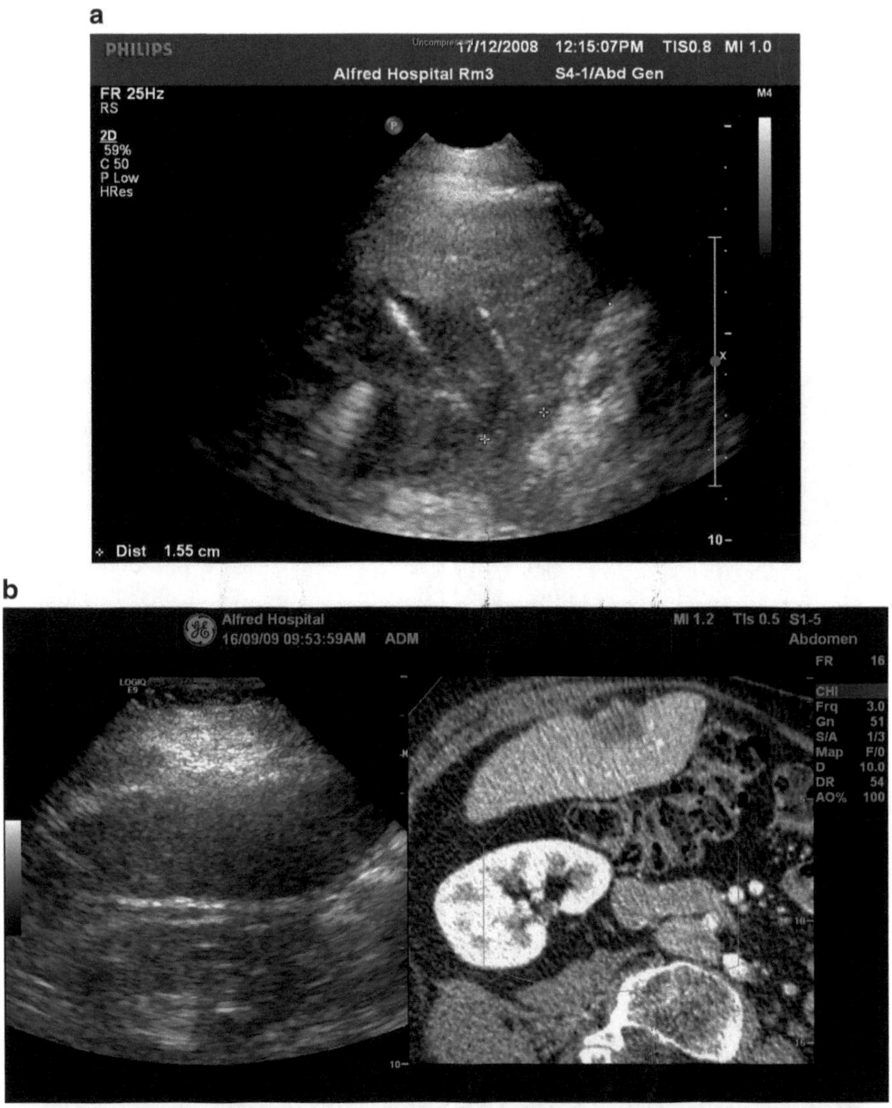

Fig. 21.3 Ultrasound imaging of IRE. (**a**) Ultrasound imaging during IRE demonstrating a high signal around the electrode produced by gas bubbles and low signal within the zone of electroporation. (**b**) When ultrasound imaging is unsuccessful, CT/ultrasound linked image guidance may be helpful. *Left* – ultrasound image; *right* – prior CT image. As the ultrasound probe is moved, the CT image scrolls to match the calculated position of the probe. However, it does not provide help with how much of the tumor has been treated

Definity™ contrast enhancement was used in order to provide confirmation of a satisfactory ablation (Fig. 21.4).

The CT imaging protocol used was a precontrast scan with triple-phase (arterial, portal venous, delayed) postcontrast scans. Apart from visualization of gas bubbles, noncontrast CT imaging did not demonstrate the area of electroporation. With contrast CT imaging, in the arterial phase, there

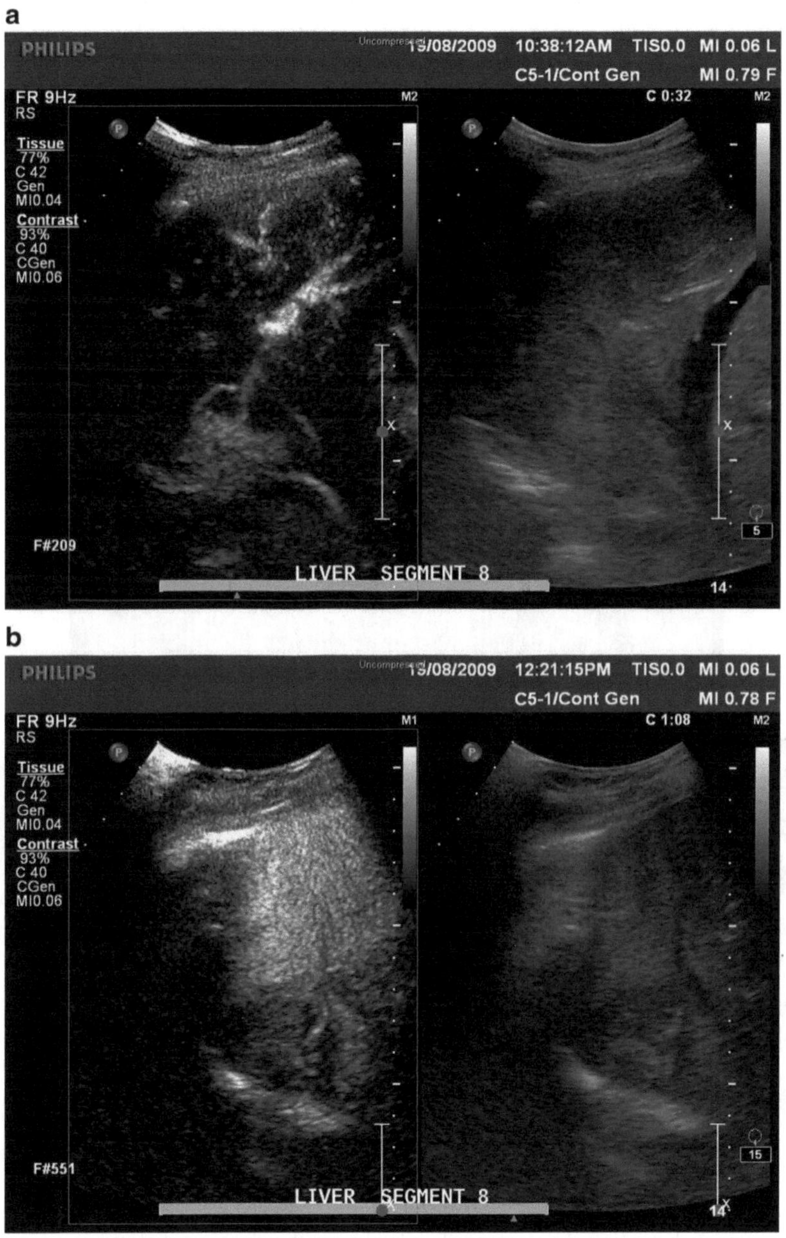

Fig. 21.4 Ultrasound contrast imaging for IRE. (**a**) Ultrasound contrast is useful for the identification and localization of tumors that may be difficult to image with ultrasound alone. *Left*: following Definity™ contrast. *Right*: without contrast. Unfortunately not all liver tumors were enhanced to this extent. (**b**) During the IRE procedure, repeated contrast injections allow monitoring of the IRE procedure until the tumor is no longer enhanced by the contrast (*left*). In the *right*, the typical low echogenicity at the site of IRE is seen

was nonenhancement of the electroporation area with a rim of increased enhancement being seen, but the rim enhancement disappeared in the portal venous phase and in the delayed venous phase (Fig. 21.5), while the nonenhancement persisted. This is consistent with capillary obliteration. Additionally, large portal vessels (>1–2 mm) could be identified crossing the zone of electroporation. In some cases of large volume electroporation there was delayed enhancement of adjacent segments until the late venous phase.

Clinical follow-up of these patients showed that the IRE was extremely well tolerated. Only one patient who had 15 separate punctures for electrode placement developed any pain requiring treatment. The virtual absence of "unwellness" and the ability to perform the IRE ablation anywhere in the liver, even adjacent to large blood vessels (Fig. 21.6), was a remarkable feature of the IRE treatment.

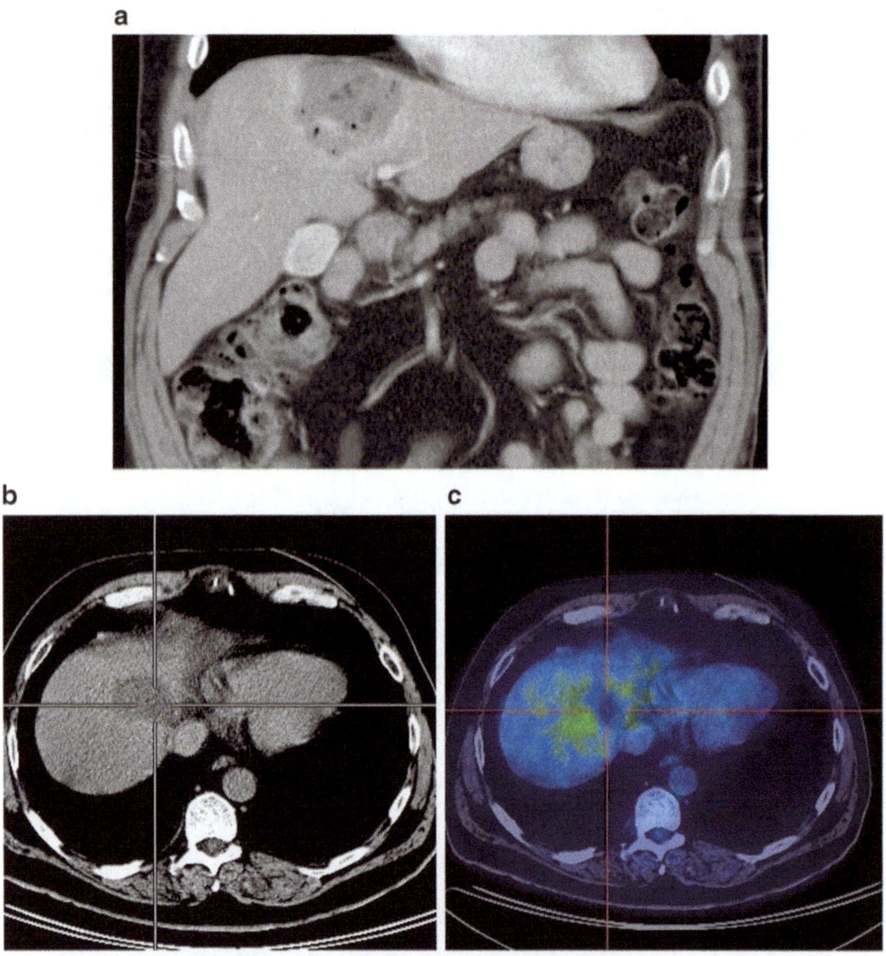

Fig. 21.5 CT imaging post-IRE. (**a**) Following IRE, CT shows an area of low attenuation with a rim of increased attenuation in the arterial phase. Note the presence of air bubbles within the zone of electroporation. (**b**) Noncontrast CT prior to a PET scan shows that the area of IRE has not decreased in size in a 3-month follow-up. This appears to be normal with colorectal carcinoma metastases. (**c**) The PET scan of the same area treated shows no activity in the IRE zone, indicating a successful outcome. There is low level activity in the remainder of the liver and at the 6-month follow-up, further metastases appeared elsewhere in the liver

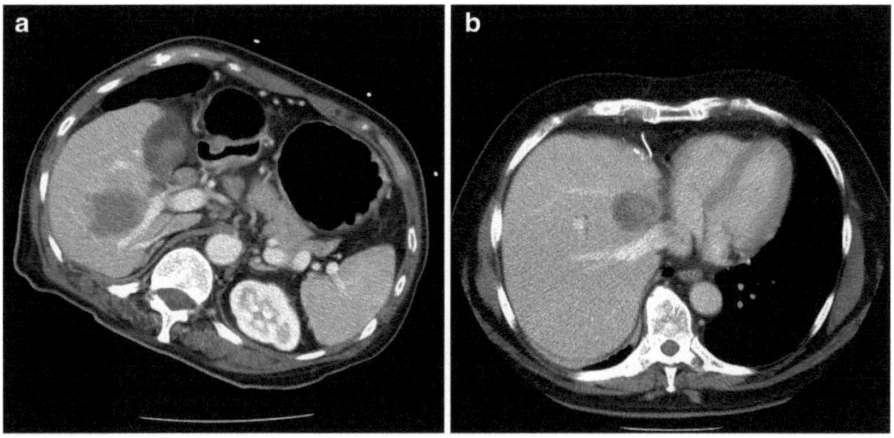

Fig. 21.6 IRE is not limited by adjacent structures. (**a**) A large hepatocellular carcinoma arising next to and displacing the portal bifurcation was treated without incident. (**b**) A metastasis adjacent to the hepatic vein and inferior vena cava close to the right atrium is not a contraindication for IRE

Liver function tests 24 h after the IRE showed an elevation of the alanine aminotransferase (ALT) from baseline levels (Fig. 21.7) but no significant procedure-related change in alkaline phosphatase (ALP) or bilirubin. Patient acceptance was high and IRE was preferred by patients who had prior experience with RFA.

CT follow-up at 1 and 3 months was performed in all patients and no other complications related to IRE were detected. In particular, no evidence of biliary stricture, biloma formation, or vascular occlusion has been revealed by CT imaging. The complications reported for thermal ablative techniques [5] were not evident. Moreover, core biopsy reveals "coagulative necrosis" with ghosted outlines of anuclear cells (Fig. 21.8).

In terms of tumor control, IRE has been variable (Fig. 21.9). Many of our patients had multiple lesions which could not be treated at one sitting while others had metastatic malignancy or multicentric hepatocellular carcinoma in a setting of Hepatitis B and cirrhosis. Consequently, follow-up revealed new lesions beyond the areas treated with IRE.

Although animal studies suggested that there would be regeneration of normal liver with disappearance of the IRE ablation zone, this did not uniformly occur in our patient cohort. The ablation zone either remained stable or decreased to a variable extent depending on the size of the area treated and the underlying state of the liver. Many of our patients previously had RFA, cytotoxic drugs, hepatic surgery, cirrhosis, and chemoemolization.

We will shortly (as of early 2010) be commencing a randomized controlled study of RFA versus IRE in tumors less than 4 cm in maximum dimension to assess the place of IRE in the treatment of liver tumors. The biggest challenge is the difficulty of ensuring adequate electrode spacing and confirming that the entire tumor and a suitable clearance margin has been electroporated irreversibly. It is hoped that segmenting software (Intio Inc.) will be available in the procedure suite to control the ablation.

Until these issues are addressed adequately, IRE faces stiff competition from thermal ablative techniques [6].

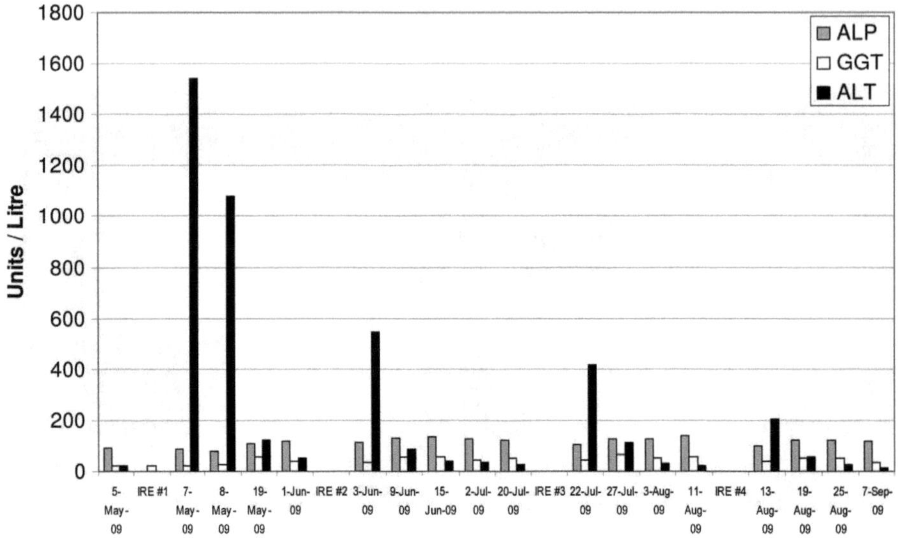

Fig. 21.7 Liver function tests after IRE. Data from a typical patient who had IRE on several occasions. Plots of alanine aminotransferase (ALT) and alkaline phosphatase (ALP) show that the ALT rose and fell rapidly, while ALP did not change significantly (see Table 21.1 for data table)

Table 21.1 Liver function tests after IRE

		GGT	0	38				
		ALT	9	36				
		AST	12	42				
	5-May-09	6-May-09	7-May-09	8-May-09	19-May-09	1-Jun-09		
	-	IRE #1	1d	2d	2w	1m		
ALP	90	0	88	80	107	116		
GGT	23	23	22	28	57	38		
ALT	23	-	1541	1078	121	54		
	-	-	-	-		-		
		2-Jun-09	3-Jun-09	9-Jun-09	15-Jun-09	2-Jul-09	20-Jul-09	
		IRE #2	1d	1w	2w	1m	7w	
	ALP	-	112	130	136	126	121	
	GGT	-	33	57	55	43	50	
	ALT	-	546	86	39	34	25	
		-	-				-	
		21-Jul-09	22-Jul-09	27-Jul-09	3-Aug-09	11-Aug-09		
		IRE #3	1d	1w	2w	3w		
	ALP	-	106	126	127	140		
	GGT	-	43	64	52	56		
	ALT	-	416	114	30	22		
	AST	-	417	36	33	32		
		12-Aug-09	13-Aug-09	19-Aug-09	25-Aug-09	7-Sep-09	20-Sep-09	8-Oct-09
		IRE #4	1d	1w	2w	1m	6w	2m
	ALP	-	100	122	123	117	99	98
	GGT	-	37	54	52	35	30	33
	ALT	-	202	55	26	15	15	12
	AST	-	259	30	40	23	24	22

These results are from a patient who had four separate IRE procedures
Data from a typical patient who had IRE on several occasions. Plots of ALT and ALP show that the ALT rose and fell rapidly while ALP did not change significantly (see Fig. 21.7)
GGT Gamma glutamyl transpeptidase; *AST* aspartate aminotransferase

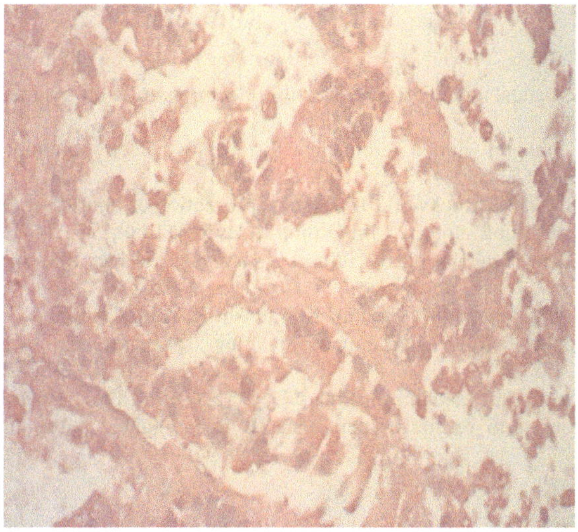

Fig. 21.8 This biopsy taken 1 month after IRE consists of fragmented cores of tissue showing extensive coagulative necrosis, and a small amount of skeletal muscle. Within the necrotic tissue, there are ghosted outlines of tumor composed of closely packed glands lined by columnar cells. The adjacent tissue shows reactive fibrosis with a mixed inflammatory cell infiltrate and a focally prominent bile ductile proliferation. There is no viable tumor, and no viable hepatocellular tissue is seen [Colorectal carcinoma metastasis]

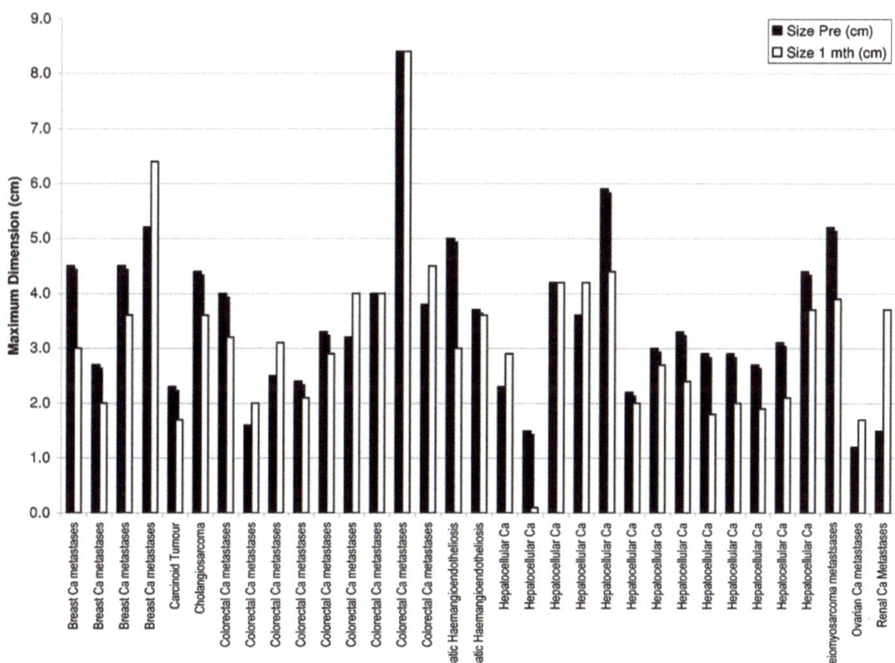

Fig. 21.9 RECIST plots. These data show the maximum tumor dimension for this cohort of patients treated by IRE. Results are shown pre-IRE and 1 month later. Because of the IRE ablation margin, the abnormal area increased in size as a result of IRE. Only those patients with a decrease on the 1-month follow-up showed continued reduction in the treated tumors

References

1. Edd JF, Davalos RV. Mathematical modeling of irreversible electroporation for treatment planning. Technol Cancer Res Treat. 2007;6:275–86.
2. Lee EW, Loh CT, Kee ST. Imaging guided percutaneous irreversible electroporation: ultrasound and immunohistological correlation. Technol Cancer Res Treat. 2007;6:287–93.
3. Cooper DE, Jenkins RS, Bready L, Rockwood Jr CA. The prevention of injuries of the brachial plexus secondary to malposition of the patient during surgery. Clin Orthop Relat Res. 1988;228:33–41.
4. Po BT, Hansen HR. Iatrogenic brachial plexus injury: a survey of the literature and of pertinent cases. Anesth Analg. 1969;48:915–22.
5. Akahane M, Koga H, Kato N, Yamada H, Uozumi K, Tateishi R, et al. Complications of percutaneous radiofrequency ablation for hepato-cellular carcinoma: imaging spectrum and management. Radiographics. 2005;25:S57–68.
6. Lencioni R, Cioni D, Crocetti L, Franchini C, Pina CD, Lera J, et al. Early-stage hepatocellular carcinoma in patients with cirrhosis: long-term results of percutaneous image-guided radiofrequency ablation. Radiology. 2005;234:961–7.

Index

S.T. Kee et al. (eds.), *Clinical Aspects of Electroporation*,
DOI 10.1007/978-1-4419-8363-3, © Springer Science+Business Media, LLC 2011

H

I

MIX
Papier aus verantwortungsvollen Quellen
Paper from responsible sources
FSC® C105338

If you have any concerns about our products,
you can contact us on
ProductSafety@springernature.com

In case Publisher is established outside the EU,
the EU authorized representative is:
Springer Nature Customer Service Center GmbH
Europaplatz 3, 69115 Heidelberg, Germany

Printed by Libri Plureos GmbH
in Hamburg, Germany